GRACE, GRIT & GRATITUDE

TARA COYOTE

The
WILD BEAUTY
Foundation

As you'll discover in my story, I share about how one very special mustang assisted me in a powerful and a profound manner. Wild horses are a symbol of free, majestic beauty in North America, but the reality is that they are being violently taken out of their natural habitat at an alarming rate.

A portion of the sale of each book will be donated to The Wild Beauty Foundation, an organization that works to raise awareness for the wild horses of North America. As Tara's mustang, Comanche has had a profound impact upon her life, she is passionate about supporting this important cause!

The Wild Beauty Foundation is a nonprofit organization dedicated to illuminating key issues wild and domestic horses are facing today, while also bringing the incredible, therapeutic world of horses to children and families. Founded by filmmakers Ashley Avis and Edward Winters, WBF seeks to raise awareness through film, education, and adoption.

For more info & for how you can get involved, please visit:

https://wildbeautyfoundation.org/

For cancer thrivers and those of you facing your shadows
May this story be a beacon of light through your darkest night

Contents

In Grace, Grit and Gratitude, Tara has gifted us with an honest account of a journey none of us would choose yet she has found a way to dance through it both physically and metaphorically. Spurred on by the turmoil of a life-threatening disease and major life changes, she invites us all to join in to find the grace that is available to us beyond even living and dying. From the gritty details of her healing protocol to understanding the larger lessons life presents, this book left me full of gratitude and inspiration to find the opportunities to taste the sweetness of life.

STORMY MAY – CREATOR & AUTHOR OF
THE PATH OF THE HORSE BOOK & FILM

The moment I met Tara, I knew she was special. The warmth of her smile, her beautiful presence, and her cheerful outlook on life is rare and almost always comes as a reward of a tough trauma. Having gone through cancer myself, I can very much relate to Tara's journey, especially about coming out whole on the other side. This is a book worth reading!

FABIAN BOLIN - CEO & CO-FOUNDER OF
WAR ON CANCER

A journey of incredible honesty, vulnerability, bravery, power, and ALOHA. One of the most profound things Tara teaches us through the embodiment of her journey is the lesson of perspective. I am grateful for her ability to affirm how perspective ultimately designs the experience, and the outcome of an experience. This is how Tara has most inspired me!

KE'ONI HANALEI – POHALA BOTANICALS

It would take a whole other book to detail my awe and appreciation for Tara Coyote's journey and her dedication to the truth. As she cultivated the power of intuition to listen to the messages her body sent through the medium of cancer, and the power of her mind in order to re-program her body to express 'health', and the power of vulnerability to surrender to the care and treatment she had feared the most, she embraced the power of the truth. Grit and Grace is the perfect description of Tara's truth and what it means to heal, body and soul.

SCHELLI WHITEHOUSE, AUTHOR OF,
THE BUSINESS OF COACHING WITH HORSES ~ HOW TO REACH MORE CLIENTS, FEED YOUR HORSES, AND CHANGE THE WORLD!

For anyone who craves the inspiration of a true living miracle, meet Tara. Her wisdom, light, and relentless courage in the face of life's most challenging circumstances shows us all an undeniable truth: anything is possible with an open mind and heart. I've had the privilege of knowing Tara personally throughout her miraculous cancer journey and what has impressed me the most is her ability to question her belief systems around western medicine and re-frame cancer and treatment into a healing nectar that's here to help her grow, evolve, and live life to the fullest. Her book, Grace, Grit, and Gratitude found me at the perfect moment – right when I learned my breast cancer had metastasized to Stage IV. Because of Tara and her powerful story, I now have the confidence to fearlessly join the sweet sisterhood of MBC Thrivers. I am forever grateful!

BETHANY WEBB, MINDSET COACH & AUTHOR
OF *MY GURU CANCER*

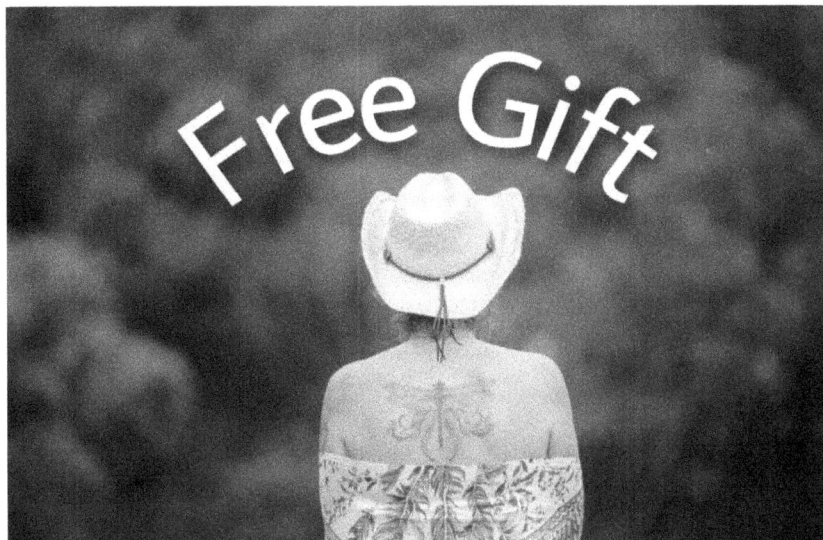

DOWNLOAD YOUR FREE GIFT!

Are you critical of yourself?

Would you like to have more of a sense of love and acceptance for yourself?

Read a piece I wrote called "The Beauty Trap".

Here's an excerpt:

"As another birthday approaches, I find myself reflecting upon the relevance of age in our culture that values beauty above wisdom in our youth obsessed world."

My piece is an encouragement to recognize your own inherent beauty, which is separate from what society calls 'beautiful'!

Download it here:
https://www.cancerwarrioress.com/book

Foreword

Tara Coyote has lived what most people only glimpse through myths of transformation. Sometimes these power stories chronicle heroic quests, outrageous tests of strength and endurance that involve encounters with mysterious beings, fantastic beasts who like Medusa can immobilize you with a glance.

In that timeless time beyond history, even the gods and goddesses are not immune to alchemical trials that strip away the ego's defenses and turn weakness into soul's gold. Of these many stories cross-culturally, the goddess Inanna endured one of the strangest, most brutal of these life changing encounters. As you'll learn in this book, her story helped Tara to not only make sense of her own underworld journey through the dark night of body and soul, it provided a map to return to the surface, renewed, empowered and more committed than ever to the beauty and sacredness of life.

Tara's encounters with close friends and family who received a devastating diagnosis mirror what so many of us face as we move through life: the suffering and possible loss of loved ones. With that comes a sense of helplessness. What can we possibly say to be of comfort? How can we support someone who has been suddenly thrust out of the predictability of conventional life into a hero's journey no one ever asks for?

In this book, Tara most certainly shows us how she was able to be present for others. And then she ups the ante. She gives us an intimate look at the thoughts, feelings, challenges, and decisions she made when cancer threatened her own life. It is ultimately an uplifting story, filled with an artful combination of realism, wisdom and hope.

I met Tara before the major trials she outlines in this book began. During the in-depth training she undertook to become an Eponaquest Instructor, I could see that she had the talent and discipline to help people explore their deepest challenges and access their hidden gifts. Back then, Tara herself was a bit like a mythical being. She radiated a compelling combination of purity of spirit, intelligence and loving engagement with life that became more pronounced as she gained confidence and skill in the field of equine-facilitated learning. We all recognized that her presence had a touch of magic to it that can't be taught. Somehow, Tara simply knew how to provide a solid, unflinching container for experiences to unfold, gracefully moving between empathetic support, compassionate discernment, emotional courage, and spiritual transcendence. That combination was a blessing to her clients, for sure, but it also turned out to be what she needed to embark on her own healing journey into the unknown, into the depths of suffering and sacrifice, and finally rebirth at the very edge of death.

Tara is not just a heroine willing to face the supernatural trials of the goddess Inanna, she is my hero. Through this book, I learned so many things I will use when supporting family, friends and clients through the kinds of challenges that always leave me feeling tongue tied and hopelessly inept. Just as important, I have gained confidence in facing my own mortality as it arises through circumstances that offer the gift of transformation whenever we, like Tara, embrace the deeper wisdom of life, with all its imperfections, challenges, and, most importantly, intense moments of beauty every step along the way.

Linda Kohanov
Author of *The Tao of Equus, Riding between the Worlds*, and other books on the healing potential of the horse-human bond

Foreword

The title of Tara's book could not be better suited and more fitting for her personal healing journey.

Grace can be defined as ease and suppleness. Anyone who has been in Tara's presence can feel the ease and suppleness of her personality and energy. As challenging as her healing journey was, Tara always displayed such ease and calm energy.

Grit is unyielding courage in the face of life's challenges. Tara's journey hasn't been an easy one. From metastasis to the bones and a weakening of her body's energy, Tara had the courage to keep seeking and not give up in the face of the progression of the "dis-ease" in her body.

Gratitude for the smallest of details allows us to live in the moment and appreciate the beauty of life. From the energy of gratitude, our bodies find the capacity to heal. Tara has always grounded herself in the energy of gratitude. Even when she lost her beloved horse ranch that was so near and dear to her heart, I remember her telling me that it was time to let it go so she could focus on her healing. She felt so grateful for having experienced the ranch and knew that, one day, she would be surrounded by horses again.

I had the privilege of meeting Tara in person at one of my Healing Diva Retreats. Everything about her radiated love and joy. Yes, she had the "deer in headlights" syndrome that most women have when they embark on a healing journey with breast cancer. But as she settled in, I saw her embrace her healing with a sense of curiosity. This was an opportunity for her to learn more about her body and ALL the available therapies that could potentially support her healing.

From bee venom to Amazon frog poison, to evidence-based natural medicine and eventually traditional medicine cancer therapies, she was willing to do whatever it took to heal her body and emerge on the other side a healthier and happier person.

As Tara so beautifully describes in her book, healing the physical body isn't just about getting rid of the physical cancer but more about the emotional cancers that lie deep within us and prevent us from living up to our human potential.

My heart swells with gratitude to have had the opportunity to play a small part in teaching Tara about healing her body. I'm so proud of her and for her. I know that her story, through the pages of this book, will be an inspiration to countless women around the world.

Dr. Véronique Desaulniers
Breast Cancer Conqueror
Author of *Heal Breast Cancer Naturally*

Introduction:

Aloha readers,

I hope my story of healing with the horses inspires you to know that great beauty, wisdom, and growth can be gained by facing your most daunting fears. As Wayne Dyer said, "We're spiritual beings having a human experience." This is what I remind myself of when I know my days might be limited. I tell myself that to be in an earthly body is a blessing. Although my body has been battered, I'm truly fortunate to be walking, dancing, swimming with dolphins, and daring myself each day to face my fears. It's all temporary. This human dance is just a dream, a game, a performance on the stage of life. I adore my son, my family, my friends, the furry creatures I'm blessed to live with and the red earth 'aina I call home. I remind myself that I'm just passing through, as we all are.

The structure of this book is woven around the story of Inanna, one of the first recorded goddesses from ancient Sumer culture, which originated from southern Mesopotamia (now southern Iraq). You will understand the relevance of this 5,000-year-old tale to my healing story as this fable unfolds.

I ask that readers try to have an open mind when reading my story. Through my health journey, I came to understand that in regard to cancer treatment both natural (non-toxic) medicine and standard treatment has value. I had to travel through hell and high water to understand what works for me.

Unfortunately, there is a vast division between the viewpoint of "healing cancer naturally" versus allopathic medicine. The gap between the two is as divided as the political system. My message is that there is a path between the two that can serve humanity. Both methods of healing cancer whether allopathic or natural medicine have their place. This is called: complementary medicine.

I believe that healing ultimately happens when the forces of duality come together. Life does not have to be in black or white.

Sadly, I saw too many friends die young from adhering to a path of "natural medicine." This is one of the reasons I am motivated to share my story. I hope this book can be an inspiring guide and resource whether someone is choosing a natural or conventional path of healing cancer. If my story helps even one person open their mind to a new possibility of healing, then I have done my job.

I have created a Hawaiian word reference guide as part of this story is told in Kaua'i, Hawaii with a strong island flavor. There is also a general word reference guide, resource page, end notes, and appendix. Don't miss these treasures in the back of the book!

Keep living. Keep shining. Each breath is a sacred reminder of what is precious.

Māhalo (thank you) for journeying with me,

Tara

SWEAT:

I woke up this morning covered in sweat. This makes me happy as it means I'm alive! This is a cause for celebration in itself.

In this moment, I feel so fortunate. I never forget my dear friends who died young, merely years ago. Their shadows walk by my side. When I do the things I fear, like swimming in deep waters with dolphins, riding on a boat that tumbles in the waves, and sharing vulnerable truths that scare the shit out of me, I remember them. I feel them encouraging me to live, since they cannot!

I choose to live big! I do the things that scare me, like telling someone I have a crush on him, even though it makes me totally vulnerable. In the end, it doesn't really matter. What truly counts is living from my heart and sharing my love. I don't really care about outcome; I just care about being real.

In The Beginning

How the Horses Saved my Life:

2007 – 2014

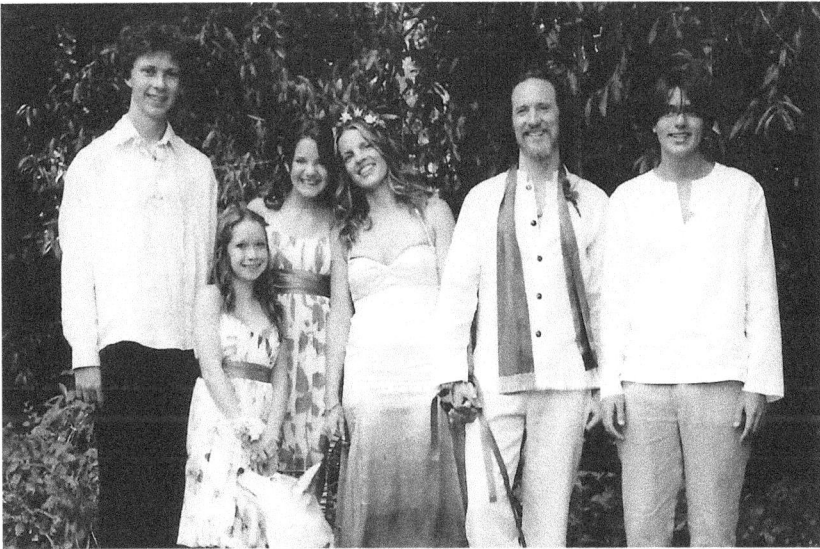

Zach, Makenna, Leilani, Jasmine, me, Tom & Willow
Photo by Shelly Garrish

I was blessed to become a single mom at the young age of twenty-two when I was gifted with a son; obviously, the single mom part wasn't easy.

As I raised my son mostly by myself, my ultimate dream was to meet a partner at some point in my future and share in the journey of having another child together. This wasn't something I readily admitted to, but the dream always lingered in the back of my mind. As I tend to be the picky type, I had high expectations for a partner, yet I knew, eventually, I would meet the right person.

When my beloved son Willow was fourteen years old, I was living in Fairfax, CA. I was single and so was Tom, a handsome musician, who was the father of one of Willow's close friends named Zach. Willow and Zach had been best buds for years. Tom also had a lovely daughter named Makenna who was ten years old at the time. I loved Tom's artistic style and how he was a committed father for his children.

Lo and behold, could he be the one? Tom's heart was open to possibilities, and we seemed to be blessed with the divine connection of love. We were both around the same age and had a lot in common. We courageously dove in. As I've never been one to tarry when I want something, after being together for one year, we were engaged and decided to blend our lives together. We joked that we were the modern-day Brady Bunch. When Tom and his two teens packed into the small house that Willow and I already lived in, it was certainly a jumble of different lifestyle habits and patterns. From the outside world, we were viewed as the "perfect, golden couple." This projection from others certainly had no pressure to live up to it!

We moved fast and, within two years, were married, as someone's biological clock (mine) was ticking loudly! Years passed in an ambiguous, seesaw conversation about whether to have another child or not. Our small house contained two adults, one home-based Pilates and Gyrotonic business, three teens, one blue-eyed frenetic husky named Leilani, two kittens (that the husky wanted to inhale in one gobble) and looting racoons trying desperately to steal the dog food. We had a full house!

As we both had our kids young, there were some layers to work through regarding the past trauma of young parenthood. Through therapy and intense inner dialogue, I independently came to the decision that I was ready to have another child. Tom, however, didn't arrive at the same conclusion.

At this point we were five years into the relationship and three years into the marriage. We were both forty-two years old.

On a fateful Valentine's Day morning, as I was hurrying to eat my breakfast and getting ready for my morning Pilates clients, Tom broke it to me that he definitely did NOT want to have another child with me.

The floor fell out beneath my feet.

Thus began the slow untangling of years spent building the picture-perfect life.

Looks can be deceiving. It's so easy to judge another's life as perfect. What isn't seen is the scars, the wrinkles and the glitches of what doesn't work. Even the most manicured mansion houses have mice in the cellar.

Tom's and my illusion of perfection cracked apart, like brittle guitar strings nearing the end of their virtuoso career. My hard-won Pilates business, cute house, family, and all I dreamt into creation seemed to fall apart at the seams once the reality of not having another child sunk in. This was all due to faulty communication of the most hormonal kind.

To add insult to injury, as I was a bullheaded woman bent on getting what I wanted, I had decided to remove the IUD (birth control method) I had within my uterus as there was no use having it there. It's not that I was going against what Tom wanted, but I realized it was time to free my life force energy of the IUD within my womb. Since I had had the IUD within me for almost ten years it had become embedded in the folds of my uterus. When I was in the medical office to get it removed, the nurse briskly yanked it out! I immediately felt harsh searing pain tear through my body. As the next few days unfolded, I felt like my insides were torn out. I had always been a healthy person and I figured the pain would eventually go away. The pain didn't disappear.

As time went on the discomfort became worse till eventually, it progressed to be like throbbing, hot fiery pokers burning me from the inside out. This agony left me moaning and crying in bed while in massive discomfort. I finally went to the doctor to find out that I had a uterus infection, which led me to take antibiotics. It eventually healed, but I ended up feeling a dull, tender soreness for about five months after the initial incident. It took deep psychological, emotional, and energetic healing to finally let go of the physical ache I experienced.

Physical pain and emotional discomfort go hand in hand. I realized many months later that I was infertile due to the uterus infection and the internal scarring that occurred after the harsh removal of the IUD. This was a grating blow. Not only was I not going to have a child with my husband, but I would never again birth another child in my entire lifetime.

My world started falling apart.

As the next year unfolded, I could have been mistaken for a fire breathing, emotional wreck of a creature. I tried to hold it together the best I could. I still had my clients, taught classes, and attempted to be the best stepmother and mother I could. I ran wildly in the woods with my husky dog to release the strong turbulence and heartache I felt. Leilani, the icy blue-eyed rescue dog matched me with the same crazed intensity that I had. I understood her wildness and she understood mine. My dogs have always been the sacred healing balm for my shattered and wounded soul.

Thank goodness for the wildness of the feminine that embraces both the dark and the light. How else can we be born again if we're not brave enough to dance in the darkness? Ultimately our most tender light is birthed from the bleakest moments.

In the ancient tale, the Sumerian Goddess Inanna travels into the layers of the Earth to visit her sister, the queen of the underworld, Ereshkigal. In order to find herself once again she must let go of the safety of her previous life in order to be born again. Through facing her fear and releasing the security of her possessions, she metaphorically opens herself up to the ultimate resurrection of spirit.

In retrospect, I see that I could have communicated better at the beginning of our relationship with my husband about my urge to have another child. If I could go back in time, I would have been crystal clear with myself and Tom about what was important to me. I see in retrospect how I wasn't honest with myself and Tom about what I truly wanted.

I had created a successful Pilates and Gyrotonic studio called Studio Equilibria and I owned and ran it for seven successful years. I had a vibrant group of loyal clients whom I cared for dearly. I worked hard to create this reality, but my world had to fall apart for the next transformation to occur.

I was fiercely committed to Tom and our family, but we had completely different visions for the future. How was I supposed to keep the structure of my life intact when my dream was ripped away? It was impossible.

I gradually slid into an empty abyss. I was depressed, angry, and shut out Tom, who was doing everything in his power to glue our fractured hearts back together again. At times, my mood fell so low, I didn't know if I could continue living. With every passing day, my emotional state became heavier. I was caught in a quicksand of depression. I couldn't understand how I had worked so hard to create my picture-perfect life and then it was slowly ripped to shreds in one single decision.

It was a torturous process, like ripping the layers of illusion away to leave a raw, bleeding wound that refused to heal.

I wallowed in intense self-pity and rage for about nine months. It takes nine months to grow a child. It took me that long to find the shards of myself again. When my ass finally hit the bottom and Tom was worried I might kill myself, I knew I had to do something. It was time to be proactive and claim my righteous light.

Tom and I took a last try-to-save-our-relationship trip to Bali, Indonesia without the kids. Sometimes, trying to salvage remnants of a relationship is like trying to reverse the process of fruit rotting on a vine. It's virtually impossible to bring decaying fruit back to life. The fruit must be allowed to compost and return to the soil. Once it encounters the verdant quality of earth it can then be born again into its next creation. Death brings quality to life.

Life's ebb and flow must be recognized for the gifts to emerge. You can't force the magic of life.

In the bustle of overwhelming tourism amidst the gentrified busy streets of Bali, we gave our relationship one more noble try.

When we went to the exotic Gili islands off the coast of Bali, the shift occurred. We were staying in a tropical treehouse, a place that was the perfect idyllic romantic location for honeymooners.

One morning on our magical treehouse trip, I missed breakfast and didn't eat on time. I was born with a sensitive body; so, if I don't properly care for it, I'm often slammed into a reactive state. The missed breakfast caused the side effects of low blood sugar to hit me hard. I was dizzy, weak and in a serious altered state of mind. Perhaps my body was evoking a warped mental framework to give me a new perspective? Maybe the Balinese gods and goddesses had temporarily visited me to guide me through the darkness.

It's always darkest before the dawn.

This extreme mental experience was like a psychedelic drug trip. To find my way through, I started praying for guidance. One of my spiritual teachers taught me to "ask for help" from my guides when I needed assistance. (Guides can mean angels, healthy ancestors, animal spirits animal spirts/Aumakua, God, Goddess, Jesus, Mary, Great Spirit, or whatever higher power you're drawn to.) I was metaphorically on my knees and praying for help. I yearned for a spark of light to assist me through the mental gauntlet I was stuck in.

I knew I couldn't sustain much more of this. My life had crumbled to the extent that I could barely work, my relationship with my husband was severely challenged, and I was in a sorry, dismal state. I was exhausted from the sadness and loss of my dream.

I lay curled up in a fetal position with the morphing of images gliding like a slideshow through the corners of my mind. The cacophonous screeching sound of monkeys, tropical birds singing, and waves lapped gently outside the treehouse.

I prayed for a long time.

The answer came...

I heard a voice say, "Be with the horses."

What? My mind didn't understand what that meant.

"Be with the horses."

The statement, "Be with the horses" made absolutely no sense. It was completely arbitrary. Why on Earth would I spend time with horses?

Poor Tom didn't know what was wrong with me and was trying to do what he could to bring me out of my strange stupor. My big-hearted Leo husband was fiercely devoted in his love toward me and always gave generously to help others in need. I was often the Piscean wingnut emotional tempest that the patient guy endured.

Tom climbed up the treehouse steps and brought me a plate of scrambled eggs which brought my blood sugar back to equilibrium. As I slowly came back to consciousness, I stored this strange comment about spending time with horses in the far chambers of my mind. The Balinese gods and goddesses had successfully delivered their message.

When the Bali trip ended, I tucked this singular sentence in the chambers of my heart as a guiding light to pull me through the shadows. Tom and I arrived back home to our perfect suburban home, and I decided to make a shift.

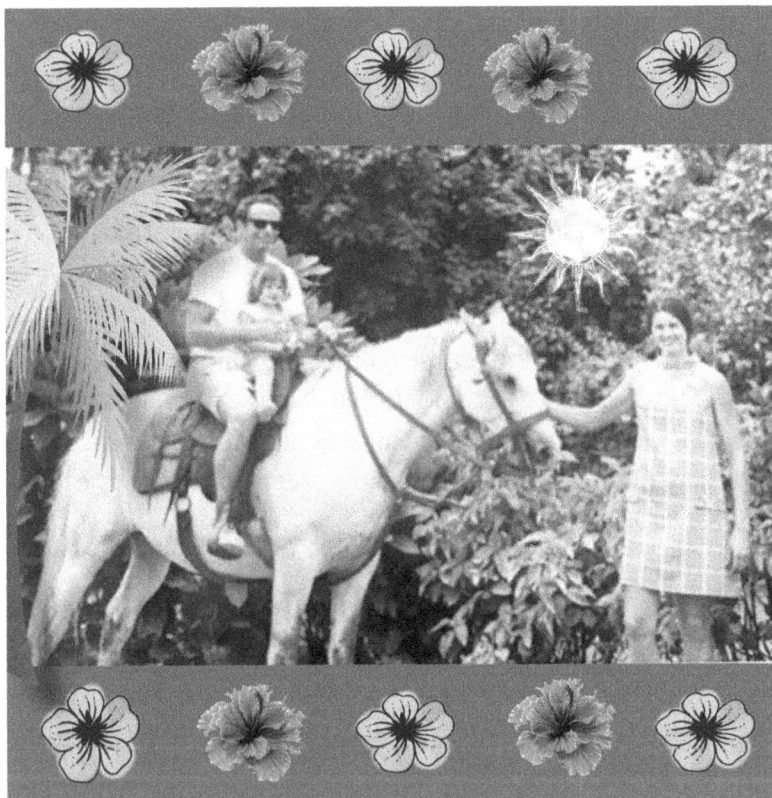

My father, me & mother in Kaua'i, Hawaii - First horse photo!

I was so far down that I would do anything to feel a spark within my soul once again. When I was a child, I was fortunate to spend to summers in New Hampshire with my cousins who had horses. I would occasionally take riding lessons while growing up in California. I was a horse-obsessed young girl and begged my parents for my own horse but never had one. I hadn't been with horses for twenty-six years when I received the message "be with the horses," which is why the message felt so bizarre.

I listened to that inner voice of wisdom and found an equine therapist who offered sessions nearby. I ended up having a handful of sessions with her.

Through time with the horses, I found a way back to myself again. In time, the grief slowly released. Through the equine therapeutic process, I could understand what the horses were reflecting to me. With the horses' assistance, I could find a pathway for my own self-growth and healing.

As I rekindled my love of horses, I recalled that Linda Kohanov's books, *The Tao of Equus* and *Riding Between the Worlds* had a profound effect on me the year before. Her ground-breaking books had planted the subconscious seed idea that the horses held a key of awakening for me.

At this point, I had nothing left to lose. My Pilates business was slowly dissolving as I had lost my love of teaching. My marriage was hanging on by a thread. I couldn't afford the expensive lifestyle in an affluent area, which required constant work to maintain. I had lost everything.

I did what any sane person would do in this situation.

I decided to save my own life.

Putting a hefty charge on my credit card, I flew to Arizona to attend an Eponaquest workshop with Shelley Rosenberg. Eponaquest is the organization created by the talented author, Linda Kohanov, who wrote the books that rekindled my love of horses. Eponaquest utilizes the practice of Equine Facilitated Learning to help promote humans healing with horses. Shelley is one of Linda's advanced teachers at Eponaquest. She is an accomplished teacher, equestrian, and author. She has quite a potent story to share which she writes about in her book, *My Horses, My Healers.*

The workshop with Shelley was my first taste of the Eponaquest work and was powerfully transformational. The experience with the horses gave me something to hold onto and gave me back the piece of my heart that was ripped away when I realized I wasn't having a second child. The equine tribe breathed life back into my soul again.

Horses have an incredible ability to mirror humans. It's possible to rapidly drop into the core issues that require healing while being in their magnificent presence. In my own experience of talking with an equine therapist about the trauma with Tom, one session with a horse was equal to six sessions of traditional talk therapy.

The equine work can be challenging to explain to people who haven't experienced the depth of this work. Here is a description from my website:

Equine Facilitated Learning (EFL) provides an opportunity for participants to discover authenticity and promote self-awareness. When doing EFL, both passive, self-reflective exercises are utilized as well as active leadership-based ones.

The Emotional Message Chart is a chart that explains the meaning behind emotions such as anger, grief, sadness, frustration and much more. Once you unlock the messages behind emotions it's much easier to cycle through feelings in a healthy manner. Emotions are meant to be temporary. Doing this work allows a clear pathway to truly listen to what our bodies are trying to communicate to us.

It's a remarkable fact that 90% of all communication is non-verbal. Horses naturally dwell in the non-verbal realm of genuineness and intuition. When partnering with horses, it's normal to find the horses behavior reflected in your own emotional experience. Horses offer a non-biased sounding board for the participant to travel to the root of the issue, identify it and then release it.

Above all, after your time with the horses, you'll leave with skills to support you in your everyday life. Spending time with the horses can be incredibly magical and profound, but ultimately you are equipping yourself with life tools to assist you in every moment with or without horses.

A few months after the first workshop with Shelley, I went back to Arizona to take an advanced workshop with the fabulous Linda Kohanov herself. What a profound experience and honor it was to learn from her! She is indeed as spectacular as one might imagine through reading her books. She is truly an intelligent, loving, aware and kind soul.

It became increasingly clear that I had to make a drastic change. I wasn't happy with life in the suburbs where my dream had deteriorated. I needed to be with the horses. It was time to embrace the new life that was calling me. I had no choice; it was literally do or die. I leapt, even though it scared the hell out of me.

In March 2013 I wrote:

"Structure falling: What the hell am I doing? I'm throwing out everything I've worked so hard for. It wasn't working as it was, but I will be okay. Soon everything will become apparent, or will it? I'm so scared, but I must trust and have faith in it all!"

Something very beautiful happens to people when their world has fallen apart: a humility, a nobility, a higher intelligence emerges at just the point when our knees hit the floor.

—MARIANNE WILLIAMSON

Unfortunately, I knew my marriage was going to be sacrificed. At this point, there wasn't much left of it.

When I was cultivating faith in my future unknown path, the experience of taking a workshop with Linda was pivotal in realizing the next chapter in my journey. On the plane ride back from Arizona to Northern California, I had a profound conversation with a young man who was lost, confused, and struggling with addiction. During our conversation, I realized that I had a gift to help others heal when they were in the depths of their darkest shadows.

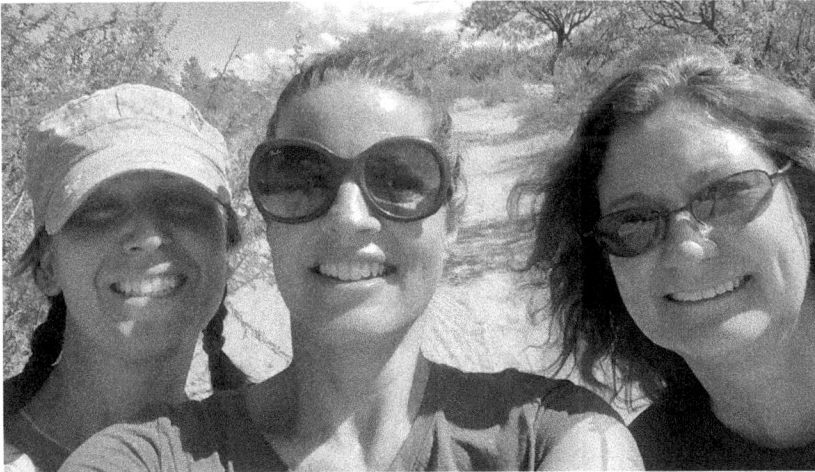

Lucinda Vette, me & Linda Kohanov

The lesson of Chiron, "the wounded healer" is to teach what we most need to learn. Only through diving into the extreme darkness of the soul is it possible to help others navigate their own shadow dance. You can't help others if you don't know the territory.

Experiencing trauma is a great opportunity for growth. From our greatest wounds we're born again.

I believe this is what happened to me. I had survived a journey to hell and back. As I was slowly finding my way back from Inanna's underground world, I was able to hold space for the young man on the airplane.

I decided to take a daring leap of faith. I decided to become trained as an Eponaquest Equine Facilitated Learning instructor with Linda Kohanov. Spending time with the horses had lifted me out of the dark night of my soul and I was inspired to help others in the same capacity. I dove headfirst into the arduous, potent teacher training, trusting my gut instinct that this new direction would take me where I needed to go.

The training was wonderful, complex, overwhelming, thorough, and required all my attention to learn. I was a relatively new horse person, which was an extra challenge. I wasn't just learning basic horsemanship skills, but I was also being trained to teach the insightful, complicated EFL material in Linda's course. It was vitally important to learn how to facilitate in a clear manner so my workshop participants could be safe around horses.

It was a huge learning curve for me to understand how to hold my energetic boundaries with horses, and I grew immensely from the process. The blessing of my newbie horse skills was that I didn't have to unlearn any bad habits and patterns of being around horses that didn't truly serve the relationship between horse and human. I was fresh, malleable, and open to learning Linda's material. Other students in the training who were seasoned horse people had to learn a new approach to being around horses that was horse centered, not human centered. I could see some of my colleagues challenged by this new way of being.

For me, it was a massive amount of material to learn in a relatively short time. My tendency is to jump fully into a new idea and then wonder after the fact what the heck I committed myself to! It was the case with this chapter of my life as well. In general, I would rather challenge myself with an arduous educational experience than take the easy route with a path that takes less time. This perspective has served me well in the various trainings I've done. The training with Linda was the same and the commitment to complete the Eponaquest training took years.

While I was in the Eponaquest training and desperately trying to untangle the shards of my suburban life, I volunteered for six months at a facility that used horses to work with developmentally disabled adults and kids. I was trying my darndest to continue teaching my students at my Pilates and Gyrotonic studio while still feeding my new focus of being with the horses.

The only thing that was certain during this confusing time in the chrysalis cocoon was that I had to be around horses. The horses were slowly pulling me out of the depths of the darkness I had fallen into. It was essential to keep going forward. It was the only thing that made sense.

During this time, I was instinctively called to spend time in the Nevada City/Grass Valley area. These two towns are also called the "sister or twin cities" and are right next to one another in the lower part of the Sierra Nevada mountains in Northern California. In the 1840s, these historical small towns formed the birthplace of the Gold Rush in Northern California. It's said that only 40% of the gold of the area was excavated during the Gold

Rush. The twin cities have a long, fascinating story with tales of the "Old West" woven through the fabric of its brick buildings.

I was drawn to this area, as it was close to the majestic Sierra Nevada Mountains and the magical Yuba River. The Yuba River felt as holy as the River Ganges in India to me. Near the Yuba River, the earth is rich with gold and other minerals, such as quartz and serpentine, which is the California state rock. Spending time in this area was genuinely nourishing and powerfully grounding for me. The vast beauty of the Yuba River was phenomenally healing for my soul.

Another benefit of spending time in these mineral-studded hills was that Stormy May, the filmmaker and author of the groundbreaking book/film, *The Path of the Horse*, lived in the area. I was learning how important my new, wild, bold horse-loving women friends were in my life.

After the turbulent last few years, spending time in GV/NC was an awakening, healing experience for my soul. I would pack Leilani in my blue Subaru Forester, and we would frolic around the gold-studded hills of this wondrous area. For the first time in a long time, I was starting to experience joy again!

It's common for me to make drastic changes when I choose to reinvent myself. This was no exception. I still managed to run my Pilates studio part time while also exploring this exciting new spot. It became increasingly clearer that it was time to let go of my old life and completely embrace my new horsewoman lifestyle. As time went by, I slowly dissolved my Pilates studio. The hardest thing about letting go of my business was saying goodbye to the clients who had become loyal, wonderful friends for the many years I ran it.

During this time of awakening, I was blessed to meet my horse soul mate, Comanche. This gorgeous fellow was an eleven-year-old mustang taken out of the wilderness near Reno when he was a yearling. Comanche was indeed a gift from spirit who breathed life back into my dismal heart once more. His grounded, calm, and wise old soul gave me the courage to make these immense changes. I ended up selling one of the pieces of exercise equipment to buy this noble gelding. I was so excited to finally be able to have my own horse!

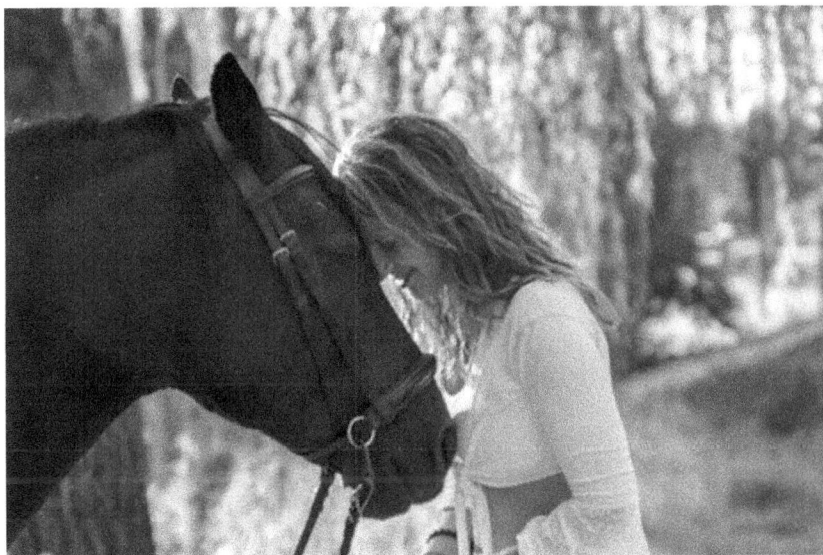

Photo by Meridian Brady

Leilani and I went back and forth from Marin to the GV/NC area for about a year and a half. After this, I took the final leap of faith and sold my cute little house in the suburbs to fully commit to living in the twin cities area. It was thrilling to make this change! I felt truly alive in this new country area that had an edge of alternative counterculture running through its veins. It was a fascinating area with a mixture of old hippies, spiritually aware people, artists, creative types, ranchers, and the Burning Man tribe nestled in the beauty of the Sierra Nevada mountains.

I was like the phoenix rising from the flames. It took a Herculean amount of faith to make these ginormous changes. Others told me I was crazy to give up my business, marriage, house, and the security I had worked so hard to cultivate. It was a bold and outlandish move to make. I could have fallen on my face and completely failed.

Isn't life worth risking failure in order to truly live?

Once my new life with Comanche had begun, this gentle horse gave me the courage and faith to keep going into the unknown direction I was headed. I was a little scared by these dramatic changes, but I ultimately trusted that I would be guided. Luckily, I was.

While I was rising out of the ashes after selling my previous home and business, I was fortunate to buy a ten-acre horse ranch in the Nevada City area. This purchase led to the gift of another fourteen-year-old Arabian gelding whom I named Spirit.

As I was a relatively new horsewoman, owning and caring for two horses was a steep learning curve. I had no idea the amount of time and energy owning two horses would require of me. Horses have to eat three times a day and the cost for their food, vet bills, and general care can be expensive. But I knew I was following my heart and trusted that a greater purpose was unfolding.

Let your faith be bigger than your fear.

Life on the ranch presented a whole slew of new duties. Right after I signed the ownership papers, I soon realized the massive amount of responsibility I had taken on. The property I purchased was grandfathered in to receive an astronomical amount of agricultural water. This meant there was an extensive sprinkler system on the property with eighty sprinklers and valves to maintain daily each year from April to October. The ag water made this verdant property jaw droppingly gorgeous, but it took a lot of effort to maintain. Often, the sealing of broken pipes and other endless repairs had to be made.

My goal was to turn the ranch into an Equine Facilitated Learning center where I could teach the Eponaquest work and host private sessions and workshops. I called my business Wind Horse Sanctuary. There was also a cute cottage on the property that I planned to list on Airbnb so workshop participants and tourists could stay in it. I had my vision in sight and I was determined to manifest it!

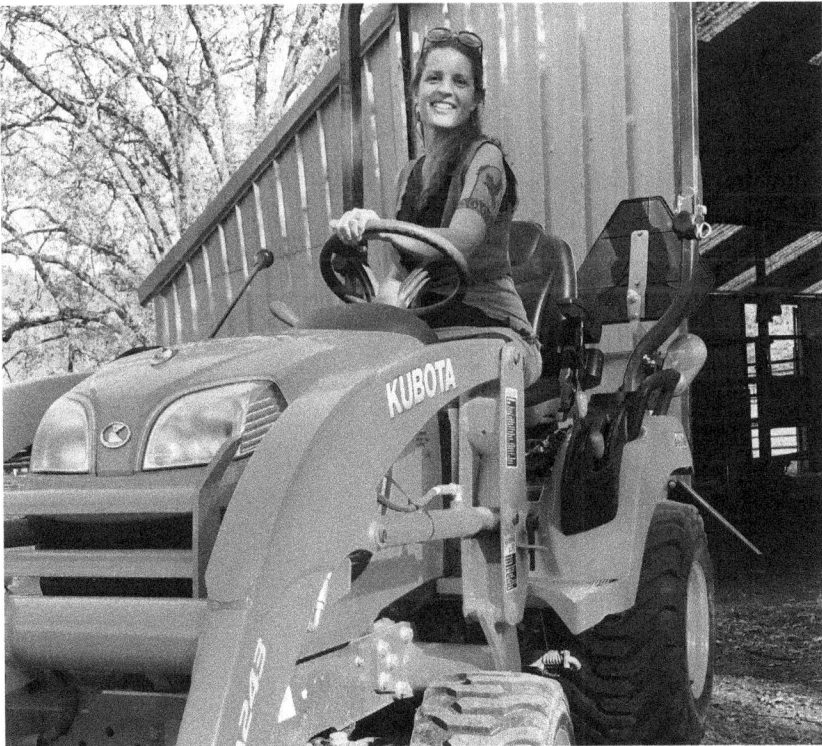

I loved my Kubota tractor!

In retrospect, all the hard work it required for the daily upkeep of the property and horse care was perfect. I needed something colossal to pour my energy into, something that was equal to the time and energy that a newborn baby required.

Sometimes, a bit of madness is what calls our soul into creation.

Often, the only way to survive is to silence the practical mind and jump feet first with blind faith.

Through this somewhat hazardous jump, trusting my intuition and listening to spirit, I was given something to live for again.

After this experience, I can say with full conviction that the horses definitely saved my life.

In every misfortune there are gifts. These gems born from great difficulty can only be found if one is courageous enough to dive beneath the surface to find them.

The horses gifted me with a direct path out of my sorrow and made it possible to witness the profound offering that the pain of not having a human gave me.

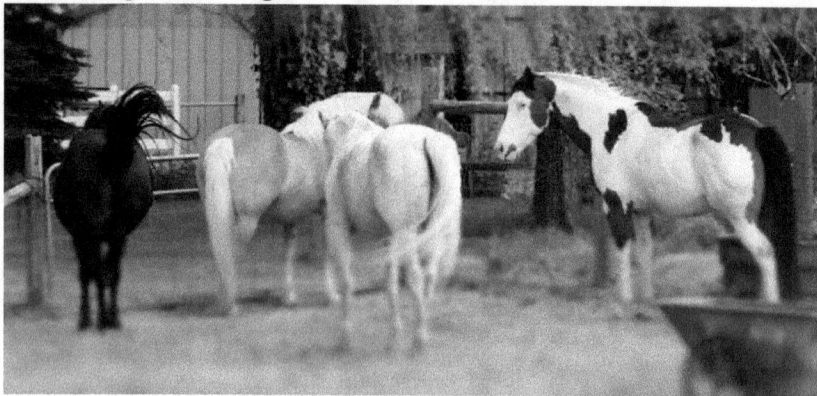

The herd - Photo by Melinda Vienna Saari

After running the ranch for a few years, I eventually had four horses instead of a child in diapers. I'm grateful, as I truly would rather have lived with these wild and strong creatures then bear the responsibility of another human baby. Besides, horse poop smells much better than baby poop!

There's always perfection in the enfoldment of the divine; we just have to stick around long enough to find out what that is.

I'm happy to share that my ex-husband and I are great friends, despite all that unfolded. Our marriage didn't survive the shifts and changes, but we both agree in retrospect that we ended up perfectly where we were meant to be. We mutually and individually grew from the dramatic experience and have come to enjoy the profound understanding between us. I have an amazing son whom I'm incredibly proud of, as well as two precious stepchildren from our marriage. We all remain close in our own way.

I bare my tender underbelly to you readers to share with you how powerful these equine beings are. I have heard and seen the horses touch others' lives just as profoundly as mine. A common theme for mothers whose kids have flown the nest is to remember their former horse-crazy selves and drop everything to be with horses again.

I've seen other profound facilitators be drawn to helping others with equine therapy due to their own experience of trauma.

Through experiencing pain, we shine the diamond of our soul. Pain is a tremendous growth opportunity.

At this point in the world's history, I believe the horses are unveiling their potent ability to heal humans during a very fragmented time on Earth.

The horses innately mirror the true authentic self of everyone the horse encounters to help transform the greater human collective.

The equine tribe is stepping forward to share their precious gifts with us humans at a time when it's most needed.

Trust your heart.

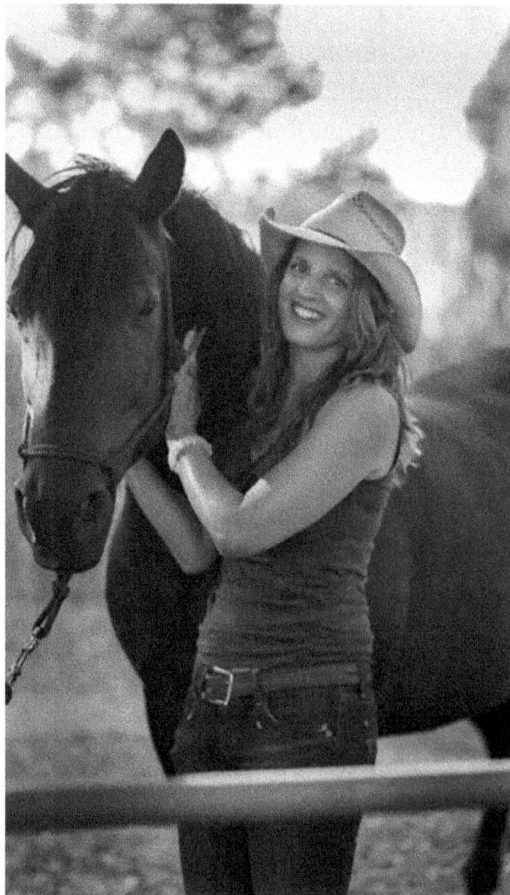

Comanche & I - Photo by Meridian Brady

Listen to your spirit.

You'll be guided.

Perhaps you'll be fortunate enough to be touched by the wisdom of the equine guides.

How I Made Peace with Death

My Tribute to Deb Hubsmith:
1996 – 2016:

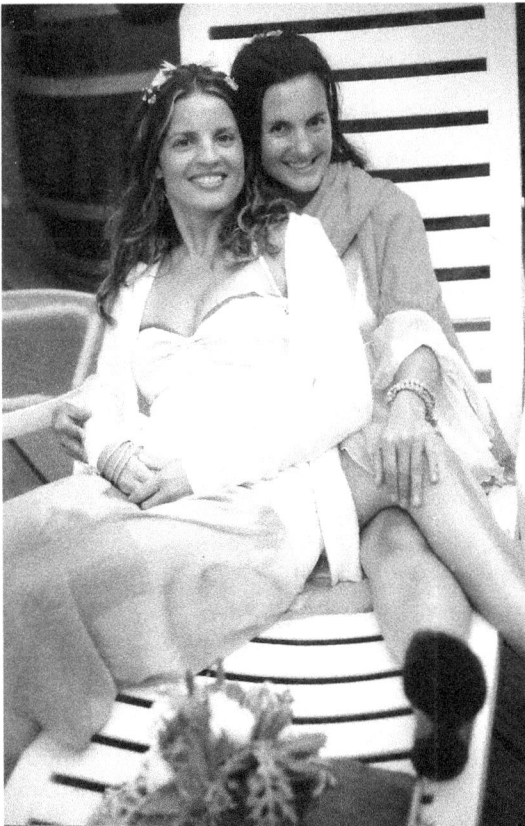

Me & Deb Hubsmith - Photo by Shelly Garrish

The path of death vividly beckons me to sit by her side, learn her mysteries and steep in her silent, elusive magic.

I met Deb when I was twenty-six years old.

I was living on the Hawaiian island of Maui in a fascinating structure called "The Pyramid House." It was a unique, pyramid-type building creatively constructed out of wood and glass in the early 1970s. To get water, there was a slight trickle of a stream that flowed through the building. After an hour of collecting water, I would bathe my young son, Willow, in a plastic tub outside that sat within a rickety old bathtub that was heated by propane burners under the surface of the bathtub. A tranquil stream ran around the hippy pyramid house.

This unique piece of architecture was down a long, bumpy dirt road on the road to Hana in a nondescript area called Huelo.

It was necessary to use a four-wheel-drive vehicle to get to the house, as the road was perilous and muddy in the height of the rainy season. Once parked at the end of this adventurous road, you took a long walk through a tropical-flower-laden pathway to get to the house. To get to the outhouse, you had to climb up a steep hill forty feet from the house.

This was a fun, fluid chapter of my life. I was a young single mom trying to find my way. My free-living jungle life on Maui might sound like the ideal lifestyle, and in many ways, it was, but my heart was calling for a more stable existence. I had dragged my son around enough during his young life.

My son Willow was four years old. He had been used to living a somewhat nomadic existence, moving frequently to different Hawaiian Islands and various counterculture hotspots like Santa

Cruz, California and Boulder, Colorado. When you're a young single mother in your twenties, it's a juggle to figure out who you are, be a responsible mother, and make sure there's enough clean clothes for your kid to wear. It wasn't an easy task, but I was fortunate that Willow, true to his name, was fairly flexible and flowed with change like the willow tree.

Ever since my mother enrolled me in "Creative Movement" classes when I was six years old, dance has always been a huge part of my life. Movement has been, in many ways, more of a comfortable expression of communication than talking. Speech can become tangled by thoughts gone awry; movement was simple and to the point. Through the telecommunication of my body, movement was the purest expression of life.

I was inspired to study "Expressive Art Therapy" at the Tamalpa Institute in Marin County, Northern California. Expressive Art Therapy is a mixture of movement, spoken word, and writing to create an effective form of healing. This therapeutic method resonated with me and I felt called to help others transform their lives through the healing power of movement. Finally, my vagabond self had a direction!

I was excited to study with Anna Halprin, the famous dancer from the 60s and 70s who had been a pivotal figure in the dance movement.

Since the late 1930s Anna Halprin has been creating revolutionary directions for dance, inspiring artists in all fields. Defying traditional notions of dance, Anna has extended its boundaries to address social issues, build community, foster both physical and emotional healing, and connect people to nature.[1]

Anna recently passed at the age of one hundred years old and inspired others to dance right up to her death.

I was also fortunate to study with Anna's daughter, Daria Halprin and the other talented teachers who taught at the Tamalpa Institute.

An ex-boyfriend, named Bo, mentioned to me that he was friends with a marvelous woman named Debbie who lived in the San Geronimo area in Marin, CA. He suggested we should meet. I was freshly back from my jungle life in Maui and newly transplanted to the dry, oak-tree-studded ground of Northern California.

While I was in the process of looking for housing, my son and I stayed temporarily at my parents' house. Debbie kindly called me out of the blue to say hello. She was immediately warm and friendly, which was a great comfort, as I was new to the area. Debbie worked at the San Geronimo Cultural Center, arranging musical events. On one of my first nights in Marin, she invited me to a dance event she had organized.

Little Willow boy and I went to the event. Willow had sandy brown hair cut in a bowl cut. I wore a long, billowing hippie skirt. Debbie would always say, in retrospect, that she met Willow when he was little and "clinging to my skirts." The dance event was magnificent, and I immediately felt like I had met a kindred spirit in this fabulously alive and sparkly being named Debbie! We became fast friends.

As the years unfolded, Debbie and I grew up together. We met each other when we were in our mid-twenties and experienced our profoundly formative years together. We shared and spoke of everything: men, jobs, clothes, spiritual beliefs, and had a great love of dancing with one another.

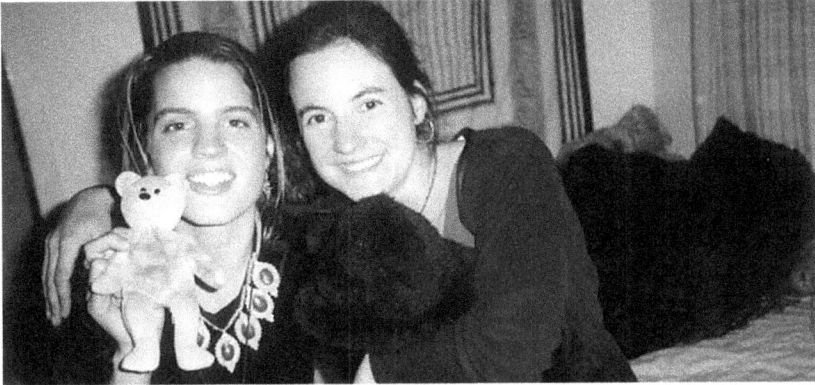
Me, Jerry Bear (featured Beanie Baby) & Deb

I felt safe with Debbie. She had a way of drawing me out of my shy, guarded self to immediately trust her. This was no easy feat, considering I had the firm armor of a resilient single mom around me. While I had always been gregarious and easily made friends, it was rare for me to let someone in like I did with Deb.

One of the keys to our close relationship was our shared love of dance. When Deb and I danced together, we were like two wild banshees freed of our humanoid skin. We were transformed into ferocious and free cats of the jungle swirling our long hair about in ecstatic joy!

Her hair was black as raven's feathers and mine was golden brown, lightened naturally by the beaming sun. I have a photo from years after we met when she visited me in Kaua'i, Hawaii showing our hair flying freely in the wind. This treasured photo lived so long on my refrigerator that it became discolored by the sun.

We matched each other perfectly when we danced. In many ways, we were like twins, sharing a deep sense of vulnerability through this mode of expression.

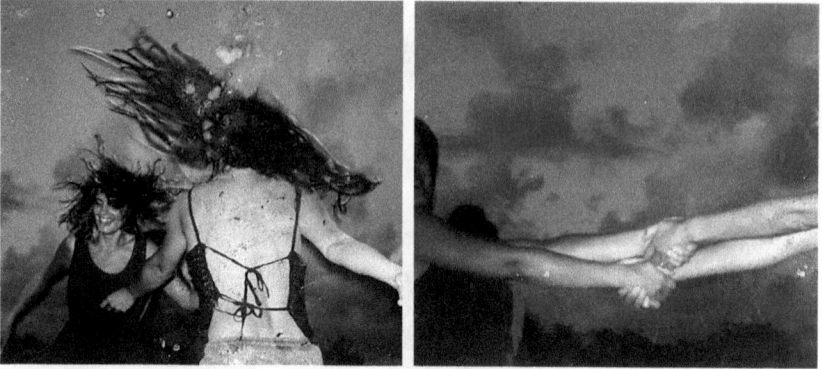
Deb & I dancing in Kaua'i

Debbie and I shared a sense of playfulness that would often have us cracking up in laughter together. She had an unforgettable laugh: loud and booming with a resonant ring to it.

We would also dive to the depths of serious topics like spirituality, reincarnation, childhood traumas, dreams, fears, and the things that would push us to the edges of our comfort zones.

Debbie called me her "secret keeper." I, in turn, told her things that I entrusted only to a precious few friends. We were bosom buddies growing up in a wild and wacky world.

Over the years, Debbie's name evolved to Deborah then, eventually, Deb. Her name morphed to fit the various places of employment she worked in.

She was a master tarot card reader. In the nineteen years of our friendship, Deb gave me pivotal card readings that helped me through difficult times.

When I was thirty-two, I fell in love with an Italian artist and his four-year-old son. I ended up dragging my protesting ten-year-old son to Florence, Italy to live. Living in Italy was extraordinary in many ways, but it wasn't the idyllic romantic life one would imagine.

It was shocking for my orderly American brain to comprehend the absolute chaos and utter disorganization of Italy. Even mailing a letter seemed complicated and a victory once accomplished! My Italian boyfriend was fairly open minded for a man raised in the Old World, but there were dramatic differences between us due to our cultural upbringing. I was from the freedom-loving Bay Area of California and he was from one of the oldest countries in the world. Even though I loved him and his son dearly, I struggled with fundamental obstacles.

In the dead of an Italian winter, I flew home to see my family, whom I sincerely missed. Deb gave me a tarot card reading to help me through the mental shadows I was wrestling with. After this influential reading, she printed photos of the tarot cards and I wrote pages of notes with my insights. Those five pieces of paper composed my guiding light in the next many months when I lived in Italy. Due to her wise reading and guidance, I navigated my way through a frustrating situation. I eventually ended up moving back to the states after giving it my best try in Dolce Italia.

Deb had an adept intelligent mind and moved mountains with her bicycle and pedestrian activism work. True to her astrological sign of Gemini, which is represented by "The Twins," she had two personalities. One side of Deb was her Washington DC self who would don professional suits and intimidate white, older politicians with her fierce drive to create safe pedestrian and bicycle pathways across the United States. The other Deb wore flowing hippy clothes; loved yoga, dance, bathing naked in the sunlight; attended community gatherings; ate vegan food; and taught contact dance.

My point of connection was with her free, artistic twin side. I'll admit, when Deb spoke about the political bills and politicians she engaged with, part of me drifted away mentally, as it was such a different world than the one I knew.

From my perspective, Deb's activism work took a toll on her sensitive body. Every New Year's Eve, her resolution would be to work less, spend more time with friends, have more down time and space to enjoy life. Like any well-intentioned New Year's resolution, it started out nobly, but as the demanding hamster wheel of the organization she created with thirty employees ramped up in the beginning of the year, she was once again endlessly busy.

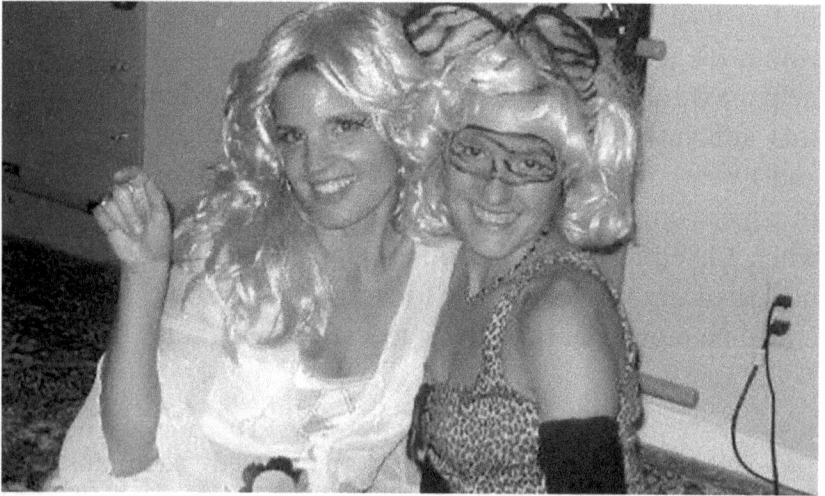

The go-go girl & blond kitty cat!

After my fairy tale Italian episode ended, I decided to move back to Fairfax, CA as my son and I both had a solid community to connect with. Deb and other close friends lived nearby, as well as my immediate family. I ended up becoming trained to teach Pilates, the Gyrotonic Exercise Method, and Yamuna Body Rolling at my business "Studio Equilibria."

I have so many playful photographs of Deb and me during this time. I have copious sweet shots that range from fun Halloween costumes to our prospective weddings, time in nature, and dance events. The Halloween photos with Deb in her usual kitty cat outfit and me in my various blue-wig get-ups are my favorite!

At a certain point, when my marriage with Tom started falling apart, I realized that I was being called to live in a more slow-paced, rural setting. The endless buzz of the Bay Area was stressful, and I craved a quieter realm to spend time in. The trees, horses, and river were calling me back to my roots.

During this time, it was difficult to schedule time to be with Deb. Both of our lives were busy. Her schedule was packed, and she would travel regularly back and forth across the United States for work. When I moved to Nevada City/Grass Valley I was determined to create a life that I loved! I craved a life closer to the earth to nourish my fragmented heart. Unfortunately, that choice took me farther away from Deb, but I was aware her life was busy and had a cadence of its own.

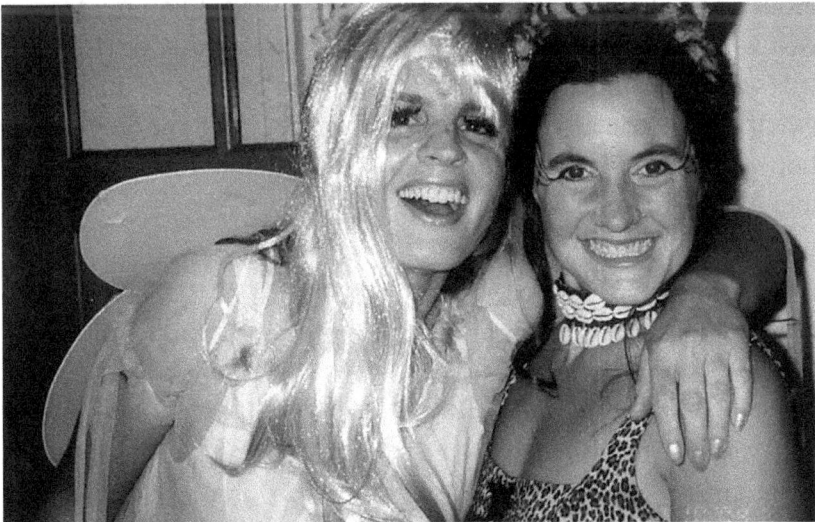

Fairy & kitty cat

Tragically, a few months after Leilani, the husky and I moved to Grass Valley to mend my tattered soul, Deb was diagnosed with Acute Myeloid Leukemia.

Acute Myeloid Leukemia (AML) is the most aggressive form of blood cancer there is. Deb was only forty-four years old when she was diagnosed. I was stunned that someone so vibrant who was also a vegan, organic and conscious eater could receive such a severe diagnosis. When I realized the seriousness of what her diagnosis meant, I was shocked. I knew I had to drop everything to be with her.

I was fortunate to have space in my life to be present with her. At this point, I had already consolidated my Pilates business and was in the midst of a huge career transition to the horse work. Life had lined up where I could devote precious time to her. It was a privilege and honor to be present for her during such a heart-wrenching time.

Due to Deb's diagnosis, I put my plans on hold to make the full move to the Grass Valley. For a year and a half, I had my foot in two worlds: Marin and Grass Valley. I remained solidly by her side and was honored to be one of her main caretakers during her twenty-two-month journey with leukemia. Her mother (Mary Lou), husband (Andy), another close friend, and I were the main members of "Team Deb."

Nine months after Deb was diagnosed with AML, she received a bone marrow transplant from a generous donor who lived in Europe. After the transplant, Team Deb waited anxiously to see if it worked. It seemed to be successful! We were relieved and ecstatic to know that Deb would live and thrive! She had surmounted incredible hurdles to get to this point and it was justified that she would live. During these blissful six months when it looked like Deb was recovering, we relaxed a little bit and

I made the permanent move, selling my house to buy the ranch that would become Wind Horse Sanctuary.

Some days, I would drive for seven hours in one day (three and a half hours each way) to see Deb for a few precious hours. The time spent with her was sacred beyond compare. It was also exhausting to be giving so much while running a 10-acre ranch, caring for two horses, and trying to build an Equine Facilitated Learning retreat center by myself!

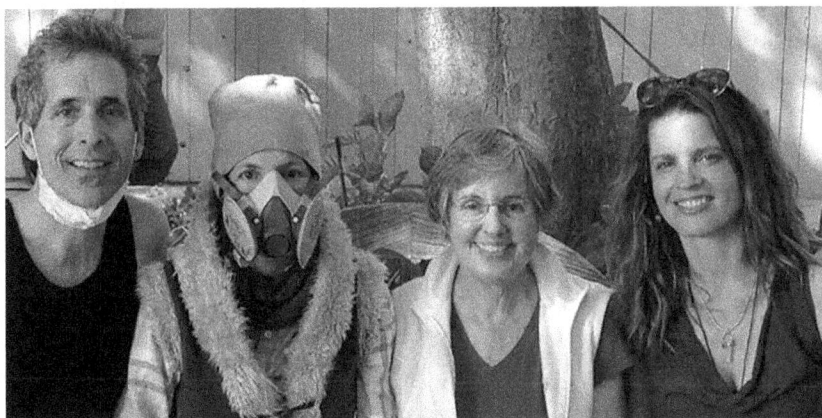

Right after Deb's bone marrow transplant - Andy Peri, Deb, Mary Lou Perry & me

Here is a piece I wrote in tribute for Deb on her birthday the first year after she died. On June 5, 2016, she would have been forty-seven years old:

> In Deb's short life, she accomplished feats that were only possible through her dedicated sense of service and love for this world. While her focus was bicycle/pedestrian advocacy, she was also an advocate for health, safety, and the well-being of our communities, especially our children. She helped to bring over $1.1 billion to create safe pathways, bike lanes, and programs that have positively impacted hundreds of thousands of Americans in all fifty states. The organization she

founded and directed "Safe Routes to School National Partnership" was an inspiration to many. If you go to Marin County, Northern California you'll find dedications to her at the Cal Park Hill Tunnel and the pedestrian bridge south of the tunnel. Both of these tunnels would not be open for cyclists and pedestrians if it were not for her inspired committed work and vision. There is also a beautiful bench dedicated to her in front of the "Good Earth" health food store in Fairfax. Her body is gone, but her spirit lives on in all of us who loved her so dearly!

One of Deb's realizations during her leukemia journey was that it was time to unite the two Debs, the powerhouse activist and the fun-loving free spirit. Sadly, she died before she could do so, and after her death, many people were surprised to learn about both aspects of the amorphous Deb.

We were like twins in the way that we would often meet one another wearing the same exact clothes or color schemes without planning beforehand. I was her "secret keeper," and for nineteen years straight, even while she was in the depth of her sickness, she was present for me like no other.

Being with Deb through her illness and death was a tremendous heart-breaking gift of immense proportion. From the moment she was diagnosed on October 17, 2013 with Acute Myeloid Leukemia to the moment of her death on August 18, 2015, with her skinny body curled up on her bed, I was transformed through intimately meeting death.

Of course, I would never have chosen to see my most precious girlfriend be slowly extinguished by blood cancer, but I'm actively choosing to be grateful for the gifts the experience has given me.

Only through embracing death can one truly live.

In the twenty-two months of Deb's illness, there were various stages of realizing that my petite firecracker friend might not survive her leukemia journey. I didn't want to acknowledge it at first because the reality that she might die terrified me to my core; therefore, I did everything in my power to try to save her. I loved her so much, how could I not?

Two years before Deb's diagnosis, another young thirty-nine-year-old friend of mine named Morgan had died from cancer. I learned from this experience that life is impermanent. After Morgan passed, I got a large dragonfly tattoo between my shoulder blades to symbolize the ephemeral quality of life. In this lesson, I knew I had to be present for Deb.

I was fortunate that I was able to be one of Deb's main caregivers for most of her leukemia journey. I dropped everything to be by her side. I visited her daily in the hospital, helped her shop for wigs after she lost her hair, gave her rides for blood transfusions, helped to figure out how to get the vegan, gluten-free, nut-free, dairy- and corn-free food she needed in a corporate hospital system, and created a fundraiser for her which raised $50,000 to cover the costs of her not working. I showed up with all my heart for her, as I knew she would do the same for me.

Love is meant to be shared.

Once you grasp love, it slips precariously through your fingertips.

Love is like an amorphous butterfly that can metamorphosize shape countless times.

I learned from Deb's death that the greatest gift is to give from the heart when you have the capacity to give. Through the experience of showing up for Deb, I now understand the true meaning of love.

I loved Deb fiercely, but in the end, the greatest lesson was to say to her, "I love you, and I will let you go."

As Deb was dying, I heard Andy and Mary Lou tell Deb, "We love you. You can leave now." Although our hearts broke to say goodbye, it was necessary to release her from the suffering her earthly body was in.

This is true love.

There is our love for our children, partners, family, and friends, but nothing can be held onto. The only constant in life is change. To hold onto what is a continuously changing form will only cause suffering.

"No one gets out alive" —JIM MORRISON

For months Deb struggled with the reality that she might die. Some people are almost relieved that they have an excuse to die when they are given a life-threatening diagnosis. Deb was the opposite. She fiercely clung onto life with both hands. She had a grandiose vision of life. She loved her husband, family, and friends and tried every medical possibility Western medicine offered her to extend her life. In the end, she had to accept the truth that she was only given forty-six brilliant, short years upon this Earth.

You're given a choice.

What are you going to do with your one precious life?

In Deb's journey with leukemia, I saw her spirit come to life. With the proclamation of her illness, she realized how passionately she wanted to live.

As her beautiful 110-pound frame slowly diminished to 65 pounds, her spiritual wisdom became radiantly bright. Her eyes would shine as she divulged the knowledge she had earned.

Life is a journey.

We all make mistakes and stumble. It's what we choose to do with these mistakes that shows the true nature of our soul.

Can you humbly apologize to those whom you've hurt? Can you bravely speak from your heart? Can you show your soft vulnerable side to those you love?

These are some of the lessons I learned from this tender dance with death.

Coming face to face with death is truly transformational. It rips your heart out. If you have the courage to look into its hollow eyes, it will forever change you. It can be difficult to relate to people in the same way you did before grief came to visit. In this realm, nothing feels "normal" anymore. If you have the tenacity and courage to feel your grief, you'll extract the dazzling treasures of loss, but it's certainly not an easy process.

Even though it's been years since her death, I still dearly miss Deb. From the ages of twenty-six to forty-six, Deb was my rock, closest confidante, dancing partner, and best friend. Boyfriends and husbands would come and go, but our friendship was solid and dependable. Sometimes, I'm tangibly aware of her spirit but the reality of not being able to reach out to her physical form can cut like a knife. Her radiant presence is gone. It's the most painful transition I've ever experienced, and the tremors of grief still occasionally tear me apart.

Throughout the pain of loss, I'm grateful for the lessons I learned. This experience led me to assist others with their grief process through the "Grief Rituals with Horses" I created and lead at my retreat center. It's an honor to hold space for others on their grief journey.

I learned that pain can be the greatest gift for true transformation of the soul. To turn our trauma into our dharma is embracing the magical power of alchemical metamorphosis.

Every loss we experience in our lifetime has the capacity to deepen us, to widen the channel of soul life flowing into us.

—FRANCIS WELLER

DESCENT

To see magnificiant colorful photos that correspond with the story in this book, please go to: https://www.cancerwarrioress.com/pictures for special access!

TRUSTING MY INTUITION:

When Deb died, a series of other tragic events slammed me on the head like a sledgehammer. Within the month of Deb's death, my cherished Siberian Husky Leilani died, and I found my boyfriend Mark in bed with another woman. It was a brutal wake-up call.

Mark was a solid support for me after my husband Tom and I split up. I met Mark during the time I was adjusting to the overwhelming reality of running a ranch by myself. He had a solid earthy nature that was calming after all the stress I had gone through. We both shared a past of being "Deadheads" (part of the counterculture movement that listened to and followed the Grateful Dead band). We had similar friends and lived in the alternative community of Nevada City. My life revolved around Deb during this time, as her health was continually up and down. Mark was already familiar with death, as both his dad and brother had died from cancer. He understood the intensity of being with a friend who was seriously ill. Many didn't have the capacity to understand, but he did. I was immensely grateful for his support.

My relationship with Mark was healing after the struggle I had gone through with Tom. He felt safe. In retrospect, I realized that I had my blinders on to certain behaviors due to the consuming reality of running a ranch, building a business, and being present with Deb. Mark would go to Santa Cruz, CA for work and would be out of touch for a few days and difficult to reach on the phone. I would ask him what he was doing in Santa Cruz besides work, and he would elusively change the subject. This felt suspicious to me, but my life was so full that I didn't give it much attention.

The ironic part of this situation was that when Mark and I got together, I vowed to myself that I would trust him. In past relationships, I had inherently mistrusted the partner I was with, fearing that he would be going behind my back with another partner. This fear was based on trauma from past relationships and childhood experiences. The fact that I vowed to not instinctively doubt Mark like I had other past partners was a huge deal. This wasn't a light decision!

After Deb died, my world fell apart. Days after she died, I experienced an ugly incident when Mark lost his temper toward me in a public setting. This was embarrassing and terribly traumatic. It was a boundary violation that led me to tell him I needed breathing room in our relationship. Two weeks passed without seeing him.

One morning before the sun came up, I got a strong instinctual hit to drive to his house. The impetus to leave the cozy nest of my bed seemed insane, but I had learned to trust my intuition. If my inner voice told me to do something, I listened! I jumped in my car at 6 am and drove to his house. As I was driving there, I had the sense that either 1) he wouldn't be at his house, 2) he would be alone, or 3) he would be in bed with another woman. I was incredibly nervous driving to his house, as I had no idea what to expect. My intuition was guiding me to see the full truth of the story. My worst nightmare was about to come true.

When I arrived at his house, I stood outside his window and peered in. I saw a woman with messy, long red hair in Mark's bed looking disgruntled at me. Mark was sitting up stunned next to her, gazing at my shocked expression. My heart was pounding. My body was shaking. I couldn't believe my own eyes. How could the man I trusted the most in the last year be in bed with another woman? I was completely dumbfounded!

I'm an extremely loyal person when I commit to someone in a relationship. If I say I will be solidly by someone's side, that's a promise I won't break. Of course, I expected others around me to operate in the same capacity. Since this incident, I learned to never assume another has the same moralistic viewpoint as me.

Mark invited me in, and I sat stunned on the sofa with him and the mysterious red-haired woman.

I found out that he had been seeing her all along when he was going to Santa Cruz for those secretive trips. In true enigmatic fashion, both of us women didn't know about the other one. He was playing both of us all along. I didn't understand how I could be so oblivious of the situation! Obviously, I was so distracted by my full life, so I couldn't recognize the deception in front of my eyes.

This was the worst possible reality to occur, especially after I decided to blindly trust him at the beginning of the relationship. Mark was my core support. To find him in bed with another woman added insult to injury.

Within the week after discovering Mark's red-headed girlfriend, it was clear my precious eleven-year-old husky dog Leilani was dying. She had been dealing with cancer for years, but it had become much worse during the last few months of Deb's decline. The toxic load was just too much for her body to handle. She had large tumors prominently sticking out on her gaunt elderly dog frame. Realizing that my dog and best friend Deb were dying at the same time was downright mentally catastrophic. Leilani ended up dying exactly one month to the day after Deb died, on September 18, 2015.

That period was a terrible shock to my body. I spent the next few months after that reeling in a frozen state of grief.

GRIEF:

"Our silence about our grief serves no one. We can't heal if we can't grieve; we can't forgive if we can't grieve. We run from grief because loss scares us, yet our hearts reach toward grief because the broken parts want to mend. We can't rise strong when we're on the run."

—BRENÉ BROWN, *RISING STRONG*

As I was deep in the throes of grief, I realized that grief wasn't an emotion that was culturally accepted. The general reaction I would get from others merely months after Deb's passing was, "Aren't you over it yet?"

Even when a death is expected, it still rocks your world. The mind and heart work as two separate organs. The mind can try to argue that you're fine, whereas the heart can viscerally feel the horrifying loss of someone precious to you.

We all carry grief, whether it be from the end of a relationship; losing a beloved to death; the loss of a pet, job, house, or an idea that didn't come to fruition; and/or the reality of our current environmental and social conditions. Even though you might not be aware of it, it's common for it to lurk under the murky surface just waiting for a chance to rear its ugly head.

Our modern-day culture would be much healthier if it acknowledged grief as a normal expression. When an emotion isn't expressed and released, it can become stuck and a source of toxicity in the body. Toxicity can lead to disease.

Disease equals dis-ease. Disease begins when there's a sense of discomfort in the mind. In our Western cultural conditioning, we're taught from a young age to stuff our emotions.

THE MESSAGE BEHIND GRIEF:

When I was certified at Eponaquest by Linda Kohanov, part of the training was to learn the Emotional Message Chart, so I could then teach clients how to use it as a handy tool for making sense of emotions many people find troublesome. This useful key to understanding the messages behind emotions was developed by Linda through extensive research that included pivotal insights by Brene Brown, Harriet Lerner, Daniel Goleman and other writers active in the field of emotional intelligence. The structure of the chart, and more specific insights into several of the emotions listed, were inspired by the work of Karla McLaren who wrote the book *The Language of Emotions: What Your Feelings Are Trying to Tell You*. While the Emotional Message Chart (EMC) is certainly helpful in personal relationships, Linda explains the wider implications of the EMC beautifully in her book *The Power of the Herd*:

> *The Emotional Message Chart and commentary presented here offer brief examples of how the meanings behind potentially volatile signals can help you manage your own and others' emotions in professional situations at work, at school, in community organizations, and in political and social activism contexts.*

The emotions that are covered in the Emotional Message Chart are: fear, vulnerability, anger, agitation or anxiety, frustration, guilt, shame, envy, jealousy, disappointment, sadness, grief, depression, and suicidal urge.

Each emotion has a message behind it. If you listen to the message, then you'll understand the valuable lesson behind the emotion. McLaren recommends asking specific questions of each emotion. This helps you tune into the meaning behind the emotion. She also observed that if the emotion isn't attended to and is ignored, then you will experience an "intensification" of the emotion.

For example, McLaren finds it helpful to distinguish between sadness and grief. By her definition, sadness is more of an emotion associated with transitions where you have a choice of when and how to let go of something that no longer serves you. Tears help you "release" your attachment to a job, a home, or a relationship so that you can move forward with energy and enthusiasm. According to McLaren, grief does not involve choice: a significant loss or death has occurred, usually due to circumstances beyond your control.

The question she recommends asking of this emotion is: "What must be mourned?" Linda also realized that a second question is also helpful: "What must be memorialized, appreciated or celebrated?"

If grief isn't paid attention to, one of the intensifications of the emotion is: "depression."

Linda writes in *The Power of the Herd* about grief:

> *Grief doesn't involve a choice. Through an accident, illness or change in the economic climate, you may lose a spouse, a job, physical health and so on before you're ready, if you ever would have been. Because something valuable has been taken against your will, there is also an element of anger in grief, it is the ultimate boundary violation to have your life*

turned upside down by outside forces beyond your control. Crying tears that often feel like a mixture of deep sadness, loneliness, anger and vulnerability allows you to slowly let go of an important relationship, job or other part of your life. Memorializing what was lost adds to the constructive expression of this emotion: finding ways to remember, cherish and, at times, even celebrate the gifts that this person, job or stage of life provided you is healing and over time restores your appreciation and enthusiasm for life.

I created "Grief Rituals with Horses," as I wanted others to have a place to safely express their grief. As I was already doing the EFL exercises, it made sense to combine them with the grief ritual work.

These events were a great success! It brought me tremendous joy to witness others' inner transformation. Many people found a voice for grief that had been repressed since childhood. For example, participants would come to the rituals, thinking they were going to grieve the loss of a spouse. Deep in the bowels of the ritual, they would suddenly realize that grief over a lost pet from childhood was never expressed.

Grief is multilayered. If you don't take time to clear your energy channels of grief occasionally, it can build up, creating depression and other emotional distortions.

Grief is also shared within community. We all experience similar grief. There's grief about environmental destruction and societal injustices such as expressed through the Black Lives Matter movement. This is all common shared grief that's important to name. Once it's named, it can be acknowledged, witnessed, and then released.

In my grief rituals, I found that when one person spoke of a topic that was bothering her, others would chime in with a common shared experience. This leads us to feel less alone in the mutual experience of grief. It's important now-a-days to feel a connection to one another rather than the vast sense of isolation that can be debilitating.

The sensation of grief can be tremendously isolating. It's normal to feel totally alone while suffering a loss. Gathering with others to commemorate a tragic loss can be remarkably healing.

I wrote this piece a year after Deb died:

SIX WAYS TO BE AUTHENTICALLY PRESENT WITH GRIEF

When loss is experienced, grief can create fundamental shifts that will manifest over a long period of time.

These developments ebb and flow. The current of grief is at times prominent and at other times, it is subtle. The direct impact of grief upon the soul is clear and transparent to the experienced eye.

One year ago, my closest girlfriend of nineteen years, Deb, died after a twenty-two-month journey with AML. I was one of her main caretakers, witnessed her slow decline and was fortunate to share the last couple days of her life with her. Through the heart-breaking incident of losing her, I have walked the stark landscape of grief and I feel inspired to share what I've learned.

1. When hit with the reality of grief, it is easy to lose the ability to make small talk. The things that seemed

important before undergoing a loss fade away in importance. When put in the perspective of life and death, topics such as scrutinizing your personal appearance can become trivial. For example, I witnessed my closest friend's stunning young body starved to skeleton size. The experience of seeing her whittled to the bone gave me a great gratitude for being alive, regardless of my shape and size.

When going through loss, it is difficult to relate to others in the same way you did before. The subject matter has changed. If you've witnessed the dark depths of death, it is hard to swim on the surface of life and pretend that the shadowy world that has become your norm doesn't exist. It is helpful to surround yourselves with those that have bravely traversed through the darkness and who understand your reality. Otherwise, it can feel common to feel like a stranger in a strange land.

2. When one speaks of your beloved who has passed, it can feel like an anvil upon the heart. This could possibly open realms of pain that might not be known to the casual conversationalist. Please be gentle around this subject matter if you know someone who is dealing with grief. It is not a light conversation matter. Having awareness and compassion around the subject can go a long way.

3. Be aware that holidays and anniversaries of the death and birthday of the beloved are all potentially rough days. On my own birthday this year, I was surprisingly swept up in a wave of grief when I realized that this was the first birthday in nineteen years that I would not hear from Deb. Luckily, I had her voice recordings on my answering machine to listen to. In general, there can be an acute absence felt on these sensitive dates.

4. Pockets of Grief: Things that might seem small can be potentially huge triggers for grief. A photo, something that reminds you of your lost one, or a random memory can trigger a flood of tears. Even the slightest reminder can send you back into the bowels of grief. Even months later when you think you've been through the worst of the storm; a small trigger can provoke a hurricane of a reaction.

   To aid in the healing process, it is optimal to feel the emotion that arises to release it. Tears and emotions need to be released for the inner momentum to flow on through. Grief rituals are profoundly powerful for this reason as it allows the grief to be freed in a safe, intentional container.

5. It is common to feel extremely alone in the grief process. Even if you have a strong support system, the gaping wound created when a beloved departs can be inexplicably crippling. When one of the above-mentioned storms hit, it can be a stark reality that your beloved's physical presence is no longer with you. There is no way to call, email, text or see them ever again. This realization can be brutally difficult to comprehend.

6. Please be careful to not say statements such as these to someone going through grief:

"What you've experienced is no big deal."
"You'll feel better sometime."
"Your beloved is in a better place."
"Time heals all wounds."

I realize that these words of comfort derive from a place of good intentions, but statements such as these are belittling and a dismissal of the grief process.

The best way to show up for someone going through grief is to share compassion, love, and understanding. Simply saying, "I'm sorry for your loss" and giving an authentic hug speaks volumes more than a statement that makes sense to the head but might not resonate with the heart.

Those of us who are traveling the road of grief might seem normal to the outside world, but keep in mind we are trained to mask our emotions. There are usually subtle layers of grief hiding below the placid looking exterior.

Grief is not a linear process. At times, it can be crippling and at other times subtle, but it lurks beneath the surface until it has worked its way through. A little bit of compassion, understanding, and awareness to what the griever is experiencing can truly aid in the healing process.

> Grief that praises life shows the depth of our appreciation for having been given life enough to begin with.
>
> —MARTIN PRECHTEL

2016

IN THE TIME OF THE FISHES:

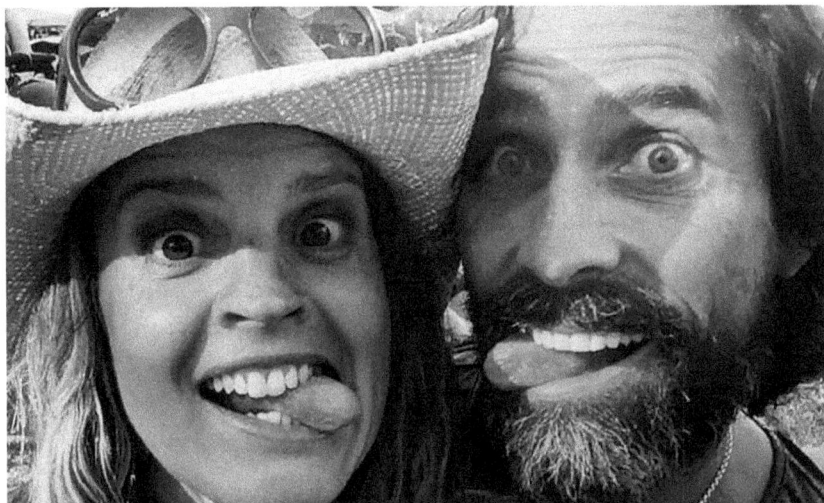

A goofy moment with Syris

Around the time I was creating "Grief Rituals with Horses," a magical man named Syris came into my life. Syris was a deep blue-eyed Pisces man with an air of mystery around him. He was true to Pisces form with his intelligent, spiritual, and ephemeral qualities. When we met, I was totally overwhelmed with running a 10-acre ranch by myself. As he didn't have a place to live, he ended up moving in fairly quickly to help me with the ranch. He became my boyfriend. Syris helped me run my workshops, did daily chores, tended to the horses, and helped to fix the never-ending list of things that broke on the ranch.

XARIA:

Five months after my dear husky dog Leilani died, I brought home an adorable 10-pound Australian Shepherd puppy. After Deb and Leilani's death, my life felt terribly empty without a dog.

I put a lot of intention into the idea of getting a new dog. In the past, I had adopted rescue dogs with a fair amount of trauma. As I was running a ranch where guests paid to vacation and spend time attending horse workshops, I realized it was best to get a dog whose entire history I was aware of. It didn't bode well to adopt a dog and have her attack a customer, terrify the horses, or kill the neighbor's chickens. My aim was to create harmony in the neighborhood.

In the past, the only dogs I had were Alaskan Malamutes and Siberian Huskies. I was fond of these fiercely intelligent, wild, and untamable fluff balls. I adored their love of freedom, though it also drove me crazy.

Malamutes and Huskies are the closest breed to wolves; hence, they're the most difficult dogs to tame. These breeds have an inability to listen if the scent of another wild creature is picked up while in the wilderness. Often, Leilani would suddenly disappear into the wilderness for thirty minutes or more if she caught the scent of a deer. This would be very frustrating!

Owning Malamutes and Huskies is hard work; they're highly energetic and total escape artists! When I bought the ranch, Leilani was getting up in years. As the surrounding neighbors had chickens, goats, and other tasty animals, I couldn't take her off the leash as her prey drive was so strong. As I was wanting to foster healthy relationships with my neighbors, it was best not to let a gorgeous chicken killer dog loose!

When Leilani finally passed from her multiple bouts with cancer, I chose to get a breed of dog whose life purpose was to stay glued to my side rather than run wild and free.

For some reason, I have a love for blue-eyed animals. Leilani had icy light-blue eyes. Often, when in public, people, even police officers, would stop and comment how stunning she was.

The paint horse that I acquired a few years after getting the ranch was renamed Blue for his one light blue eye and his other half blue and brown eye. Native Americans would call horses with magical eyes like this "Medicine Horses." Blue was the David Bowie of the horse world.

I decided it was wise to get an Australian Shepherd puppy. Aussies were nicknamed "Velcro dogs." I was told they were excellent ranch dogs and worked well with horses and other animals. Australian Shepherds are fiercely intelligent, loving, and great companions.

During this incubation time of deciding what to do, I went deep into my heart to ask for guidance. I often prayed for advice when I most needed it. My heart was broken from the loss of Deb, Mark, and Leilani. I actually prayed to the spirit of Leilani, my last dog to bring me a similar spirit to her in puppy form.

Once I decided to get a puppy, I felt a newfound sense of hope, faith, and anticipation about the future. I was excited to have a little fluff ball to train and entertain me with goofy puppy antics. The idea of having a new dog was a hand to help lift me out of the shadow of grief that I was submerged in.

I started researching Australian Shepherd breeders. Two friends suggested a breeder near Middletown, CA. When I checked into it, I found that it was family-run business that cared deeply for the animals. One weekend, I took a visit to meet Shari (the breeder) and her dogs. That day, I was introduced to a very pregnant mother dog and the sire. I was in love! I put a deposit down for one of the pups to be born.

When the pups were a month old, I was excited to make the three-hour drive to meet the three pups and pick one out. Of the three pups, two had brown markings and brown eyes. One pup, a female, had mostly white marking and icy blue eyes. Her personality seemed gentle yet determined. This little white pup seemed remarkably like Leilani's spirit. She was the one. It felt like Leilani had reincarnated into this little pupsicle body.

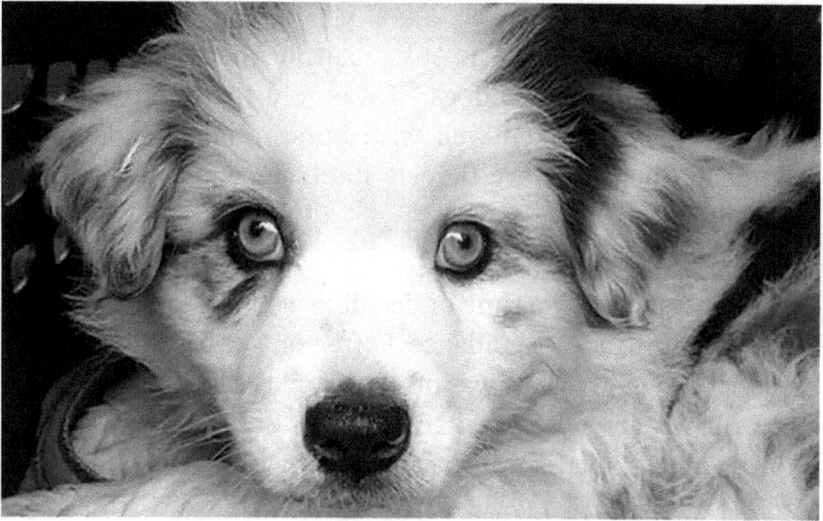

The day came to pick her up. I had all the proper puppy materials picked out for her in preparation for this exciting day. I was so excited to bring home this precious little niblet! I had certain names picked out for her, but once I got her, none of the names seemed to fit. Intuitively I felt called to search names online when I got back to the ranch. I stumbled upon the Persian name "Xaria," which meant "Gift of the Heart." Xaria was her name! I loved how it sounded: playful, spunky, with character and upbeat. She fit it perfectly.

As Xaria grew up, it felt like she was the Australian Shepherd version of Leilani. Thank goodness she didn't have the urge to wander like Leilani did, but had a loving, gentle, smart similarity to my husky friend. I felt like my prayers had been answered. Xaria truly was a "Gift of the Heart."

As Xaria got older and her little puppy face morphed from a squished furry ball to having a definitive snout, it was amusing to see how her quirky, cute, and loving personality developed. She was a true healing force.

ROWEN:

Life continued. The next many months consisted of grieving the death of my best friend Deb, running horse workshops, grief rituals, hosting guests at the Airbnb cottage, doing private sessions with clients, and everyday ranch life. During this time, I studied equine-assisted coaching and facilitation with Equine Alchemy. During that program, one of the women I trained with was Schelli Whitehouse (who was an Equine Alchemy EFL teacher at that time). Later, Schelli became my business mentor, coach, colleague, and friend.

Six months after Deb's tragic death, my former sister-in-law, Rowen was diagnosed with stage 3 colon cancer. Rowen was the mother of my niece Jasmine. To hear about another person in my inner circle having cancer was heartbreaking. When she was diagnosed, Rowen and I weren't as close as we had been twenty-one years earlier when she became pregnant with my niece. Rowen was the only person in my family I could talk to who would understand the emotional and psychological dynamics that others outside our family wouldn't understand. It was shocking to find out that another one of my closest friends was affected by cancer. My world was rocked yet again.

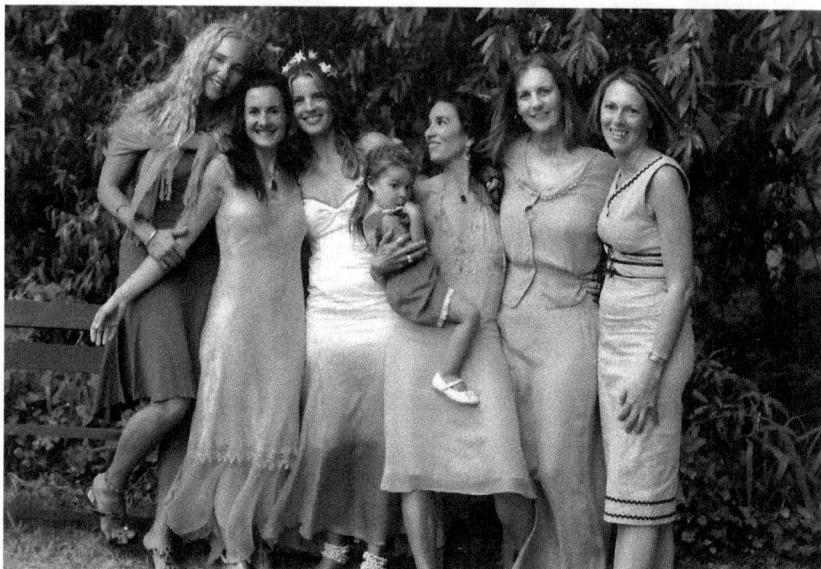

One of my favorite photos taken from my wedding. Anny Owen, Deb Hubsmith, me, Zenobia, Michelle Russi, Siena McCarthy & Rowen Holland - Photo by Shelly Garrish

In my wedding photo from 2009, I'm surrounded by four of my closest friends. This particular photo is dear to my heart as it illustrates the love that I have for my closest girlfriends. Three out of six of us in this photo have been affected by a late-stage cancer diagnosis all within our mid-forties. It's uncanny. We're living examples of canaries in a coal mine.

Those who get cancer at a younger age represent a wakeup call for humanity. The sad reality is that environmental and food toxicity is affecting the human population at an alarming rate. My hope is that we wake up to the fact that we're killing ourselves with our fast-paced industrial lifestyle, all in the name of profit. (I speak about this topic in my environmental short film titled *Honor the Earth*.)

Rowen lived four hours away from me in the Bay Area. After her diagnosis, I went down a few times to see her, but due to the distance and my responsibilities at the ranch, it was difficult to see her often. I was happy to raise money for her cancer healing fund. I had already done this for Deb and was familiar with the nuts and bolts of running a health-oriented fundraiser.

My already fragile heart took a greater pounding with the reality of Rowen's life on the edge.

The troubles affecting you serve to carry you to your next
plateau of growth.
Each challenge is an opportunity for expansion.
Rise beyond each breath.
Seize your sword.
Your light will not be extinguished.

A PREMONITION:

In the late spring of 2016, I started noticing a lump in my breast that wasn't going away. As I had fibrocystic (lumpy) breasts in the past, I didn't pay much attention to it. For years, I had been heavily occupied being Deb's caretaker and with excessive ranch and business duties; so, I neglected my own self-care.

Ancestors on both sides of my family were from hardy stock. My mother and father both grew up close to the earth. My mother is from Conway, New Hampshire and grew up on a farm with her three sisters and one brother. My father is from the exact opposite of the United States on Kaua'i, Hawaii. They both grew up in a rural location where hard work is a necessary virtue. They both were taught to be strong, stubborn, independent, and never give up. Of course, I inherited this sense of resilience as well!

If there was a challenge, I was happy to jump at the opportunity. If someone told me I couldn't do something, that was an invitation to prove them wrong! Deb, my dear friend who had recently died, was wired similarly.

With my skepticism toward standard medical care, I rarely went to a Western doctor unless it was a real emergency. Due to my beliefs and stubborn adherence to natural medicine, I never got regular mammograms. I believed that mammograms could cause cancer due to the high radioactive content in the scans. After seeing what Deb had endured with countless months in the hospital, I was convinced that standard medicine was dangerous.

As the months rolled by, I noticed that the lump in my left breast was getting harder and bigger. When it started silently screaming its prominence, I mentioned something to Syris about it. When he said he had noticed it but wasn't sure how to ask me about it, I knew I had to check it out. Reality started creeping in around the edges of my periphery.

Scheduling a medical appointment when you don't have insurance can be a conundrum to navigate. My first attempt to schedule an appointment for a breast exam was in July 2016. It took until September, two months later for a basic screening appointment to be made.

In August, Syris and I took a trip to Oregon to commemorate the one-year anniversary of Deb's death on August 18. I knew I had to do something special to honor her. If I didn't take time to commemorate her, I feared I would drown in a pit of sorrow. It's vitally important in the process of releasing grief to honor and celebrate those you love.

"Grief is the last act of love we have to give to those we loved. Where there is deep grief, there was great love"

–ANONYMOUS

It wasn't an easy task to leave the ranch for a week as there were constant chores that needed to be done. It was worth the energy and effort to make the trip happen, though. Little did I know how important this trip would be!

On the first leg of our journey, Syris and I stopped at the spiritual town of Mount Shasta, which is one of my favorite spots on Earth. Ever since I was twenty years old, I was drawn to its snowy pinnacle. The sacred mountain has always been a powerful place of spiritual healing. It was such an incredible anchor point for me that I even named my first dog, a fluffy, precocious Alaskan Malamute, Shasta after the mountain.

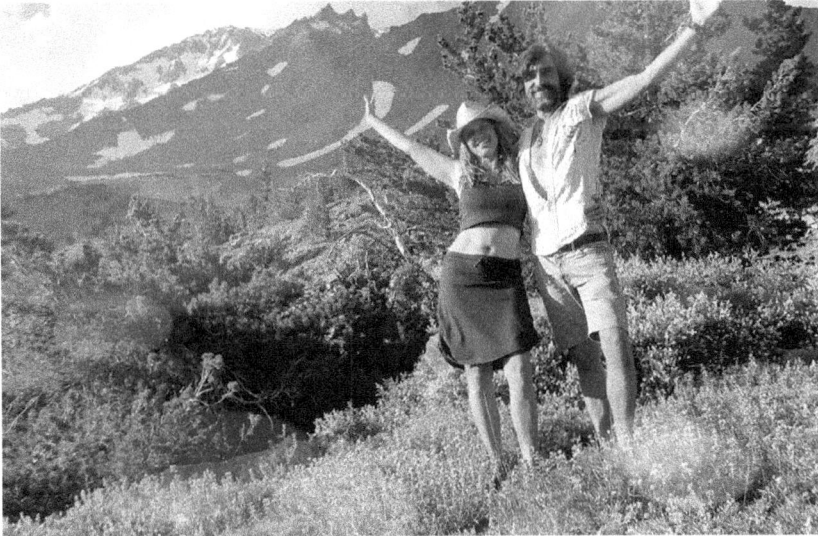

A magical moment on Mount Shasta

Many say Mount Shasta is connected to ancient Lemuria, the Inner Earth city of Telos, St. Germain, alien landings, and Tibet. It was sacred to the Native Americans for thousands of years.

This dormant volcano is not part of any mountain range. She's uniquely her own mountain in many ways. With a summit of 14,125 feet above sea level, Shasta is the second highest peak in the Cascade Mountain range. Her slopes rise abruptly nearly 10,000 feet above the surrounding landscape.[2]

We had an auspicious experience on the mountain. In the afternoon, we took a walk on the snowy ancient volcano. Soaking in the rays of sunshine, I built a small altar with my favorite crystals and sacred items to commemorate Deb.

It was a joy to be on the road with Syris. I had always loved road trips and to be able to discover the shared collaboration of a road trip deeply satisfied my freedom-loving self!

We drove up to Breitenbush Hot Springs in central Oregon to gather with our talented musician friends Jaya Lakshmi and Ananda for their "Altar of Love" event. For five glorious days we did kundalini yoga, sang and chanted sacred songs, danced, did a cacao ceremony, soaked in hot springs, ate delicious organic food, and camped near ancient trees. To be able to touch into community life like this with the backdrop of healing music was genuinely healing and rejuvenating for my soul. We made new friends and savored the harmony of this enchanted event.

During the road trip I was aware of the medical appointment that awaited me upon my return. Being an optimist, I didn't think about it that much but was vaguely nervous of the unknown reality that awaited me.

When we returned, happily greeted by bouncy Xaria and indifferently approached by our two barn kitties, I knew it was time to mentally prepare for the crucial appointment.

BLUE PAISLEY RAIN BOOTS:

When the fateful day approached, I went by myself to the appointment. I told the nurse who greeted me that I had had a lump in my breast for some time. As soon as I said that, an abysmal look of fright flashed over her face.

I frankly think that medical workers would benefit with a thorough training in how to handle potentially petrifying situations with patients. In the years of being immersed in the medical world, first through being with Deb and her leukemia journey and then my own personal health experiences, I've witnessed horrendous reactions from various health workers.

The nurse had a terror-stricken face as she proceeded to look at the lump in my breast. She mumbled something about be right back and slowly slinked out of the room.

While I waited for her, I was anxious about her reaction. If the nurse was so easily freaked out by the mention of the lump, then there must be something off kilter about the situation, right?

When she came back into the room, she told me that I would have to make an appointment somewhere else. Apparently, she couldn't give me a regular mammogram due to the presence of the lump in my breast. Alrighty then.

I was flummoxed. I had to dive back into the rabbit hole to figure out where I needed to schedule an appointment.

During this time, Rowen, my former sister-in-law and the one who was going through colon cancer had just moved up to the Grass Valley area. She wanted a change and desired a slower lifestyle away from the frenetic fast pace of the Bay Area to heal. We had planned that I would help her out with her cancer healing journey. As I had already been on a similar path with Deb, I was happy to help Rowen out. I loved her dearly. She was family to me. I truly believed that moving to the rural setting of the lower Sierra Nevada mountains would provide a much-needed healing shift for her. Little did we know what was in store for all of us.

Rowen had moved to a house in Grass Valley, and I had my appointment booked for the fateful mammogram two weeks after she moved in. Rowen had offered to come with me to the appointment and I welcomed her support. I had a great disdain and reluctance to engage in Western medicine and having a close friend by my side was appreciated.

The appointment started out with a regular old mammogram. Getting your boobs squished is a hell of a party! After the mammogram, I was told that something was detected within my breast and it was necessary to take a deeper look. My head started to spin. Thank goodness Rowen was there to hold ground for me. I was told I needed to get an ultrasound to see deeper into the tissue layers of my breast.

As I laid on the table with cold goo spread on my boob, an indifferent radiologist used his fancy ultrasound device to peer into my tissue. The prognosis: Something was there, and it wasn't Kermit the Frog.

The nurses and technician didn't look horror stricken like the previous nurse, thank goodness. There's definitely a place for aloof behavior in situations like this. With my own mind jumping to worst-case situations, I didn't need to deal with the visceral reactions of the medical staff.

The part that was truly terrifying was when I was told I needed to have a biopsy immediately! At this point, I had already been in the dreaded Sierra Nevada Hospital for two hours. I hadn't planned to be gone this long.

I never had a biopsy before and wasn't sure what to expect. I tend to have a high pain tolerance and, therefore, didn't fear the needle that would pierce the tender tissue of my boob. I already was covered with several tattoos; how bad could a biopsy needle be?

As the nurse approached with a long needle, I started to get a bit nervous about the procedure. Rowen inched up close to my feet to hold them in her warm, comforting hands. I had no idea the needle would plunge so deep into the folds of my breast. I winced in pain as Rowen lovingly squeezed my feet. No numbing solution was put on, which meant I felt all four inches of that dreaded, evil needle. Ouch!

I was told after the fact that a titanium marker was put into my breast when I received the biopsy. I was upset about this, as I was given no choice whether I was okay with having the metal marker put under my skin. It would have been nice if the doctor had said, "We usually put a titanium marker in you when doing a biopsy, so I know where I'm making the incision for future reference. Is this okay with you?" I believe it's important to be given a chance to decide what one's body wants to endure. It was disturbing to me to learn later that the metal marker can create more disease and imbalance in the body.

After this experience, I was shaken, drained, exhausted, and deeply disturbed. I was told I would receive a call from one of the hospital staff in the next week. Now, I had to go home and wait!

That day, I was initiated into the official Heroines Health Journey. Like the ancient Sumerian Goddess Inanna who dove into the darkness to face innumerable tests, my own journey into darkness had begun. The physical pain, emotional reaction of fear, plus the three hours I spent at the hospital were deeply traumatic. I had no idea what was in store for me, but I knew something wasn't right. I didn't tell anyone else what happened; only Syris and Rowen knew about it. I figured there was no need to upset anyone over a possible diagnosis.

I spent a week waiting for the news.

When I got the phone call, I was about to go outside to tend to the horses. As I was putting my wool-socked feet into my blue fashionable rain boots, I heard the phone ring. Throwing my kitschy blue paisley boots on the floor, I ran to the phone.

"Hello, is Tara there?"

"This is Tara speaking."

"Hi Tara, this is Serena from the oncology center of Sierra Nevada Hospital."

"Uhhhhhhhh, hi..." I reluctantly replied realizing this was the phone call I had been anxiously waiting for.

The nurse asked me, "Do you want to hear the good news or the bad news first?"

I stumbled on my words, "Um, the bad news?"

She replied with a caring voice that obviously was used to making these dreaded phone calls, "The bad news is you have cancer."

There was a pause, a silence that all the sand of the Sahara Desert couldn't fill.

Finally, I replied, "What's the good news?"

"The good news is that it's only stage 1."

Okay. I'm not sure if receiving news that your cancer diagnosis is only stage 1 is good news, but considering the alternative of a more serious diagnosis like stage 3 or 4, I suppose it is.

I sat there stunned, leaning up against the doorway of my beloved ranch house, my socked feet hovering over the ground.

The next few weeks were a blur, during which I had various appointments with an oncologist, surgeon, and radiologist. A week or two after the ominous phone call, I found out that I was misdiagnosed. Basically, my good news was not so good after all. I actually was diagnosed with stage 3 breast cancer, as there was a mistake with my biopsy. When the biopsy was taken, they thought that actual cancer cells were taken as a sample, but they had missed and not gotten any of the cells used to determine the proper staging. WTF?!? I had gone through that terribly painful incident for nothing?! During an appointment with a surgeon, he regretfully informed me that it was definitely stage 3.

Ugh! Deep breath.

The standard treatment suggested was a mastectomy, followed by the "big guns" of chemo and radiation. I was told that I could possibly die during chemotherapy treatment, and I would most likely be hospitalized, as the treatment would be so hard and definitely weaken my immune system.

I was scared.

I couldn't understand why there was such a prominent expression of cancer in my life in the last many years. From my dog Leilani to Deb and Rowen, it seemed impossible to escape the deadly presence of cancer. It had affected most of my nearest and dearest. Now I had my own dance with cancer to contend with. This was inconceivable! My brain was utterly baffled!

I did an immense amount of research about what path to choose for my healing journey. I ended up making a dramatic choice that I knew would create turbulent waves among those in my family and possibly those in my community. This blog post was a result of the deep inquiry. It took a Herculean amount of courage to share it with the world.

FINDING MY OWN HEALING PATH:

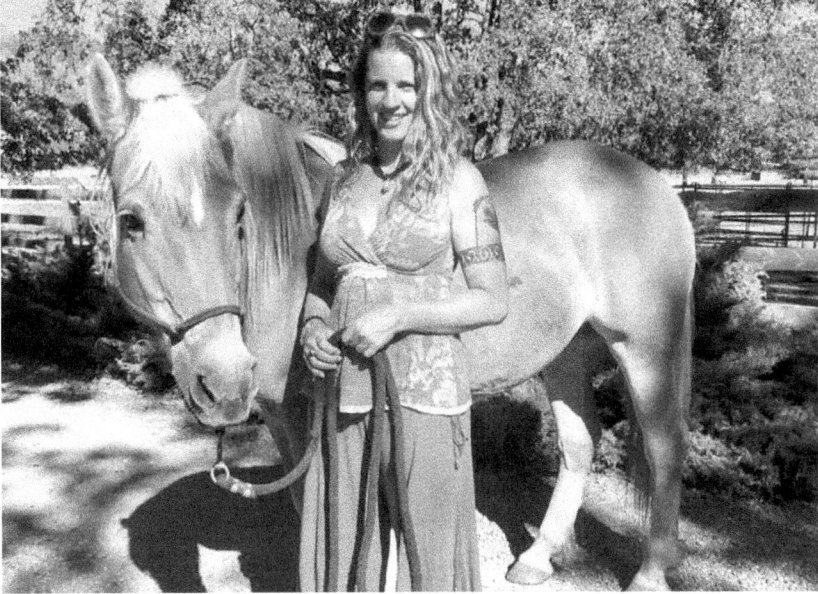

Daisy & me - This photo was taken a week after diagnosis. I can see the vulnerability in my eyes.

11/8:

I was recently diagnosed with stage 3 breast cancer. The western method of healing is prescribing four and a half intense months of a powerhouse form of chemotherapy called ACT (a cocktail of three drugs), followed by surgery, radiation, and ten years of being on a hormone replacement drug, if I even survive that long.

Side effects: My oncologist told me directly that the chemo would most definitely put me into early menopause, I would lose my hair and it would compromise my immune system. Because of my young age, they are prescribing what they call the 'big guns' of chemo, which could lead to spending extended time in the hospital with serious complications and could possibly even cause death. They say they would NOT give this high dose of chemo to an older person, as it could kill them. That makes me feel really safe!

I already have a compromised immune system due to an autoimmune thyroid condition. My diet has been gluten free for ten years. I don't eat sugar, processed foods or take aspirin. I've eaten organic all my life. My friends say I'm the healthiest person they know. I have such extreme sensitivity that I can't walk into a mainstream grocery store without being bombarded by the smells of laundry detergents and chemicals. I don't drink, smoke and everything about my lifestyle is clean. I gratefully live close to the earth with my horses and blessed beasts. In short, I know my body well.

I'm choosing a different route.

Please keep in mind that I witnessed my gorgeous, vibrant friend at the age of forty-four be diagnosed with AML, endure chemotherapy, and die twenty-two months later. I was by her side throughout her whole journey as one of her main caretakers. It was the most horrifying yet pivotal experience of my life. All the endless days spent at the hospital with her have left their mark upon me. I must choose what is right for me.

My decision is to take my own health into my hands and heal myself through alternative natural methods rather than the traditional western route of chemotherapy, radiation, hormone drugs, and surgery. I have researched this extensively and have come to this decision through deep soul searching, reading books, talking to specialists and others on a natural route of healing, watching films, and doing web research.

I know this will frighten some of you. Some of you might think that my choice is a death sentence and I'm crazy to put my trust in alternative natural healing methods. Honestly, at this point in my diagnosis, I think there is more chance of me dying by submitting to standard medicine. Blindly following the route prescribed to me would strip me of my power. I fear it would leave me with side effects that would render my spirit to silence.

Please hear me: If you have doubts arise from my decision, please keep your opinion to yourself! When you challenge me, shower me with your doubts and fears, it not only stresses me out but invalidates the process that I feel will truly heal me. We all have our choices, and this is my body! Please make your own decisions for your body and respect my choice for mine. Before you discount me, walk a mile in my shoes to understand the ginormous decision I must make.

To be given a serious cancer diagnosis is frankly a mind-fuck. I thought I had gone through hell and high water before, but this takes the cake. To face the demons in my own mind when I realize I have a dis-ease that in a short time could kill me if I don't step up and take charge of every element of my being is challenging — not to mention the reactions of everyone around me whether it be pity, fear, or sadness.

The hardest part of this journey so far has been the blunt reaction from my closest family members challenging my plan. They believe that I will die from this decision to choose a nontoxic, natural route to heal cancer. I know they are scared to lose me, and their fear comes from a place of love. They think I'm crazy to not start chemotherapy right away and blindly trust the medical system.

The best thing you can do now is to have faith in me! I'm a strong, capable woman and have a solid potential to create whatever reality I desire. I know I will be successful in my mission!

Though the doctors and nurses have good intentions, the experience of witnessing Deb in the standard cancer world and now my own experience with it showed me how disempowering the medical system can be. For example, my first day spent in the hospital where I received a mammogram, ultrasound, and biopsy left me shaky and terrified. Before they injected a 4" needle multiple times into my breast and armpit for the biopsy, I was told a small bit of titanium would be injected permanently into the two spots. I was not given a choice in the matter. I was told it was harmless and would not affect my body. Research later confirmed my suspicion that indeed those titanium markers can create irritation in the skin, and it is challenging to remove them. It is not natural to have metal in your body. Fear and the rush to move fast as there is "danger of the cancer spreading" stopped me from questioning this procedure. In retrospect, this was a complete violation of my body.

Please note that I'm grateful for western medicine and its ability to heal. I appreciate the medical advances made in certain modalities. This particular viewpoint is expressed specifically pertaining to my experience in the cancer world. I have already experienced a vast amount of trauma from being with my best friend Deb and my own personal experience. This fear prevents me from going forward with the prescribed treatment.

It is normal for cancer patients to be rushed into treatment. We are told we have to act fast; otherwise, the cancer will spread like wildfire rapidly through our body. The truth is that once you are diagnosed with cancer, most likely, you "had" cancer for years before diagnosis. Cancer doesn't materialize overnight.

Cancer cells proliferate in a body which is out of balance due to many possible causes such as stress, chemical exposure, emotional trauma, unhealthy diet, lifestyle, and a myriad of other health issues.

When an oncologist puts pressure on a cancer patient to decide to start treatment immediately, it puts unnecessary anxiety on the patient, which, in turn, can create more of sympathetic stress response within the body. Healing occurs when there is a sense of peace and relaxation in the body, not when it's paralyzed with fear.

The overwhelmed feeling that can occur when cancer patients feel pressured to start treatment immediately can lead patients to not truly question what the right form of treatment is for them. I encourage patients to take time to come to the truth of what treatment resonates for each individual. Hurrying to make a decision is never prudent. Besides, the treatment will ultimately be more effective if time is taken to feel clear about the decision.

If a patient is pushed into treatment from a sense of fear, then that same paralyzing sense of dread is carried throughout the treatment period. If I'm doing chemotherapy treatment but thinking of it as 'poison' rather than a healing elixir that will heal me, it will not have the same potent power of healing than if I was receiving it peacefully into my body.

We are energetic creatures. Our thoughts create our reality. I recommend you check out the powerful books of Joe Dispenza, *You Are the Placebo* and *Becoming Supernatural* and his transformational meditations. He offers wonderful tools to access the potential of your innate healing ability. Joe's work inspired me to shift my perspective from a place of dread, to knowing and believing I'm healing.

I refuse to buy into the fear. I know my body well. I know what I need to heal. I trust in the wisdom, food, and natural health protocols that have served me well my whole life.

I know this is my heroine's journey. I'm aware that my life is at stake. I have the power to choose what will heal me. I choose life! My body created this opportunity to manifest a deeper sense of balance in my life. I'm grateful for the lessons I'm learning!

In many ways, this is the greatest gift I have been given, to realize how precious life is. I can either choose to embrace each moment and live it to the fullest or whittle away in the illusions of my mind. I'm well aware that I must fully commit to my healing process or I might not make it to my fiftieth birthday. If this doesn't make me open my eyes to the glorious gift of life, what will?

If you were told you had a year to live, how would you live your life?

Cancer Warrioress:

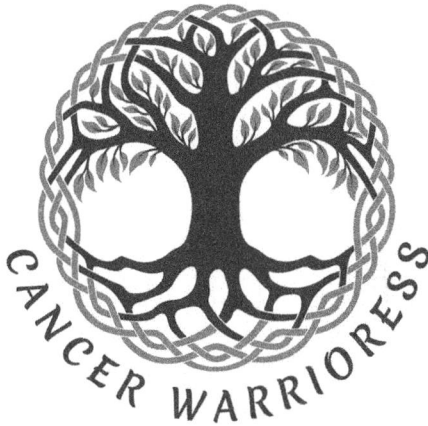

I recently created a blog page & Facebook page titled "Cancer Warrioress" with the decision to share my health journey publicly. Deb also shared her experience with AML publicly, which inspired me to do the same.

The reason why I chose the term "Cancer Warrioress" is because the courage it's taking to navigate this diagnosis is immense. Not only is it challenging within my own mind, but the choice I'm making to heal myself with an alternative healing protocol is attracting criticism from the medical world, family, and certain friends. The title CW symbolizes the conviction that's needed to face this arduous experience. Due to facing immense opposition, it's necessary to step into my true warrioress self and stand in my power.

I'm not choosing to be at war with my body and the cancer cells. I'm choosing to love the cancer, see it as a gift, and bring myself to healing through making peace with the cancer cells within my body.

Life is precious. Seize it with everything you have! From my experience of losing my closest friend and now journeying with cancer, I cannot reiterate to you enough how important it is to value each moment and your beloveds. Life is short. Health is precious. Inhabiting a human body is a gift beyond compare. Please don't waste this opportunity to shine your light and fulfill your destiny, whatever it may be.

ALTERNATIVE MEDICINE:

Unsolicited Advice, Healthy Communication & Boundaries:

As soon as I was diagnosed, my partner Syris and I dove into massive research about the best path of action to take for my healing protocol. As I decided on a natural route of healing cancer, my next adventure was to figure out what method of nontoxic medicine I was going to choose. I faced an unbelievable number of options!

Typically, when someone is diagnosed with cancer, a massive amount of information is thrown in their direction. Well-meaning people are uncomfortable with the topic of cancer, as cancer represents death. Whatever you do, don't mention the word "cancer" in a death-phobic culture! Those with a cancer diagnosis are staring at their mortality like two bright high beam car lights paralyzing a deer on a dark, wintery evening.

I understand that these well-intentioned people giving advice come from a place of wanting to help. Sharing naive guidance such as "using lemon essential oil will cure cancer" or "my cousin heard of someone who drank their own urine, and their cancer totally went away!" are unabashedly shared when you're recently diagnosed. It can be utterly overwhelming! It's hard enough to grapple with the reality of your mortality, the pressure from the standard medical world, and the shock of everyone else around you, while also grappling with an avalanche of unnecessary, unwanted guidance.

I've learned to clearly communicate when I post something on social media about my health and say, "I'm not looking for advice. Thank you for wanting to offer solutions, but I'm not looking for any now." I clearly ask when I actually am seeking advice by asking others opinion. This is different than a friend or family member launching into unasked for recommendations that I'm not wanting.

It all comes back to boundaries. If someone gives me unsolicited advice, a boundary is crossed that can be very uncomfortable. I love it when friends and family ask me, "Are you open to hearing my advice?" before launching into their opinion. In my mind, that's a respectful way of sharing information. If I say, "No thank you, I'm not open to hearing it," then the friend can understand I'm not receptive to their opinion. This creates a healthy way of communicating and fosters a balanced relationship for both people.

The same respectful way of communication can be applied to any challenging conversation topic. Healthy interactions can go a long way to creating harmonious and loving relationships with others.

DOCTOR V & RGCC/GREECE TEST:

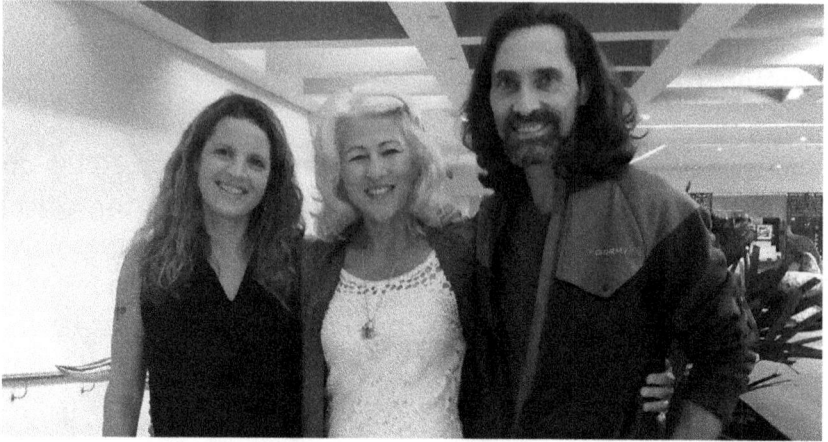

Me, Doctor V (Véronique Desaulniers) & Syris

As I was bombarded with tons of advice from friends and people I had never met on social media, Syris and I soon devoured loads of information. I read books, watched movies, and talked to others to find out what they had done to treat cancer. During that time, I was fortunate to stumble upon a book by Véronique Desaulniers (AKA Doctor V) called Heal Breast Cancer Naturally. A light bulb went off when I found this book on Amazon.

From the first moment of my diagnosis, being submerged in the medical system felt extremely off kilter for me. I immediately sensed the fear, dread, and inherent pushiness from the medical establishment in Grass Valley, CA. The experience felt completely bizarre for me.

Finding Doctor V's book was like finding a gem amid garbage. I sensed that her book would provide a path that would offer great comfort in a time of utter confusion. I immediately ordered it and devoured it cover to cover after it arrived in my searching hands. Her book is well organized and holds a plethora of information about how a healthy lifestyle prevents or heals cancer. It addresses diet, supplements, herbs, and modalities that will aid in the healing of breast cancer.

Doctor V has healed herself naturally from breast cancer twice using her "7 Essential Systems" of healing, which she created and discusses in her book. She teaches workshops and provides coaching to women needing guidance during a cancer experience. Her book is a valuable resource for people wanting help with an exclusively natural path of healing cancer or an integrated treatment plan.

The term "natural" is a loose definition and is the new hip catch phrase. Healing oneself naturally from cancer generally means without receiving chemotherapy or radiation. There are gradients of this term as well.

I immediately appreciated Doctor V's viewpoint about bringing in emotional healing, as it has always felt intrinsically connected. Mind, body, and spirit act as one. If you're suffering from a traumatic situation, then your body is invariably going to act as a buffer to absorb the emotional shock.

I was immediately drawn to Doctor V's coaching program and decided to sign up! I absolutely adored the coach I was assigned to work with. She was such a loving source of support, kindness, valuable information, and hope during a frightening time in my life. It felt good to have a direction to go toward on my healing journey.

Through Doctor V's coaching program, I heard about and took the Oncotrail RGCC test, which is also called the "Greek Test." It's a blood test where your blood is withdrawn, sent to Greece and the amount of circulating tumor cells in your bloodstream is tested.

This seemed like a brilliant way to test the amount of cancer I had in my body. It was extra appealing to me, as I had the unfortunate experience of the hospital staff in Grass Valley being extremely pushy toward me. This was a shame, as I didn't feel comfortable being monitored by standard medicine.

Another test the RGCC company offers is the Onconomics Extracts test. This test tells the patient which particular natural medicines are helpful in the treatment of the particular cancer diagnosis. Before I took the test, I was spending a lot of money on supplements, shoving all sorts of pills in my mouth, drinking disgusting teas, and shooting blindly in the dark with my choice of treatment. Ultimately, I wasn't sure if it was helping me or not! The appeal of this test would be to actually know what supplements were directly effective with my own diagnosis.

It's also important to mention that there is also a version of the test called the: 'Onconomics RGCC." I ended up using this test later, which was extremely helpful for me:

When I first took the Oncotrail RGCC test, my score result was 8.2, which was on the high side! It's said that anything over a 5 is advanced cancer. How did I get the high number of 8.2? The high score was intimidating and definitely whipped my bootie in gear as I took the results seriously. I was determined to get that 8.2 down to below 2 in record time!

After I got my test results back, I also received a detailed supplement recommendation list from the Onconomics Extracts test. Herbs and exotic tinctures like iodine, pork liver enzymes, curcumin, and mushrooms to an expensive yet disgusting fermented soy drink named Haelan from China were recommended for my protocol. I had my hands full navigating where to get this long supplement list. I wasn't sure how I was going to pay for it all, though. At this point, I had a thriving horse retreat center business with full workshops and a year-round booked Airbnb cottage. All the money I earned was going directly to running my 10-acre ranch and feeding/caring for my four horses. Running a ranch was expensive with the costly repairs and unexpected expenses. I didn't have extra thousands of dollars to put into a pricey supplement list.

I had loads of experience doing fundraisers. I had helped Deb raise $50K for her healing journey and played a strong hand in helping Rowen raise $20K for her cancer treatment. If I could raise money for them, couldn't I do the same for myself?

I dove full on into creating an online fundraiser. Friends generously organized various events to raise money for me as well: dance parties, Kundalini Yoga workshops, a clothing sale, a silent auction. My community from Nevada City to Marin rallied to help me fund my mission to heal cancer naturally. It was unbelievably therapeutic to realize how loved I was and how people truly desired to assist me in my healing. I had always been the giver and helped others in their time of need; now, it was my lesson to learn to receive. Over a period of two and a half years, through various sources, I raised about $50K. My friends loved me and wanted to show up for me. I realized how incredibly blessed I was to be so loved!

Due to the generosity of my community, I felt confident to be able to fund my healing cancer naturally journey.

TARA'S BOOT CAMP:

I decided to call my extensive health protocol "Tara's Boot Camp" as it was a serious regimen with an organized and somewhat arduous schedule.

November:

I intend to dive deeply into my healing process. This means that I will sift through past emotional wounds that still fester and affect me in my daily life. I will honor the need to care for myself. This means I will not push myself so hard and will examine my tendency to be constantly busy. I plan to step back from the hamster wheel of society. I know I have behaviors from past childhood patterns and my false, conditioned self which have contributed to my tumor growth. I'm choosing to see them as opportunities for my healing growth.

I'm committing to a serious daily regimen of natural therapies. I have been doing this protocol for weeks already and I'm seeing results through detoxification.

I've gotten a baseline of where the tumor growth is now, due to doing an ultrasound and other tests. After a period of my boot camp, I plan to check my tumor level again. I will get a second opinion at UCSF to see what protocol of healing the doctors there would prescribe for me. In this time of healing, I will constantly check and realistically assess if my plan is effective.

For those of you who want to support me in my healing journey, PLEASE TRUST MY ABILITY TO MAKE THIS DECISION FOR MYSELF. Prayer is powerful! Instead of focusing on doubt and fear about my decision, please transcend the fear and visualize me being radiant and healthy. Please picture me living a long, healthy life, witnessing Willow thrive in his and hopefully meeting my grandchildren one day. See me continuing to do the transformational work I do with my horses. I love my life and I intend to keep living. Thank you. Your prayer and intentions are greatly appreciated!

Instead of feeding a future vision of me with fear, please focus on the abundance of love and the infinite healing potential within me!

***

One month later, I shared this update about the health protocol I had chosen. These updates are snapshots of the time I was in. My viewpoints and beliefs might have changed since this was written. You can see the mindset I was in and what my experience was at this time. This was my path with the cancer guru. I hope my experience can help guide yours in some way.

If you have a different viewpoint of what works for you, I support you in whatever resonates for you. Whatever you choose must be right for you. No one can make the decision for you. I encourage you to truly drop down and listen to what your authentic voice says. You have the right to make your own self informed decision!

In the Land of Detoxification:

It's been a month since my last update. During this time, my body has been doing an immense amount of detoxification due to the cleansing diet I'm on.

Generally, I've been feeling pretty good. There are days when the effects of detoxification kicks in, which causes me to be tired and need to rest. Overall, my body is adjusting to the extreme amount of vegetable juices, nutrition, supplements, and herbs I'm consuming. I often am met with surprise when someone knows I've been recently diagnosed with cancer and sees me out in the world. I regularly hear, "Wow, you look so healthy and vibrant. You don't look like you have cancer at all!" I realize I'm breaking the paradigm of what's expected of a cancer patient.

It's a common assumption that with a stage 3 cancer diagnosis, one should look sickly and depleted. This judgment is based on the belief of how a cancer patient is supposed to look because most patients with cancer choose the standard route of healing of chemotherapy, surgery, and radiation. A patient receiving this treatment is usually processing such a massive amount of toxins that it's common for the patient to look exhausted, underweight, sick, and depleted. Chemotherapy attacks the cancer cells but also affects the immune system. My choice of healing is to build up my immune system rather than break it down.

To be clear, I wasn't feeling sick when I received my diagnosis. Besides the tumor in my breast there was no other sign of cancer in my body. As I'm choosing to load myself up with an extreme amount of nutrients, there's no way I cannot look healthy!

I know I have a road ahead of me. Healing takes time. I had a sense this diagnosis would be tough, but now I get it on a deeper level. This experience is making me dig deep into my inner strength. Put one foot in front of the other.

I plan to do the RGCC test again in ninety days so I can accurately monitor my healing progress. I'm choosing to do a blood test, as it's non-invasive. Other monitoring methods such as PET and CT scans can be damaging to the body through being exposed to a massive amount of radiation and toxic material. Biopsies require cutting into the tumor, which can possibly spread the cancer. I'm choosing a nontoxic method of healing cancer.

My conclusion from witnessing my friend Deb on her twenty-two-month journey with AML and my own experience after being diagnosed is that standard cancer medicine isn't focused on the health of the patient but is sadly all about profit.

I know I will ruffle some feathers with this statement. I don't discount the individual oncologist's intention of healing; this statement is addressed at the pharmaceutical companies rather than any single doctor. I'm choosing to respect my body and treat it well with natural medicine. I would rather do this than to give a fat pay bonus to the resident oncologist for a prescribed dose of expensive chemotherapy. There's a rumor that every time oncologists give certain prescriptions, there's a large kickback from the pharmaceutical companies for prescribing their particular medicine. I say, "No thank you!"

In the past five years, this is just a taste of what I've experienced:

1. My husband and I divorced.
2. I gave up my thriving Pilates studio and started a horse retreat center.
3. I uprooted my life and moved 250 miles away to a new community.
4. I was one of the main caretakers for my best friend of nineteen years through her twenty-two-month journey with AML. I went through immense grief after she died.

It's said that cancer usually knocks on someone's door within two years of experiencing great grief, going through a major life transition, moving, changing jobs, or going through a divorce. I went through all these huge transitions!

I had many hoops to jump through. I've learned that an "attitude of gratitude" serves me rather than feeling sorry for myself and staying stuck in the victim mentality. I see every challenge as an opportunity to polish the diamond of my soul. Although I would love to not have a serious cancer diagnosis, I'm choosing to embrace and use it as a route for unbelievable transformation!

I'm fortunate to have found Kundalini Yoga three years ago, which is a powerful practice to bring me out of the quagmire of my mind.

My healing protocol is rigorous, which is a ginormous time commitment. It takes dedication and hard work, but it beats chemotherapy, which would completely annihilate my immune system. I don't want to deal with the nasty side-effects of chemo.

Gerson Therapy:

I'm following a rough version of the Gerson diet. I'm seriously considering committing 100% into this strict diet and healing protocol to achieve the maximum benefits.

The Gerson health protocol was created by German born Max Gerson, the author of *A Cancer Therapy: Results of 50 Cases* in 1918. He suffered from persistent chronic migraines and created his own health routine to heal his condition.

After 2 years of an elimination diet, he finally was able to completely halt his migraines through a specialized diet of fruits and vegetables with no fat, salt, alcohol or spices.

In 1918 his "migraine diet" became somewhat well-known and widely used by his patients and others. Then, as fate would have it, a patient returned to Dr. Gerson and reported an observation that not only did the "migraine diet" cure his migraines, but his skin tuberculosis was also cured. This was a miraculous report considering tuberculosis was incurable at the time. The news of this miracle spread quickly throughout the medical community.

When Nazi Germany threatened the Jewish population, Max was the only one of his 7 siblings to escape alive. He left Germany in 1933 and ended up in New York City, NY. In 1938 he started his own medical practice in New York where he remained & cured many patients of cancer and other diseases until his mysterious death by arsenic poisoning induced pneumonia in 1959.

The Gerson dietary regimen consists of a low salt, low fat, and high carbohydrate diet plus oral administration of minerals and vitamins to supplement those vitamins missing in the diet. The diet is chiefly made of large amounts of organic fresh fruit and vegetable juices and doesn't allow any meat, milk, alcohol, canned or bottled foods. Tobacco in any form is prohibited.

The diet burns down to an alkaline ash and in general is a combination of many well-known and approved dietary nutritional discoveries by many other workers. The therapy also includes a liver detoxification procedure via coffee enemas.

Max assumed that the closer one's diet is to nature and the soil with fresh fruit from the trees and fresh vegetables directly from the garden, the nearer one is to normal health.

This new approach to the cancer problem is of fundamental importance because it is the first promising method which treats cancer as a systemic disease, that is, a disease of abnormal chemistry of the whole body.[3]

After Max Gerson's death, his daughter Charlotte Gerson continued to promote the therapy and started the Gerson Institute in 1977. She created a healing institute in Tijuana, Mexico where cancer patients visit for two weeks and participate in a proficient health program.

Gerson's diet appealed to me and everything about it made sense. I was happy to find a pathway that appealed to my mind, body, and spirit.

Healing Protocol:

To see how committed I am to my healing routine you can see my daily regimen:

- Kundalini yoga sadhana – KY helps me focus on healing, energetically clearing away any blocks and staying mentally clear. I'm grateful to be able to learn and take classes in person with my wise friend Jai Dev Singh. (See Life Force Academy link in Resources)

- Daily Coffee enemas

- Freshly made veggie juices

- Exercise: jogging, rebounder, walking

- Infrared sauna

- Colonics

- Digestive Pork Enzymes taken hourly

- Food: veggies, bone broth, no grains, no solid meat, simple foods

- Cannabis products

- Positive visualization, time for contemplation, centering, clearing away the doubts and mind gremlins when they come my way

- Castor oil packs

- Rest when needed, although I must admit this is difficult for me

- Nature and horse time

- Various healing modalities: chiropractic, acupuncture

- Puppy play because Xaria is just the most delightful little ball of fluffy joy!

Vitamins and Supplements List:

- Curcumin (Turmeric)

- Zinc

- Resveratrol

- Enzymes (Pork)

- Probiotics

- Se-zyme forte (Selenium)

- Mushrooms

- Vitamin D

- Vitamin C

- Multi vitamin

- Dried desiccated liver capsules

- Tinctures for cleansing: Dandelion, milk thistle, and mistletoe

- Two drops of iodine a day

- Essiac tea
- Ayurvedic ghee drink
- CBD oil

In the Public Eye:

For some indescribable reason I was called to share my healing journey publicly. Deb did the same thing years before me. I never stopped to question if I should NOT be public with my journey, it just seemed right.

I was aware when I openly shared about the breast cancer diagnosis that I would be closely observed, like a specimen under a microscope. As I chose a less traveled path of healing cancer naturally, I knew that my social media posts would be of great interest to others. Friends, family, and social media acquaintances would be watching from the sidelines asking: Is her treatment working? Is she healing? Is she dying? WILL SHE LIVE? If I put up a less than positive post it could evoke fear of my impending death.

Western culture fears death. The word cancer evokes terror as it's becoming a frightening epidemic due to our toxic world. How many young people do you know who have announced a stage 3 or 4 cancer diagnosis in the past year? I knew I would be a mirror of others' mortality with my diagnosis announcement.

My almost daily vulnerable sharing of my journey was incredibly cathartic. To share my heart so openly helped me move through the challenges that came my way and gave me the support of others who might not have known I needed help.

The experience of being in the public eye on the cancer journey has been a deeply transformational experience. I found that sharing a challenging experience helped to transcend it. In the process of sharing, I'm seen, witnessed, and heard. I've been told by others that seeing my experience helps them feel less alone. Knowing I can help others by my own experience brings me deep joy and, in some funny way, makes all the difficult moments so worth it!

When I shared with the public about the diagnosis, I was prepared for the well-meaning advice, stories, messages, and attention that Deb experienced. I didn't know I would be receiving so much encouragement, support, and adoration. At the age of forty-seven, I found myself learning the art of self-love. Thank you, cancer, for this valuable lesson.

2017

The Wheel Turns

Months went by and I was solidly committed to my healing regimen. In January 2017, President Trump was inaugurated into office. This created a sense of upheaval among most of my friends and family members.

FACING THE GREAT UNKNOWN:

1/30:

What a powerful time this is! I know many of you feel a sharp unsettling jolt with the current political paradigm. It occurred to me today how similar these dramatic changes are to someone who has a cancer diagnosis.

In this time of facing the great unknown, it's easy to become swept away by fear. When I'm faced with unsettling anxiety, I find what helps me is to surrender to whatever situation I'm in. The idea that I have any control at all is really an illusion. When I stay stuck in the past, I prevent the possibility of a brighter reality to emerge for me.

I know it's not easy, but I encourage you to have faith. There's certainly a greater plan unfolding here; of that I'm certain. I believe that we can create a brighter world if we all unite, joining forces with our collective vision!

As far as my healing protocol is concerned, I'm solidly committed to it. I've started new supplements. The biggest addition to my healing protocol is doing high-dose Vitamin C infusions.

Based on the results of my RGCC Oncotrail blood test I've been prescribed a three-month supplement plan from one of Doctor V's coaches.

This test shares with me specifically what supplements work most effectively to shrink the tumor and free my body of cancer. (At the end of three months, I will do a similar blood test to test my tumor markers.) I also have the support of other alternative doctors and am being closely monitored through other blood tests. I'm in excellent hands! This plan of healing was created through my extensive research of what cures cancer and through the support of these angels on my team.

I'm grateful to be on this path of healing. I'm consciously building my immune system through these healthy protocols. I feel deep in my body that I'm indeed healing!

My health regimen each day is a full-time job. My protocol with Doctor V has me swallowing about twenty-five pills three times a day at mealtimes, six enzymes every hour (which comes to be about forty-five enzymes a day!), Haelan (a nasty fermented soy drink from China which tastes like dirty socks!) and Vitamin C infusions twice a week (it takes hours to do one infusion).

The Vitamin C infusions have been the biggest transition for me. The detoxification effects can be extreme. Immediately after the infusion I feel a dynamic burst of energy. I'm like the energizer bunny bouncing enthusiastically around the ranch performing endless tasks! I'll have so much energy that it's hard to sleep at night. Then the exhaustion hits, and I experience bone-tired fatigue for days.

Cancer proliferates in an oxygen-deprived body. Linus Pauling, a Nobel Laureate proved that high doses of Vitamin C could heal many diseases, including cancer. Vitamin C creates "oxygen blasts" in the bloodstream, which annihilates cancer cells. Blast those babies! Unfortunately, Paulding was labeled a "quack" in his lifetime until his death in 1984. Now science has confirmed that his studies were right; Vitamin C does help to heal cancer!

Lo and behold, do you see a trend with alternative doctors being discredited and silenced by the pharmaceutical industry?

I learned that the extreme exhaustion I felt after the Vitamin C infusions was totally normal. Max Gerson of the Gerson Institute would call dramatic bouts of tiredness "a healing reaction." This means that the protocol is working, and the body is doing its job to find balance. When the body kicks into healing mode it's bringing the body back to homeostasis. I believe the body's innate wisdom knows how to mend itself if it's given the proper tools to do so.

I've seen a vast difference between the standard and alternative viewpoint of healing cancer in the past months that I've been doing research. From the perspective of my alternative naturopathic doctors and my own personal research, I think I've discovered what triggered my cancer cells to be active. (By the way, everyone has cancer cells in their bodies; mine decided to come to life to grow in me in exponential ways.)

I've seen that the alternative path of medicine digs down to find the cause and treats it. My observation of the standard path of medicine is that it treats the side effects rather than the cause.

I'm deciding to build my immune system and actually treat the cause of why I was blessed with the lessons of breast cancer.

The topic of what caused the cancer never came up with any of the standard doctors! It would have made sense to me if the oncologist analyzed my blood to see the imbalance of what caused and fed the cancer to prevent reoccurrence. Along with the lack of understanding of why cancer began in the first place, the fact that I have an autoimmune thyroid issue (Hashimoto's) was never considered as well! This makes absolutely no sense to me.

You ask, what caused the breast cancer? I can't know for sure what it is, but this is the information I'm gathering:

My naturopathic doctor helped me discover that I have two mild forms of Epstein Barr and Chlamydia Pneumoniae (both viruses). These two viruses can distract the body into fighting them, which takes the attention away from the cancer cells that are developing. Say, isn't this a clever military tactic?

The other cause that makes logical sense is that I was exposed to high doses of chemicals at the age of thirty-one. As a young, single mom, I worked on a flower farm on Kaua'i. To ship the exotic tropical flowers to California it was necessary to dip the flowers in a chemical solution to kill the pests. As time went by, I was struck by migraine headaches that would become increasingly worse with time. After I was knocked out for twenty-four hours in bed with a splitting headache, I realized the culprit of my headache was the deadly flower chemicals I was exposed to. Once I figured this out, I immediately stopped working there. One year later, I began to have serious hypothyroid issues and was diagnosed with Hashimoto's disease, an autoimmune condition. There's much to be said for avoiding chemicals!

The year before I was diagnosed, my closest friend of nineteen years died from Leukemia. I was one of her main caretakers for twenty-two months and her death was a heartbreaking loss. It's a common tendency for people diagnosed with breast cancer to be natural caretakers for others. The breasts represent mothering. A mother's milk flows out of the breasts to nurture her tiny baby's life.

In the article: "The Energy Medicine Perspective of Breast Cancer," Phylameana Lila Desy writes:

> *Breast Cancer is one of the physical dysfunctions associated with the heart chakra. Barbara Brennan states in her book 'Hands of Light: A Guide to Understanding Human Energy Fields' that a torn chakra indicates cancer.*

> *"A torn chakra... has appeared in every cancer patient I have ever seen... A chakra can be torn, and the cancer will not appear in the body for two or more years later."*

> *Issues concerning love and nurturing affect the health of a woman's breasts. In an energy analysis of a patient with breast cancer in women, medical intuitive, Caroline Myss wrote:*

> *For some women, cancer develops in response to an inability to nurture, which results in guilt feelings and self-hate. Others experience fear and identity crises as a result of not accepting the natural closure of the cycle of motherhood when children leave the home.*

> *Christian Northrup, M.D., a visionary of mind-body wellness and cofounder of 'The Women to Women Health Care Center' writes:*

Energy dysfunction often arises when a woman is confused about how to use both her loving (fourth chakra) and her creative (second chakra) energies optimally. The major conflict within women is that most of us still believe that in order to be loved, to receive love, and to guarantee that someone will need us, we must care for loved ones' external physical needs.

Cancer survivor, author, and one of the founders of the self-help movement, Louise L. Hay is well known for her healing affirmations. Hay on the breasts:

The breasts represent the mothering principle. When there are problems with the breasts, it usually means we are 'over mothering' either a person, a place, or a thing, or an experience.... If cancer is involved, then there is also deep resentment.[4]

Louise Hay speaks about breast cancer:

Louise states that she has noticed a consistent pattern in every woman suffering from breast cancer. According to Louise these women have a tremendous inability to say no. Breast represents nourishment, and women with breast cancer seem to always be busy in nourishing everyone in their world except themselves. These women find it extremely difficult to say "NO." One of the reasons behind this may be that they were raised by parents who used guilt and manipulation for discipline and now they have become people pleasers, surrounded by people who are constantly asking them to do more than they can comfortably do. These women are seen to keep straining themselves for others and saying "yes" to demands that they really don't want to do. They keep giving until there is no more nourishment left in them to give.

It can be very difficult to say "NO" for the 1st time because the people around you have become so used to you saying yes to their demands. When you first say "NO" you receive a very angry reaction from them. Louise advises to accept this reaction and says that "anybody who is learning to say "NO" has to put up with anger for a while." Louise also recommends not to make excuses once you say "NO." This gives the other person a chance to talk you out of your excuse. Louise says, "Just say NO. No, I can't do that." "Not anymore." "No, I don't do that anymore." – any short statement that sends a definite "NO" message will do the trick. The other person will get angry, but you have to be confida\ent that it's not because of you. These people get angry because now you're not giving. They can even call you selfish. You don't lose your confidence and self-respect. After all, you finally got it.[5]

I'm breaking the pattern of putting others before myself. One of my most valuable lessons is learning I'm worthy of receiving. It's an act of kindness to give myself the same love and adoration I give others. I'm worth it! My beloved friend Kim calls this concept "Selfullness." I love this term! Instead of being selfish, it's an act of selfullness to learn I'm worthy of love!

I got a third opinion from a local oncologist and had a wonderful surprise! He told me he would support me in my alternative healing path and help me in whatever way he could! His clear encouragement of me was a refreshing surprise after the close-minded responses I had received from other oncologists. It gave me hope!

As my healing protocol is costing me a ridiculous sum of money each month, I've had to step up and ask for financial help. Since I've spent my entire life being a strong Amazon, this is challenging and uncomfortable. I'm so grateful for all the donations, love, and support!

For me to learn I'm worthy of receiving is one of the greatest healing gifts. Thank you to every one of you who has stepped up to help. This abundance allows me to relax and be present in my healing experience. I hope to be able to return the gift through sharing awareness, helping others navigate their cancer journey, being a cancer thriver, and telling my tale!

YOUR ONE WILD & PRECIOUS LIFE:

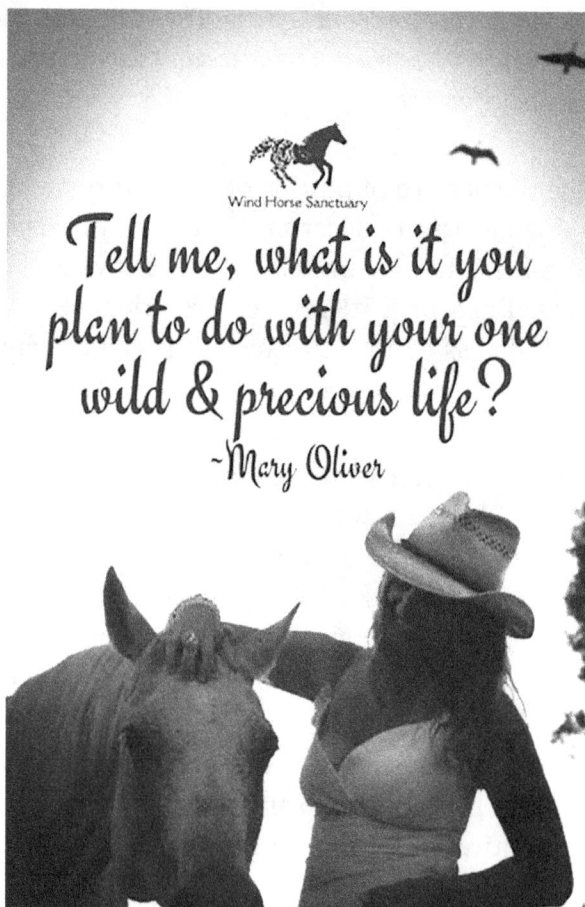

Wind Horse Sanctuary

Tell me, what is it you plan to do with your one wild & precious life?
~Mary Oliver

A poem which has always captured the elements of how I truly felt as far as living life to the fullest is this Mary Oliver poem.

The Summer Day

Who made the world?
Who made the swan, and the black bear?
Who made the grasshopper?
This grasshopper, I mean--
the one who has flung herself out of the grass,
the one who is eating sugar out of my hand,
who is moving her jaws back and forth instead of up and down--
who is gazing around with her enormous and complicated eyes.
Now she lifts her pale forearms and thoroughly washes her face.
Now she snaps her wings open, and floats away.
I don't know exactly what a prayer is.
I do know how to pay attention, how to fall down
into the grass, how to kneel in the grass,
how to be idle and blessed, how to stroll through the fields,
which is what I have been doing all day.
Tell me, what else should I have done?
Doesn't everything die at last, and too soon?
Tell me, what is it you plan to do
With your one wild and precious life?

CANCER THRIVER!

1/18:

What if our so-called adversities were really calls to action to actualize our full potential?

Have you noticed how much fear & terror circulates around the word "cancer"? Since my diagnosis I've witnessed two kinds of reactions: avoidance and utter compassion.

Avoidance: When I see friends and acquaintances who haven't seen me since the diagnosis, I have occasionally witnessed an acute sense of discomfort from them. People don't know what to say or do in the face of a cancer diagnosis. It can be incredibly awkward.

Then there are those who are suddenly disappearing from my life. If you're one of those people, I love and forgive you. I'm well aware that I'm a symbol of your mortality now.

Compassion: I've received an unbelievable amount of support and love that touches me beyond words. Those of you who've stepped up and have showered your unconditional love upon me, please know this is an incredible healing balm that brings me through the challenging moments.

I'm happy to report that the instances of compassion are higher than the avoidance!

There's the danger with a serious health diagnosis to fall into a victim mentality. I struggle with this daily. The negative self-talk is something like, "Poor me, I have cancer; therefore, I can't

_____ (insert whatever fun thing you used to do before your fateful diagnosis)."

Even the term, "cancer survivor" conveys that if a patient makes it through cancer treatment, they've just trudged through the most horrible nightmare! Fuck the victim mentality! Maybe whatever terrible hand we've been dealt whether it be a health diagnosis, break-up, death of a loved one, job loss, or change in the political climate serves us for our growth? Maybe mining the seeds of adversity will grow us into our most vibrant selves?

I love the term "cancer thriver" and am choosing to use it! Honestly, cancer has been a gift to awaken me to potent healing, which I'm grateful for. Yes, there are shitty days, but the gifts I'm discovering far outweigh the hardships.

How can you rise above and transform the challenges in your life?

**

In February 2017, I noticed that I was corresponding with about 30 different cancer thrivers dedicated to a healing cancer naturally journey. Many of these connections were through Facebook and various channels of social media. I got the brilliant idea that it would be wonderful to connect everyone together in a secret Facebook group for cancer thrivers. That same month, I birthed a group called "Conscious Cancer Collective"!

This group was a wonderful place for others on the cancer journey to connect with one another, exchange ideas, support each other, and share the experience together. As time went on, the group slowly expanded as word got out among the various communities of people on a cancer healing journey. I enjoyed being the leader of the group, as I saw the value of the shared connection of the journey.

2/13:

My seventy-nine-year-old father told me recently regarding my recent cancer diagnosis, "Tara, I wish I could have your diagnosis instead of you. If it's your time to go, I wish I could go instead of you." His words touched me deeply, and, honestly, I know exactly what he meant. When I watched my closest friend of nineteen years slowly decline over twenty-two months from Acute Myeloid Leukemia, at times I wished I could take her pain and suffer instead of her. I did everything I could to save her, started a fundraiser that brought in $50K and showed up to the best of my ability. Unfortunately, it wasn't her fate to live beyond her short forty-six years.

My dad's words sparked the inquiry about why we young people are selected to embark upon a journey with a life-threatening illness while others skirt easily to their eightieth year without their roots being shaken by sickness. Why did my dearest friend die so young? Why is another close friend of the same age struggling with a serious cancer diagnosis? Why have our worlds been turned upside down to find the solution to living beyond our fiftieth birthday? Life is indeed mysterious, and there often seems to be no rhyme or reason why we're selected to walk a certain path.

In the challenging times, I curse getting to know the grim reaper so intimately. I choose to be grateful to realize how precious life is, even with death dancing so close to my face. My astrologer friend tells me it's no wonder I'm becoming friends with death, as I have four major planets in the house of Scorpio (death, sex, transformation); there's no avoiding this path in this lifetime.

COGNITIVE DISSONANCE:

3/10:

In psychology, cognitive dissonance is the mental state when a person holds contradictory beliefs, ideas, or values, and is typically experienced as psychological stress (discomfort) when they participate in an action or are confronted with new information that goes against one or more of them.

Since my cancer diagnosis, my decision to treat myself using natural and alternative methods has challenged those who believe in conventional medicine and put them and myself in a state of cognitive dissonance.

It threw many of those closest to me and myself into a stressful tizzy as the issue of mortality was staring straight into our faces. Those who believed I would unquestionably follow the prescribed route of standard treatment were shocked and deeply perturbed when I announced I would follow an "unproven" route of alternative healing. Immediately, I faced not only having to swim through my own fears but the incredible terror of those closest to me. (I understand that their fear came from a place of love and not wanting to lose me, but it was a lot to navigate.)

Thankfully, after two months, due to continually setting my boundaries and their acceptance of my "crazy" path, the dust began to settle and the debate about my healing plans quieted down.

Very early on in my cancer journey a friend mentioned the term 'cognitive dissonance' to me and I realized this would play a significant part in my choice to heal cancer naturally. We're raised to think, behave, and operate in a certain manner in our society and are formed by our cultural, family, and religious values. In the Equine Facilitated Learning work I teach, you find your "Authentic Self." The Authentic Self is the you that's found at your absolute core separate from social or family conditioning. Horses easily mirror back the beauty of your true self, which is why they're excellent facilitators for this work.

When a member of society goes against what the commonly held belief system is, it's usual to be questioned, doubted, threatened, and generally projected upon by another's perceived fear. When I stated I wasn't going to rush into dousing my body full of chemicals, I immediately got the reaction from some people close to me that they were going to prepare for my death. If I weren't following the prescribed path, how could I possibly survive? Now here I am five months later, feeling better than I have for years!

The ironic thing is that if I had chosen the conventional route of healing, some of my friends would be urging me to question chemotherapy and try the alternative methods! The truth is you can't please everyone; all you can do is choose what's right for you and be clear in your boundaries with the naysayers.

I know that I've ruffled feathers by stating my beliefs so openly about the way the modern cancer industry operates, and it's not my intent to offend anyone. I apologize if I might have offended you by my bold statements. I own my beliefs as I own my body and it's my choice to heal my body how I choose to. I have no judgment toward others who choose a different path and I wish them well in their own healing journey.

I choose to speak my truth to inform others who might not know they have a choice in their healing modality, as having a diagnosis like this breeds instant fear and many doctors use intimidation to push you into treatment right away. The truth is that if you have a tumor, it most likely has been growing in you for 5-10 years;

so, taking a few weeks or a month to decide your best course of action is a prudent idea.

I see how my decision to choose a different route of healing shakes the belief system of those who put inherent trust in what a conventional doctor prescribes. If one belief system is shaken, it can ripple out and affect the other held beliefs of what our "normal reality" is. I see this also playing out with our current political system. Since Trump's inauguration, many feathers have been ruffled with his unconventional methods. The new president plays the wild card in what looks on the outside to be a safe and organized structure, yet at the root is an unbalanced and corrupt system.

Maybe the best solution is to surrender and know that nothing is predictable, as it seems to be a time of chaos and uncertainty. Perhaps the more we cling to our belief systems the harder it will be to flow and bend with the turbulent tide. The truth is that nothing is for certain and this is all we can be certain of! I know when I drink in this truth my fears dissipate and I put my trust in being present with what's real in the moment. All we really have is NOW; why not try to live it to its full potential?

Surrender to what is. Let go of what was. Have faith in what will be.

–Sonia Ricotti

BEE VENOM THERAPY:

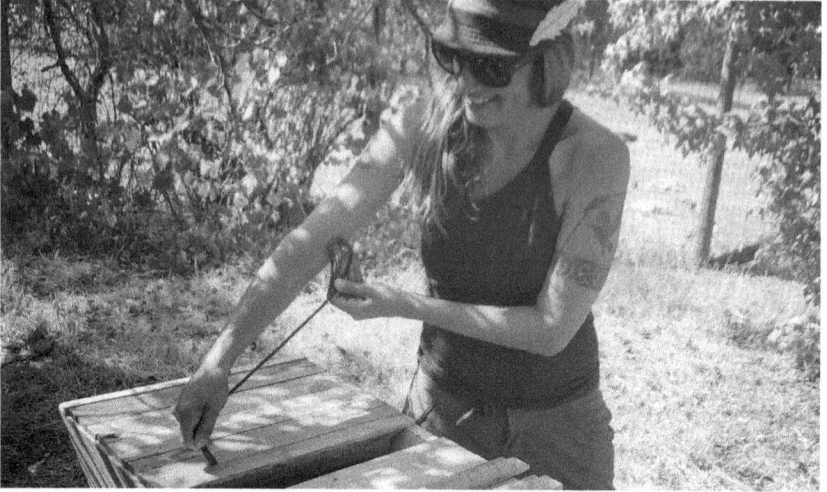

With my top bar bee hive

This piece was originally published on HoneyColony.com (in resource section)

The keeping of bees is like the direction of sunbeams.

–Henry David Thoreau, Walden

I would never have imagined that healing breast cancer would involve stinging my own boob with live bee venom daily. Ever since my serious breast cancer diagnosis, it was necessary to make courageous decisions regarding my health. I now consider bees and their venom an integral part of my radical self-healing journey.

I witnessed and supported Deb as she made difficult decisions related to treatment. It felt right to her to choose a conventional, allopathic route. In watching Deb endure the endless rounds of chemotherapy and bone marrow transplant, I experienced the grit and trauma of standard medical treatment.

Deb's courageousness was inspiring, but her end was tragic. So, when facing cancer myself, I knew I couldn't follow the year of chemotherapy, radiation, surgery, and hormones prescribed to me. As I already had a deep distrust of conventional medicine, a natural route seemed the best option to honor my unique spirit.

Healing Breast Cancer Naturally with Bees:

After an extensive amount of research, I created a healing protocol to follow over the next several months. It consisted of the Gerson protocol (veggie juicing along with coffee enemas) and supplements such as high-dose Vitamin C infusions, Poly MVA, curcumin (turmeric), pancreatic enzymes, and others. I also tried infrared saunas, a myriad of strange tasting liquids such as Chinese herbs, a fermented Chinese soy drink called Haelan, turkey tail tea, and so much more! Eight months into this natural route of healing, a friend mentioned bee venom therapy to me, and I knew it was something I had to try.

I've had a long-time fascination with bees. Back in 2007, I met the talented apitherapist, Tamara Wolfson, in Fairfax, CA. I attended one of her evening classes to learn about the properties of bee medicine. Years later, I met the beekeeper, Jacqueline Freeman, author of Song of Increase. I spent several weeks studying horse Rolfing with her husband, Joseph Freeman, while Jacqueline would cook delicious meals for lunch. Jacqueline gave me a tour of her hive and a DVD about Top Bar hive beekeeping. The experiences I had while working with Tamara and Jacqueline became seeds for my future beekeeping adventures. I had no idea that a life-threatening illness would be the initiating circumstance for what has now become my profound relationship with bees.

The first step in my apitherapy exploration was to book an acupuncture/bee venom session with Tamara Wolfson, who lives three hours away, to see how my body would react to this particular therapy. After only two visits with Tamara, I discovered my body loved the bee venom! I could feel the burning sensations of the venom healing breast cancer in a holistic way.

Tamara uses a unique and rare method of micro-dosing patients with bee venom. While holding a bee with tweezers, she can gently apply multiple stings with the same bee without the bee losing its stinger. Thus, the patient gets multiple doses of medicine while the bee keeps its life.

At the start of our treatment sessions, Tamara placed acupuncture needles on specific meridian lines where she felt my body needed healing. Then, she would use the live bee on acupuncture meridian lines to deepen the session. The result was powerfully cathartic. Once the initial shock of the stings had passed, I felt my body immersed in a new level of rest and relaxation. Some of the venom's effects were mild pain and slight swelling as blood rushed to the area.

Hours after receiving the stings, I experienced an exuberant amount of energy to get a lot accomplished or go on long walks. Once that initial rush passed, I felt tired and needed to rest. I often experience a high then a crash when I use powerful medicines.

Putting Bee Venom Therapy into Deeper Practice:

After my initial exploration of bee venom therapy with Tamara, I was fortunate to find Heather Luna, who lived nearby and could assist my healing journey with bee venom. Heather is a clinical herbalist, apitherapist, and director of the Acorn School of Herbal Medicine. I spent many months under Heather's guidance, allowing my body to adapt to the full doses of venom, all the while strengthening my immune system. When I first started visiting Heather, I would start out with one or two stings around my breast. After months of seeing her twice a week, I was up to five stings a visit. Eventually, I felt confident to work with the bees directly, stinging myself. Heather patiently guided me in this process.

I learned of a wise woman who mentors others in the shamanic practice of beekeeping named Cheyanna Bone through my conscious community of Grass Valley. After meeting her, I knew she was the perfect person to guide me in this sacred art. I knew I wanted a hive to work with and caring for a wild swarm sounded more appealing than buying mass-produced commercial bees. Near the end of the swarm season, Cheyanna serendipitously found a small, delicate swarm that had gathered in a tree in our community, and she collected it for me. I had a very profound experience as the guardian of this swarm. It's been one year since I've had bees, and I now have two top bar hives. The top bar hive is the oldest and most commonly used hive style in the world. It features individual bars laid across the top of the hive cavity, which the bees then make their comb on. This set-up is healthier for the bee and easier for the humans tending the bees.

With Cheyanna's guidance, I confidently spend time with the bees without a veil, as trust is inherently present within our connection.

Stinging Myself with Bees:

A question I frequently get is, "How do you sting yourself with bees?"

Well, I very gently take a bee from her abdomen with tweezers and hold her up to the area where I want to be stung. By allowing her stinger to pierce my skin, the bee venom is administered directly to the breast tumor tissue. I usually sting myself three to five times around the breast, like a bull's-eye. The stinging does hurt a bit, but my body has adapted to the venom.

Often, I'm asked if the bee dies after I'm stung. The answer is yes; to get the full effect of the sting, the bee does indeed die. (Please note: Tamara is an advanced apitherapist and can sting without the bees losing their stinger. This is a rare skill.) I have found a healthy collaboration with the bees based on respect, vulnerability, and trust. Each time I visit the bees to use their medicine, I ask permission. Then I see, intuitively, which bees want to help me with my healing. I know they're sacrificing their lives for me. After I sting myself, I thank them each for giving their life. I'm gentle and loving with my bees and give them a safe, healthy space to live. In exchange they give me their medicine for my sacred journey of healing breast cancer.

The Endurance of Bee Medicine:

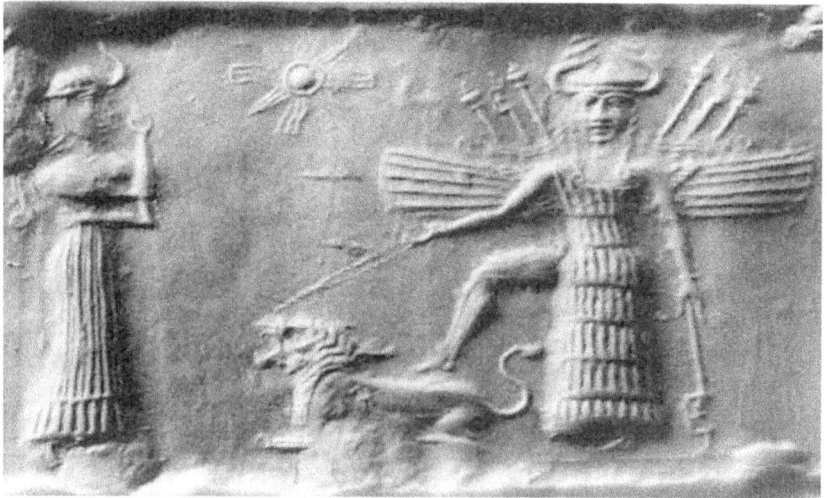

Ancient Akkadian Cylindrical Seal Depicting Inanna (in a bee form) and Ninshubur
2334 – c. 2154 BC

Bee medicine such as bee pollen, royal jelly, propolis, bee venom, and pure, raw honey have been an integral part of traditional medicine practices in ancient Egypt, China, and South America.

As far back as 500 BC, bee venom therapy was written about in the ancient Chinese text, *Huangdi Neijing*. In 300 BC, Aristotle referred to the healing property of bee venom in his book, *History of Animals*. Hippocrates, the father of modern medicine, used bee venom therapy for joint pain and arthritis. He described it as Arcanum, a mysterious substance whose curative properties he didn't quite understand.

Today, many bee products are used therapeutically for cancer. I found myself voraciously studying "Bee Venom in Cancer Therapy" from Nada Orsolic, of the University of Zagreb. Orsolic teaches in detail how melittin from bee venom works in the die-off of cancer cells. In plain language, melittin is toxic to cancer cells. As the melittin contacts a tumor, it causes the tumor to pull back from the venom. Renal, lung, breast, liver, prostate, bladder, and blood cancers have had success with the application of BV peptides. Studies show how bee venom inhibits cancer cell growth.

Blessed by the Bee Journey:

I have been blessed by many gifts on my journey of healing breast cancer naturally, and time with my beloved bees has been a highlight. It has been two years since my diagnosis. I'm still focused full-time on my healing, which requires patience, faith, and dedication. I use the RGCC test to chart my progress every few months.

Test results show that I'm definitely healing, and the cancer is contained. My biggest challenge is to face the fears that can creep in daily when living with this life-threatening diagnosis. I find it takes a huge amount of courage to believe in my ability to heal myself with my 100% natural route of healing. My bees are a force of strength on my journey. I know I'm tapping into an ancient channel of wisdom by being present with them and using their medicine. I feel vibrantly alive and recognize how precious each day is as I care for my bees, who have contributed so significantly to the strength of my immune system.

I'm so grateful to these magical insects for the recognition into what's truly sacred in this life, as well as bringing deep healing for me and many others, both physically and personally.

ANOTHER GOODBYE:

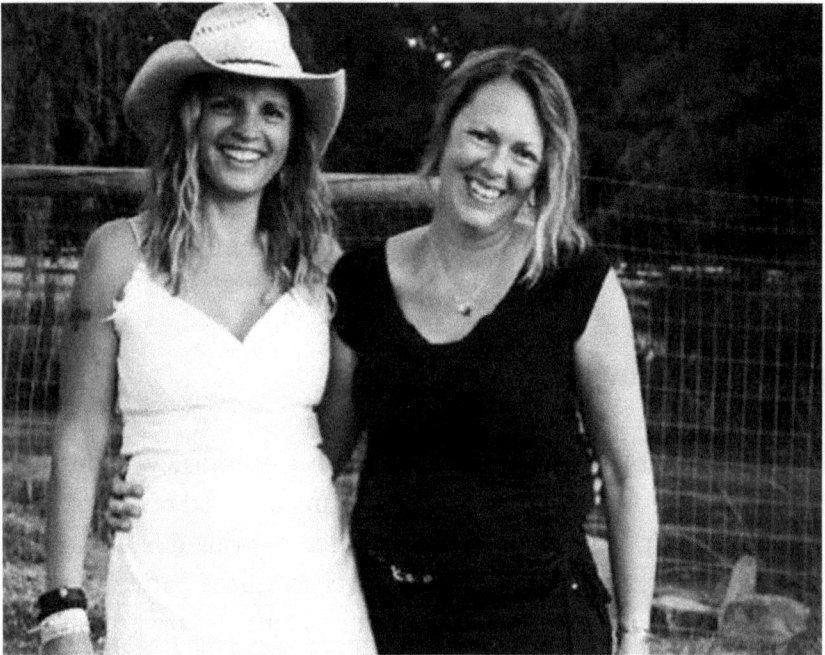

Me & Rowen - Photo by Melinda Vienna Saaria

In July of 2017, I suffered another severe loss in my life. Rowen, the mother of my niece Jasmine, died from colon cancer. I wrote this piece in commemoration of her:

This morning I woke up at 3 am and thought of Rowen. My Scorpio friend was so real at times that I would have to watch what I said to her. If my talk involved something that upset her, she would verbally sting me like a scorpion. However, when it came to her listening to the depths of my shadowy emotions, she, like the great mother, could hold it all.

We met young. Rowen was a friend of my brothers and, at that time, went by the name of Chrys. My tow-headed child, Willow was a toddler, clinging to my arms. Little did I know that she would become my sister-in-law. A few years after we met, she birthed my stunning niece Jasmine, the sweet little baby with the wrinkled nose. Chrys/Rowen loved her beyond words. We were all young parents, struggling to figure out who we were amidst the responsibilities of parenthood and making enough money to feed our tender kids.

In many ways, we grew up together. R/C and I would have long, soul opening talks. As the years went on, I appreciated how honest I could be with her. She had an East Coast tough as nails but raw as an opened wound quality about her, which was new to me. Growing up in California and Hawaii, I was used to an eternally optimistic (but not always totally real) disposition. Her personality was refreshing to me. I learned to trust her and thought of her as the sister I never had.

After years of family and friendship, she became one of my closest friends. I have many friends, but I only allow a handful of them into my heart. I'm fiercely loyal to those I decide to trust, and Rowen was one.

After Rowen was diagnosed, she struggled to redeem her life, find her joy, and claim her sovereign self. In a moment of inspiration, she decided to move to be near me. I was excited to try to help her while she struggled to find her light amidst a serious cancer journey. I realized after twenty-two months of being with Deb from diagnosis to death and then Rowen's dance with cancer, that cancer was a huge, unwelcome teacher for me. My heart reeled with sadness for my friends.

Ironically three weeks after Rowen moved to Grass Valley, I was diagnosed with stage three breast cancer. My own world was rocked, and Rowen briefly became a stable shelter from the earthquake that upended my life. The announcement of a cancer diagnosis is unparalleled, and it requires you to stand strong in yourself like nothing I'd experienced before. It can be a great opportunity for awakening, but the initial news is frightening to the core. The realization of your mortality can cause you to step up in strength or wither away in dread.

Due to the immense task of running a 10-acre ranch, the care of four horses, and attending to my own self-care with my health diagnosis, I couldn't show up for her as much as she needed. What followed was a very difficult stormy winter. There was no end to the rain, sleet, and snow that continued to pelt Northern California. Rowen had moved far from her tight group of midwife friends and the only person she knew in the area was me. She had also given up her midwife career and didn't have that to lean on.

Just as in Inanna's journey into darkness, those journeying with illness are asked to give up many of the familiar comforts the mind likes to cling to. Work and identity are often one of these causalities. It certainly was for Rowen.

I saw my beloved friend spiral into deep depression and a swift decline in her body while I also physically and mentally struggled to keep my head above water. What followed sadly was a deep fissure in our friendship. In the last four months of her life, her friends helped to move her back to Santa Cruz, CA where she could get the proper care she needed.

It broke my heart that I never got to properly say goodbye to her. I believe, in a strange way, she was protective of me and, since I was going through such a serious diagnosis, didn't want me to see her in her swift decline.

I was grateful to be in communication with her mother who asked me to come down and commemorate her body after she died. It was somewhat of a closure to at least say goodbye to her physical form after she passed. Her mother asked me to adorn her body. Similar to what Deb's friends and I did with Deb, I surrounded her with my favorite crystals, draped her with fabric and roses. This was a symbolic finale to our friendship, though there were many layers of grief to process after her death.

Here is an excerpt from one of my many pieces about Rowen:

Dearest friend, partner in cackle crime, smart as a whip, mother of my niece, brave explorer of shadows, catcher of babies, all you wanted was to just be loved and cherished. Isn't that all we ever want?

I'm so sad that you did not recognize while you were here how loved you are!! We all tried to move mountains for you, to show you how much we cared. This was not enough.

Precious angel wherever your spirit flies now, hear my voice. You are forever loved and never forgotten!

NO STONE LEFT UNTURNED:

8/28:

There's a funny thing that happens when you receive a Stage 3 Cancer diagnosis. Suddenly, the importance of life is magnified. Petty things that bothered you before are rather insignificant when staring down death's doorway. For example, part of my healing cancer naturally path is to pick apart everything that doesn't serve me. This means I examine relationships, habits, false or conditioned ways of behaving, or anything that continually creates stress. Stress feeds the tumor and exacerbates the cancer growth. It means I leave no stone unturned, however painful the process might be.

Rejecting what doesn't serve me can be an uncomfortable process. This can mean walking away from unhealthy relationships and situations. It could potentially be a heart-breaking process to realize that someone or something you love might not be good for you, whether it be a family member, friend, partner, pet, work relationship, job, or living environment.

It comes down to a choice of life or death. When you realize your time could possibly be limited, why waste your precious resource with people and situations that ultimately don't serve your highest good?

In less than two years, I've witnessed two of my closest young friends whittle down to 65-pound skeletons and die. I saw their bodies taken away to the crematorium. This is a horror that I wouldn't wish upon anyone. Doctors tell me that if I don't follow their allopathic protocol, I will probably die. I'm following my natural healing path and right now I'm healing at a rapid rate. I'm well aware that life is ephemeral and fleeting. Every breath I take is precious.

Life is painful. Growth can hurt. Being true to yourself and living in integrity means sometimes you have hard choices to make. If I were to choose between growth/life and staying stuck in patterns that don't serve me, I choose facing my demons!

Maybe fierce self-love means to bravely walk away from the circumstances that ultimately don't serve you. Perhaps that's truly the test of courage.

When staring death in the face, you quickly learn time is an illusion. I cannot assume I will live to a ripe old age. All sense of control has been ripped away with the death of my friends and my current cancer journey. All I have is this moment and I intend to live fiercely and freely. If this means I have to face an uncomfortable situation to stand in my truth, so be it.

YOU ARE LOVED:

9/30:

Do you know that there's no one else on Earth with your unique DNA blueprint and personal mission? Are you aware of the pivotal and powerful force you have upon those around you? Do you have any idea that if you suddenly ceased to exist, countless loved ones would grieve your loss? A dear friend of mine died this summer and her closest friends and I were touched at the tremendous outpouring of love, respect, adoration, and honor focused upon her after her passing. I wondered if she had any idea how much of an impact she had upon those who grieved her loss? It occurred to me, if she had known how absolutely loved she was, would that have made a difference in her own personal healing journey?

I witnessed her slide into a depression over the harsh Northern California winter that made it more challenging to do the hard work necessary to heal from cancer. It's painful to watch the suffering of someone you deeply love and feel powerless to help. I could tell her I loved her and that she was valued by countless friends, family, and the lives of people she touched, but until she believed it herself, my words would fall on deaf ears.

In the past few years, there have been more suicides in distant circles of friends. I wonder if the person who chose to take their life had known how missed they would be, would they still have killed themself? Did they have any idea how loved they were?

Are we all living our lives unaware of how much we're valued and cherished by one another?

If I told you how beautiful you are, would you believe me?

How much precious time do we spend criticizing our faults rather than praising our attributes? We live in a society of judgment, judging ourselves and others.

We choose where to direct our thoughts. Every thought, statement, and action is a choice of our conscious and unconscious brain. Our thoughts are like mantras, and each thought is a direct action of what we wish to manifest.

This summer has been tough. My dear friend and family member died, I broke my arm, and I've been journeying with healing cancer naturally including the self-discipline and sometimes nasty body detoxification that comes with it. I've noticed my mind criticizing the one closest to me, my partner, as a way to deflect the inner turmoil within me. Lately I've been trying to catch the critical pattern and recognize what emotional tide I'm bypassing by projecting it at him.

Life is short. There's no time to be caught up in blame. I encourage you to practice love. With the loss of two of my closest friends and the cancer diagnosis I received all within two years, I've been blessed with the lesson that life is oh so impermanent.

The next time you find yourself in a negative spiral of criticism, either toward yourself or another, I encourage you to refocus the thought pattern. What do you cherish about yourself or the other? If it were the last time to see them, what words would you want them to remember you by?

If I could go back in time, I would infuse my friend with the love that was expressed toward her after she died. This is impossible to do. So, instead of telling her, I have decided to remind you that YOU ARE LOVED. You are cherished. You matter far more than you think you do.

Now, please spread the message so others know how loved they are!

2018

New Zealand:

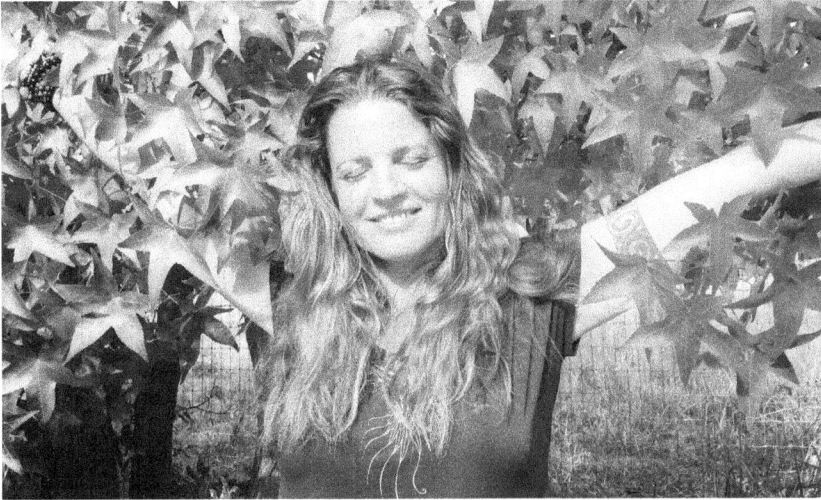

Celebration!

In the fall of 2017, I got an "almost cancer free" test result from the RGCC (Greece test) that I did.

The jubilant test results led me to take advantage of an incredible invitation to present my "Grief Rituals with Horses" work in New Zealand! Laura Williams, another Equine Facilitated Learning instructor was the creator of "Spirit Horse Festival." We became acquainted through the horse community on Facebook. She's a fascinating woman who is American but lived in Russia with her family and horses. Laura had been following my health story and was aware of the grief work I did. She invited me to present my work at the horse festival.

As I had always wanted to travel to New Zealand, I viewed this as the trip of a lifetime and decided to do it! Life was short; why not seize it with both hands? I was so excited to witness the land of the Kiwis (New Zealanders).

My plan was to spend eight days witnessing the splendor of South Island and then the remainder of my journey at the Spirit Horse Festival on North Island. I was warned that my total twenty-one-day journey would feel far too short. I was told that, ideally, one would spend a month or two in New Zealand soaking in her breathtaking beauty. My attitude was I would take what I could get!

As I was using bee venom therapy as part of my cancer healing technique, crazy me devised the plan of getting a small bee box and traveling around New Zealand in a camper van (which I named "Bertha the Bee Mobile") and to call my journey "Traveling with Bees." I was determined to keep up my healing routine. As New Zealand was the magical home of Manuka honey, I knew there would be no issue in finding bees to use for my therapy.

Before I flew on the fourteen-hour flight to Auckland New Zealand, I did some networking to locate beekeepers to find bees to journey with. I connected with a few lovely ladies who ran a biodynamic farm and had bees. They invited me to stay at their location, sleep in my van on their property, and asked me to give a talk to others about healing cancer naturally. Of course, I accepted the invitation!

Here's some excerpts from the journey:

1/29:

Traveling with Bees Day 1: Off to Christchurch, New Zealand today! Love the magical unfolding of it all: I'm honored to be invited to share my story of healing cancer naturally at a biodynamic farm tonight to a group of fifteen people. They invited me to gather bees for my journey here! (So grateful for the kind invitation from a fellow bee tribe sister!) Life unfolds in some pretty spectacular ways if you allow it to!

I'll be picking up the camper van today. Note: I'm a little nervous about this! Wish me luck on driving on the left side of the road with a stick shift. Fortunately, I had some experience doing this in December!

1/30:

What to say? Simply spectacular! I'm a bit speechless from the beauty, genuine quality of people here, and all the magic that's unfolding! Last night, I shared my story of healing cancer naturally to fifteen very curious and open-minded individuals. It was an honor to be present with them, answering questions, and sharing.

This morning, I spent time with my new friends and wonderful hosts, sharing stories and hanging out with the bees! It was a two-person job to gather bees for my tiny bee box. I'm deeply touched by the kindness of these big-hearted women.

After I bid farewell to my lovely hosts, I courageously drove four hours through hills and windy roads to Kaikoura in the camper van. Such an epic drive! Bertha the Bee Mobile is old, and it's quite a challenge to change her sticky gears. Fortunately, my arms are quite strong from hauling hay around, so I can maneuver my ancient jalopy.

This morning, I had a big emotional release when I realized that part of the reason why I'm challenging myself on this heroic woman's solo journey is for Deb and Rowen. I'm pushing myself to face some immense fears by traveling all around New Zealand in a rickety old van. My two beloved friends would have loved a trip like this. I'm doing it in the spirit of adventure because they would have wanted me to do it. You never know when you'll get another opportunity to pursue a dream!

So, on I travel, embracing the magic and carrying my two beloved friends with me.

HEALING CANCER WHILE ON THE ROAD:

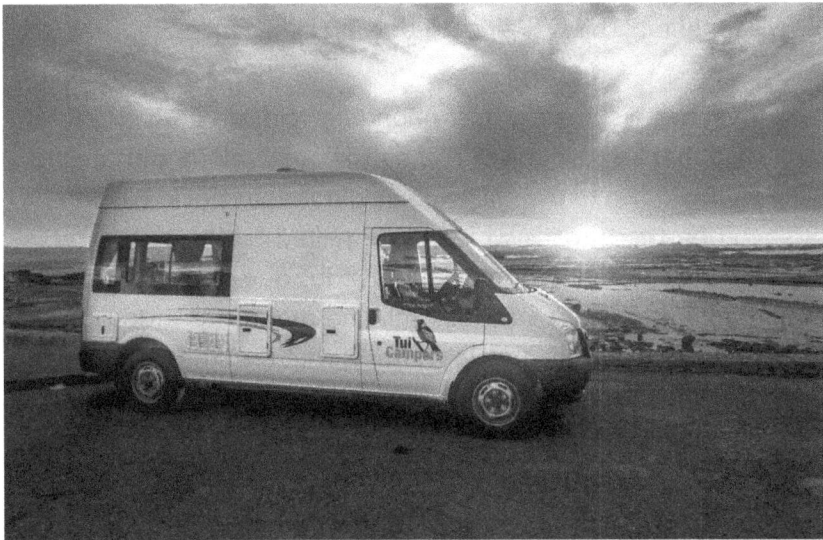

Kaikoura, New Zealand - Photo by Shawn Reeder

I tried to keep up my healing regimen while on the road to the best of my ability. The juicer I painstakingly lugged in my overweight baggage unfortunately died during the first part of my travels through South Island. I did the best I could by stopping at health food stores along the way and stocking up on already made juice. I pretty much subsisted on a diet of gluten free potato pot pies while on the road. Bertha the Bee Mobile had a small refrigerator and stove top. I managed to figure out how to partially warm up the English sludge pies. The charm of adventure often overrides the need for comfort for me!

1/31:

I had some serious angels watching over me today as I had a treacherous 5-hour drive from Kaikoura to Takaka. In the fall of 2016, there was a devastating earthquake on the

Kaikoura coastline which destroyed various sections of the road due to massive landslides. It recently opened up in early January 2017, but there's still heavy-duty road work happening. This was a death-defying experience!

Imagine this: high winds, pounding rain, portions of the road that are just gravel, and narrow roads along cliffs that plunge down to the sea. Imagine ginormous trucks passing you on these roads while you're pelted by the elements. Picture constant roadblocks and stops due to the massive road work repairs needed. Imagine me in my large Ford campervan, Bertha the Bee Mobile, with the stubborn stick shift on the left that sometimes refuses to go into gear, driving on the LEFT side of the road. I was like Mad Maxine traveling through unruly territory!

Now picture the most stunning landscape you can imagine, one that easily beats California's picturesque Hwy 1. I wish I could have taken photos, but both my hands were occupied just staying alive! Insert the music of Elvis, Emmylou Harris, Simrit, Johnny Cash, Indian pizazz, and endless kundalini yoga music in the background. Imagine the buzz of bees sweetly singing and well, you get the picture.

Suddenly something terrible happened!! Amidst the crazy drive and the winds that threatened to blow my trusty home into the frothy Pacific Ocean below. I dropped my lip balm.

Yes, it was a tragedy! Poor me had to drive twenty minutes in these intrepid conditions with my lips becoming increasingly chapped. My lips almost fell off they were so dry! I barely survived!

Luckily at the first pull off I gratefully steered Bertha the Bee Mobile safely to the side and recovered the precious lip balm from under the seat. All is well in the world! Phew!

Seriously though, I'm very lucky to be alive besides this cancer thingy as three and a half hours of the drive was a white-knuckle treacherous adventure! I'm so grateful to be alive!

2/7:

I get sudden bursts of inspiration and must record the rushing waves of words cascading through my brain.

Here's a little snippet of three random people I've met while traveling, one is a gas station attendant and two are Uber drivers:

1. This morning, I got a ride to the Christchurch airport from an inspiring Chinese man, Alan. One of the qualities I love about New Zealand folks is they're quite friendly and talkative. I truly enjoy getting to know the people who make up a place.

Alan and I got into a conversation about the New Zealand government's plans to spray out millions of tree seeds to reforest certain areas. Alan was thoroughly enjoying talking about planting trees. As our conversation unfolded, I understood that planting trees is his thing! Besides being an Uber driver, he loves to plant trees! It brought tears to my eyes (not hard to do these days) as how often do you hear about people inspired to plant trees, especially an Uber driver?! It was a profound reflection of a country that puts care and attention into its environment as opposed to the current U.S. government, which is destroying our precious resources faster than a speeding bullet!

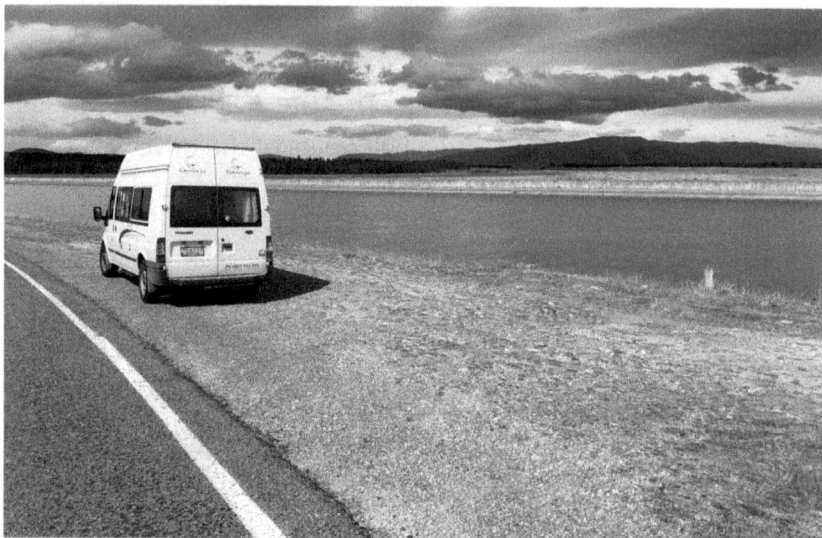

Being here and speaking with Alan is helping me see there's another pathway beyond greed, fear, and government control that's increasingly becoming more terrifying on American soil. It gives me bright hope for the future.

2. Last night, I got another Uber ride from Dixon who confessed to me that his life partner had recently sadly died from stomach cancer. He confessed that she went in for a doctor's visit and ended up dying three weeks later. He said that he had recently gone through prostate cancer. Right after he recovered from treatment, she was diagnosed. Dixon shared that he chose to spend his days giving Uber rides, so he doesn't have to be alone while feeling sorry for himself during the day. He admitted that he doesn't really need the money, but he appreciates the company.

Dixon mentioned that he's seeing an increase in cancer cases, specifically breast and prostate cancer in New Zealand. I told him about my two friends who recently died but chose not to tell him about my diagnosis. Sometimes, it's nice to be out of the limelight.

I was touched by his resilience, positive attitude, and ability to still show up in the world despite the recent loss of his wife. Hats off to you, Uber driver Dixon; you're a teacher for us all!

3. The last person who made a brief but dramatic impression on me was an Indian gas station attendant in Nelson. She was young, in her late twenties I would guess. As she pumped my gas, she asked me where I was from. I answered, "I'm from the sunshine state, California in the USA!" She told me she really wants to travel to North America but it's tremendously difficult to get a visa these days because of the current U.S. government.

She proceeded to talk in a humorous but straight-up manner how she doesn't understand why our country could have Trump as president? She blurted out that she thought he was mentally unstable. I flat out agreed with her. She continued, saying that our government is making a bloody mess in the rest of the world. I just nodded my head in agreement, feeling the ever-present American guilt.

These three Kiwi characters touched me in their own unique way. Sometimes, brief interactions can be deeply profound, as they present you with a direct yet brief snapshot of another's life.

I'm grateful to be getting another perspective beyond the normal American tunnel vision. There's something to be said for stepping out of the box and seeing the world with new eyes. It's good for the soul.

Onward to North Island!

2/7:

Ki Ora dear friends! I'm about to take a little social media break as I venture into Spirit Horse Festival land in Helensville, New Zealand. I'll be teaching two workshops: The first workshop will be a shortened version of one of my "Grief Ritual with Horses" events. The other presentation will be a multimedia show about my journey with Deb through her sickness and death and my own journey of healing cancer naturally. Of course, the continual theme for my talk is that the horses are my profound guides for traversing through the rough moments.

I saw the stunning Franz Josef Glacier on South Island. It's a glacier rising from sea level that's surrounded by a tropical environment. Pretty wild!

2/12:

This almost three-week trip has been set to the soundtrack of Eddie Vedder's "Into the Wild." I'm utterly grateful for this magical journey through the depths of New Zealand, as I explore its craggy, winding roads that are full of endless mud slides due to the tumultuous storm that almost threw me off a cliff and the delightful land and people. A profound innocence is present in its land and people that is deeply refreshing to my soul. My experience with living in the mainland USA is that there's an increasing sense of collective fear. After the last few years of being surrounded with death and cancer, roaming freely through the wilds of New Zealand was just what I needed. It was vastly liberating!

My soul felt as wild and free as a butterfly. No wonder it was named the land of new zeal!

My spirit is quenched. My body is exhausted from pushing myself to drive for 5-6 hours a day for the first nine days of my adventure on South Island. After that, I traveled to North Island and taught two workshops at the Spirit Horse Festival. I met enchantingly lovely aware horse-loving peeps!

The weather was a bit challenging for me as it poured rain for 5 days straight! Imagine staying in a camper van in the cold, wet rain, which chills you to the bone as you're innately a tropical girl. You've never been one to love cold weather. Imagine camping at a lovely festival surrounded by large mud puddles. It was a New Zealand kind of adventure!

The Kiwi people and the lush green splendor of the enchanted land made up for the discomfort of cold van life, but it did push me to my edge. When a new friend I met at the gathering offered her house to stay at for a few days, with a warm shower, bed, and heater, I jumped at the chance to be with her and her loving family!

Healing cancer naturally while on the road in a camper van CAN be done but yes, it can have trying days!

I experienced such a nurturing spirit of community while at the Spirit Horse Festival and in New Zealand in general. It's so important for all of us as individuals to come together in nurturing community to bind our fragmented society. In Western society nuclear family paradigm, it's easy to forget the value of sharing village time together.

The loving Kiwis touched my heart to the core. For this wounded bird who is still mourning the death of two beloved friends, I find my tears fall so easily here. Salty water sliding to the earth, nourishing my soul, releasing the trauma of seeing two young beauties shrink to death, their 65-pound skeletons cold and immobile to human life.

The healing wind reaches my heart and breathes new vital air within its quivering beat. I'm learning to let life in a little bit more. I allow myself to be a bit more vulnerable and shed the armor that I've been carrying for so long. This awakening gives me the promise of hope for tomorrow, for all of humanity and the future of the Earth. The key to recovery is to release what doesn't serve.

At the Spirit Horse Festival, I held a mini "Grief Ritual with Horses," which twenty-five people attended. (This was the largest group I had ever led in a grief ritual before!) The relentless rain stopped momentarily for my event; otherwise, there would have been a crowd of people with overblown rain gear shoved into a 10'x 15' tent for ninety minutes! It was eye opening to lead a group of courageous Kiwis through a grief ritual. Even though I view New Zealanders as being more evolved than the general American, even Kiwis were taught to stuff their grief. The tears and words expressed from my new friends were a lovely reflection of all that begs to be healed.

Release your tears now, and you'll laugh later. Suppress your tears, and your mind, body, and spirit will likely become numb.

For my own personal presentation, it was an honor to share my story of being with Deb through her illness and death and my own journey of healing cancer naturally. As my own journey revolves around horses, it was appropriate to share this experience with a crowd of horse lovers. It was profoundly moving to share my vulnerable story to a group of teary strangers whom I now call friends.

Thank you, New Zealand and my astounding new Kiwi friends, for opening your illustrious magic to my fragile heart. Thank you spirit for guiding me here, for being the voice that insisted I say YES to this experience. I'm forever changed and deeply catalyzed to step forward in a transformed fashion! The caterpillar has broken through her chrysalis. The newly emerged butterfly slowly unfolds her exposed, translucent wings. This healing was indeed necessary and so welcome!

Tomorrow I board a big silver bird bound for San Francisco. I'll be returning Bertha the Bee Mobile to the camper van rental company. I will miss the van, bees, environment of New Zealand, and the outstanding Kiwis I met.

The remaining bees shall be released with a prayer for their continued life with immense gratitude for this shared sacred journey, "Traveling with Bees."

Bee wisdom. Bee here now. Bee healed. And so it is!

The journey is complete.

BACK TO REALITY:

The New Zealand trip was utterly magical, yet driving for five hours a day on the edge of death-defying cliffs did take its toll on my body. In hindsight, I don't regret a moment of the trip, although I might have structured it differently to reduce the stress of travel. Twenty-one days was truly not enough time to see the illustrious land of New Zealand and take in all the magnificent beauty.

In the spring of 2018, I got the test results back from the RGCC Oncotrail test that I regularly did. I found out that the cancer cells were increasing in my body. This led me to realize I needed to step up my natural healing cancer routine. As insurance wasn't paying a dime for the expensive medicines, I realized I needed to bring in more money. The money I made running the ranch just barely covered the costs of maintaining a 10-acre ranch, four horses, and my medical expenses. If I were going to be effective with my healing routine, I needed to bring in more money.

I wrote this in my blog in April 2018:

Getting Vulnerable & Asking for Help

Life sure has its twists and turns! To cut to the chase, the "getting vulnerable" part is about me asking for help. I'm needing to step up in my fundraising, as healing cancer naturally is one pricey endeavor. I've struggled with this one, as I pride myself on being a very independent woman, and I know many of you were quite generous with me when I first started out on this healing cancer naturally journey.

I was told I was "almost cancer free" in October of 2017 with my last RGCC Oncotrail test scoring at 1.7. (Cancer free is under 1). I was so happy to be given this news, that I lived life to the fullest! My healing routine was so arduous that when I thought I was cancer free, I was excited to pour myself back into work and making money again. I couldn't possibly refuse the once in a lifetime opportunity to travel to New Zealand! I realize, in retrospect, that I went a little wild with my excitement of being almost cancer free.

I was given a health maintenance supplement protocol after I received the test results which lowered my health expenses. I could finally afford my healing routine and live a little!

I would usually do the RGCC test every three months, but due to the holiday season, DHL (the shipping company) making a mistake with my blood shipment to Greece and my New Zealand trip, I ended up testing six months later. My test score went to 3.1 which considering all that unfolded was a small slip. To give some perspective, I started with my first test at 8.2 (over 5 is advanced cancer), to 6.5, then 3 then 1.7. Ultimately, I'm back to where I was in the summer. In the big picture, it's just a little setback and could be much worse.

This is a huge wake up call for a deeper level of self-care! I'm seeing very clearly how easily I give to others rather than putting myself first. I see how my life literally depends on me giving myself the gift of self-love.

I feel like a heroine in a fantasy novel who thought after facing demons, dragons, and endless challenges that their journey was done. The main character realizes they have thousands more miles of treacherous mountains to travel through. Fortunately, the heroine (me) is well equipped with excellent tools and a fabulous map!

I've been hit a bit hard with this new mental reality of diving into the deep end again. I'm keeping the perspective that there's more I need to learn from this cancer guru, like excellent self-care. It's definitely been a bit challenging. I try to surrender the best I can and keep the perspective that it's the journey not the destination. The money piece is especially hard, as I was just getting my feet on the ground, establishing my coaching practice, and enjoying working and making money. It's hard to think of asking for help again but I also get there's a deeper level of learning to receive. Unfortunately, this is quite common for those on a natural healing journey, as it's so expensive and insurance covers nothing.

With my dedication to healing cancer naturally I was practically willing to try anything. I was determined to live!

KAMBO: JOURNEYING WITH FROG MEDICINE

7/21:

For someone who has willingly let bees sting me as part of my healing cancer naturally journey, it might not surprise you to know that recently I experimented with Kambo, a poisonous extract from an Amazon frog. I believe that nature gives us all we need to heal. I figured I use bee venom, why not frog poison?

There's a vast amount of material that shows how Kambo successfully heals cancer, shrinks tumors, and heals depression and a multitude of other illnesses.

Kambo, also known by its scientific name Phyllomedusa Bicolor, is a large green tree frog from the upper Amazon rainforest. The

Kambo frog has few natural predators because its skin secretion is poisonous to other mammals and reptiles (but fortunately not to humans!). The secretion from Kambo has many bioactive peptides and neuropeptides that are known to have positive effects on the human mind and body. Below are some of the known benefits of these peptides:

- Improved immune function

- Pain management

- Potent antimicrobial activity against bacteria, yeast (including Candida), fungi, and enveloped viruses

- Sedation/Relaxation

- Reduction in blood pressure[7]

Taking Kambo was a powerful transformational process for me. It's recommended that the minimum dose that's initially taken be three applications applied over three days. I decided to have my first experience under the guidance of Zahrah Sita, a woman whom I had gotten to know over social media and I highly respect. She brought two wonderful Chilean men up from South America to guide a small group of us for a weeklong journey. Due to my full ranch load during the summer season, three days was my maximum time I could get away.

The men who guided us were authentically trained in the Amazon rainforest to give Kambo, so I knew I was in good hands. Zahrah had healed herself naturally from a cancer diagnosis years earlier and was familiar with the realm of healing cancer. Those of us on the cancer journey can feel like "strangers in a strange land" at times, so the fact that she knew the territory well made me feel comfortable attending.

The process of taking Kambo is relatively quick (compared to other mind-altering substances) and entails drinking about a gallon of water in a short period of time, gently burning the skin of the leg with a piece of straw from the rainforest, scraping the skin away and applying the powder from the frog poison upon the fresh burn marks. Immediately after the powder was applied, our guides would start singing their sacred chants, as we were encouraged to drink yet MORE water.

Then the purging began. I never thought I would willingly sign up to spend time with strangers with a bucket and throw up together! This was certainly a bonding experience I'll never forget! With such a copious amount of water in our bellies and continuously drinking more, it was only natural for the vomit to emerge with the mixture of the frog medicine.

As we all were deep in our inner process and finding our way through the labyrinth of the journey, I wasn't aware of others purging around me. What was real to me was the inner battle I embarked upon. It was necessary for me to stay focused on my strength to face the demons that arose. One cannot hide when this sacred medicine is finding its way through your body, removing mental and physical toxins. With every release my body and mind became clearer.

The purging only lasted for ten to twenty minutes. Afterwards I was led to lie down on the ground under a wafting willow tree. My head spun as I saw concepts and beliefs that didn't serve me. I took the opportunity to let go of each unnecessary pattern, like a leaf slowly blowing off a tree. It was an emotional experience for me. I discovered trauma and grief I was still holding onto from my dear friends' deaths in the past three years. The reality that two of my closest friends had died young from cancer in such a short amount of time has shadowed over my own healing cancer journey. Even though I had worked hard to release a tremendous amount of grief, there was more to let go of.

I've been in the public eye with my own healing journey for twenty-two months. Many have reached out to me for support, and, subsequently, I've stepped into a leadership role. This piece was an essential one for me to process, as well. Being a natural giver, I willingly love to help others, even if it's at my own expense. I saw the price I've paid for helping others navigate their trauma, not only with cancer but with personal loss and grief as well.

The most profound lesson of Kambo was the extreme amount of subconscious pain that I had taken on from others from childhood through my adult life. I understood in a deep manner how much of a martyr complex I've had. My subconscious pattern has been to take on other people's pain with the belief that I can save them from suffering. Is it any surprise I was drawn to be a caregiver for my friends while they were journeying with cancer, stepped up to lead grief rituals, and have put myself out in the public eye to help others through their cancer experience? While on the Kambo journey it was clear to me why a tumor grew right over my heart. The pain of the world can be overwhelming at times.

I now realize that impeccable self-care is truly the most important piece for my continued healing. I'm learning to put myself first for my body, mind, and spirit to be cancer free. My love for life and desire to live is beyond any past contract that I made to be in servitude to an outdated belief. In this realization, I release any limiting thought patterns that hold me to suffering.

I'm so grateful for this wonderful crew and all the love they gave me. I suspect I was one of the louder participants during the ritual as I had such an intense emotional release. This emotional release was necessary for me to let go of past patterns that were holding me back from growth and healing. Zahrah, our Chilean guides, and the rest of the team were gentle and patient with me. It was wonderful to feel so safe in this process.

Each day's experience was uniquely different. I found the first and third day to be the most challenging, which were the days in which I moved through my biggest shadows.

While the frog medicine was in my body, I could feel it traveling to the places in my body which most needed healing. I could actually feel it working with the tumor in my breast!

This wasn't an easy journey, but it was extremely rewarding! The inner vision I discovered was highly beneficial for my current cancer journey. It takes a tremendous amount of strength to continuously know I'm healing a stage 3-breast cancer diagnosis naturally.

Would I do it again? Yes, in a heartbeat! I feel like I have rewired my inner circuitry and limiting beliefs that I adopted from childhood. It's a vastly liberating feeling!

The effect of Kambo allowed me to feel deeply refreshed and renewed. My body and mind feel strong and clear. The anxiety and stress that has sat on my shoulders for as long as I can remember has dissipated. While there's still stress in my life, I'm able to shake off the tension and access a state of joy in a rapid fashion.

A month after taking Kambo, I can honestly say that my relationship with my partner has improved, I'm able to access a state of love rather than fear and my ability to tap into my own innate healing ability has increased.

The three days of Kambo felt more effective than a year of therapy. I now have greater tools for navigating this heroine's journey. I'm deeply grateful to have had a chance to dance with the sacred frog medicine that hopped into my life!

MY ANGEL/DEVIL NEIGHBOR:

As I dearly needed to create more income for my cancer healing routine, I focused on what the best solution was to raise money in a sustainable fashion. I didn't want to spend an eternity doing perpetual fundraising. As I ran a retreat center and had been making steady income on Airbnb for years, it was a no brainer to get another possible structure to rent on Airbnb. I was immediately drawn to procuring a Tiny House as they were the newest rage among the alternative community! It was a no brainer to invest in a Tiny House.

I started researching the best kind to get. One of my dear friends, Lindsey Wood was a Tiny House connoisseur and had created one with her husband. She was an invaluable resource for me. Another dear friend provided a generous loan for me to purchase it and I was ready to purchase!

I found a company that had a demo model for sale and put down a deposit in May 2018. The Tiny House purchase started with a series of unfortunate events: There was a delay of a month in receiving the Tiny House. Once it arrived there were multiple issues like the plumbing not being hooked up correctly, the electricity accidently blowing out all the lights in the Tiny House and more! It seemed like everything that could go wrong did go wrong! I was about to tear out my hair in absolute frustration! Once it was finally listed on Airbnb in July 2018, I believed all my Tiny House issues were over. I was wrong!

As I was in the public eye with my healing journey and quite vocal on social media, it wasn't difficult for anyone who watched me on my various channels to follow the Tiny House escapade. I was so excited to have it, rent it and bring in more income that I shamelessly shared it all over social media and on my large email list. In my mind this was the right thing to do to get reservations and spread the word about my snazzy new Tiny House!

The moment the Tiny House was listed on Airbnb it was booked out for weeks! The Tiny House had a modern flair with its wood and metal frame. As I already knew how to decorate, it was easy to make a pleasing, aesthetic space for the guests. I was thrilled that my hunch to take out the loan and put this plan into action was actually working. My body relaxed for a week or two as I watched the reservations coming in.

Then the letter arrived.

The following are some posts from July to November 2018 that illustrate the utter bomb that was dropped upon us:

Notification from Planning Department:

7/23:

This heroine's journey has challenged me to no end the past few years. Deb and Rowen's death and the cancer diagnosis I received almost two years ago has pushed me to the edge many times now. All through-out it I have stayed strong in my belief, placing my power in love over fear and have continually seen the beauty in the challenge. Now, here's another major hurdle:

Part of healing cancer naturally is the ongoing fundraising that's necessary as insurance covers nothing. This spring, faced with the choice of selling my ranch and horses (a very heart-wrenching thought) as I wasn't making enough money to support myself, I had a brilliant idea to get a Tiny House to put on the property to rent out on Airbnb.

Later than expected and an astronomical amount of money later, the Tiny House project was complete! I happily listed it for rent on Airbnb two weeks ago. It immediately was booked out for weeks! I reveled in the fact that I could get a pricey Vitamin C infusion and not stress over the money. That was huge! It seemed like abundance and ease was at my fingertips.

Was this too good to be true? Maybe. Last week I got a letter from the county saying they were aware of unpermitted buildings on my land. I called and found out that someone had narced on me! Now I'm facing losing both incomes from the Tiny House and cottage. This means I can't house people when they come to attend my workshops. Basically, my retreat center is pau!

I work hard at not falling into victim mentality, but whoever calls in a neighbor who is facing a serious late-stage cancer diagnosis and is struggling financially is seriously fucked up. I don't use that term lightly!

I do my best to be a good neighbor and am the treasurer on the road committee. This is a job I chose to do from the kindness of my heart. Why would someone be a total shmuck and turn me in when my own survival stakes are so high?

I truly believe that everyone is innately good, but this is a direct act of sabotage that throws a wrench in my faith in humanity.

This is very real and vulnerable here. I stand to lose these beautiful horses that hold my heart. I suspect I will have to give up my retreat center and the livelihood that I have worked so hard to create.

Today, I cried big tears of surrender. Nothing is for certain, not even life itself. As I shed tears with the horses and Xaria by my side, Blue the horse sensed my agitation and came to share space with me. Anytime I'm upset I can tangibly feel the horses and Xaria present for me. They're the holders of tender sacred space.

I attempted to create a sustainable form of income where I can continue to heal.

I've been knocked down yet again.

Yet, I have faith.

I will continue on.

I will not give into bitterness toward whoever tattled on me to the planning department.

I will heal.

I surrender in the light of it all.

I trust in the greater vision.

All will be okay.

Even if I have to let go of this ranch and luminous creatures, I will be okay. It will be a hard-hitting blow, though.

8/5:

Tomorrow both my rental properties are being taken off Airbnb which leaves me with relatively no income. This means I'm seriously considering selling my ranch.

I vacillate between being in acceptance and anger. Only those of us who are given a life-threatening diagnosis knows how much courage it takes to face each day in a positive manner. I'm curious if the neighbor who turned us in is aware of how much trouble they've caused. It means I will have to most likely face the stress of giving up everything I've worked so hard to create for four and a half years. It means visitors who would visit WHS won't have the experience of being on its lovely healing lands and the powerful work with the horses. It possibly means that the four gorgeous horses will have to find new homes. This is tragic as my horses have a very good life! It could also possibly mean that this devastating change could tip the scales on my already fragile health.

On the other hand, this idiot could actually be an angel to show me a new path that might be better aligned to my healing. It could potentially be a freedom, a liberation of sorts. I'm constantly reminding myself to have faith and not to get stuck in fear.

Let your Faith be Bigger than your Fear

"Surrender is the highest power to gain all that you want."

–Yogi Bhajan, July 13, 2020

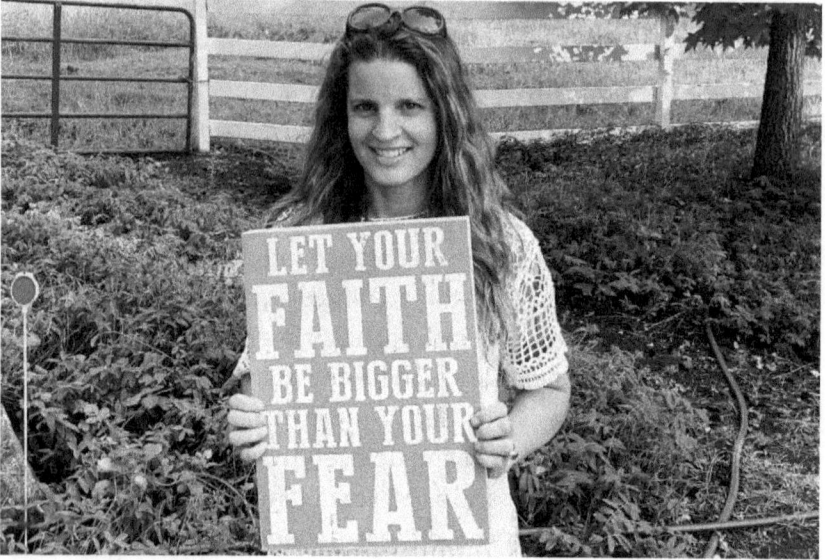

The Yogi Bhajan day calendar told me this relevant quote today and how very appropriate it is for me! The events of the last few years have taught me the more I resist change, the more I will suffer.

Release or be dragged.

I have to laugh, as life continually seems to keep me on my toes. This is the point in the heroine's story where the dark clouds circle yet again around the once jubilant main character. The viewers of the great adventure are aware of another undertaking about to unfold. In other words, Tara has yet another mountain to climb!

It seems as if existence with a life-threatening diagnosis and a tumor in my breast isn't enough. Without falling into victim mentality, I'm seeing that my very source of income is now threatened.

It's necessary for me to surrender at this point to the reality that life may have me moving in another direction. It might be in my best interest to let go of my beloved ranch. Finding balance is more important than stress and struggle. If I'm dealing with extra strain, then it will just inflame the cancer growth. I must have an environment conducive to my healing.

Surrendering is crucial to my survival. What I resist persists. The death of my two close friends and this cancer diagnosis continually remind me of this reality.

8/19:

We're ending the days of hosting guests at Wind Horse Sanctuary. It has been three and a half awesome years of hosting possibly a thousand guests from all over the world. I'm going through waves of massive release as I drop into trust that I will be provided for.

I feel sadness, as I do love hosting guests. It's been an enriching experience to witness the transformational healings that have occurred here with guests at the Sanctuary. I've put all my heart into it; however, grasping onto the past isn't worthwhile. Even the best laid plans can be blown away in an instant. Like a Tibetan sand painting, it's gone in a moment. I'm trusting that its absence is creating space for the next stunning scene to emerge.

"Life isn't about how to survive the storm but how to dance in the rain."

I've had this bumper sticker saying on my car for a few years. I have been learning how to dance in the storm through the death of my two close friends, my own personal cancer healing journey and now the latest episode with a snarky neighbor and the planning department. While I'm grateful for the wisdom, I'm ready for the shit storm to be over!

And yet I must trust. I'll keep fucking dancing as the rain, sleet, hail, and lightning bolts keep falling down!

8/25:

I'm teaching what might be my last three-day workshop at the ranch. As usual, I'm deeply humble and grateful for this powerful horse work.

The workshop I'm teaching is "Healing Cancer Naturally with Horses." These brave souls journeying through the reality of facing cancer in a holistic and aware manner are truly inspirational. Walking this path requires strength and tenacity.

I'm soaking up each moment of the experience. I have faith this work will continue in some capacity. The meaningful elements of life will always endure in some form.

My time at WHS has truly touched and changed my life as well as the hundreds who have stayed here and engaged in horse work. All I have is gratitude and reverence for the horses, land, and people. Even though it's ending in this form, it was still a success!

Thank you to all of you who stayed here, participated in workshops, and shared your vulnerability with me. I have such love and respect for all of you.

9/7:

I'm up late at night being with the total uncertainty of my future. I have no idea what will happen with this beautiful herd. My plan is to list the ranch for sale in October. Part of me knows this is for the best, as my healing is the most important thing now. The less stress the better for my body. The other part of me is devastated, as I love this land, the horses, and the life I created. This is a dramatic loss.

I'm needing to trust that this renunciation is for my highest good.

Bless these gorgeous horses. May they be protected and nourished with whatever the Universe has in store for them.

11/10:

Last night, I had a powerful dream that I was being tossed and turned in a huge, frothy wave. I grew up partially on Kaua'i, Hawaii. Therefore, I spent a good part of my childhood being tossed by waves. Throughout my childhood, the lesson the waves taught me was to surrender and to trust my lungs would find the earthly air again. I would eventually be tossed upon the ocean floor with sand in my ears, water up my nose, and sand all in my bathing suit.

The dream was similar. In the dream, I knew that if I struggled against the current, I would drown. The key was to let the epic wave toss me about like a rag doll until eventually I came up for air. I knew I would feel the ground under my feet at some point and could blow the saltwater out of my nose.

The dream ended as I was deep in the heart of surrender and trust. I woke up knowing this is the perfect metaphor for my life now. Giving up my ranch is like being tumbled by a huge wave. The key to find my way through this disaster is to let go. It's not always easy to do but has its rewards on the other side. I look forward to that moment of crawling out of the maelstrom and being on the safe sandy ground once again.

Perhaps all sense of safety is merely an illusion? Perhaps the sheer bliss of life is to be contained in the endless wave of life. Surrender is key.

HEARTS WITH WINGS:

One of the things that was particularly difficult about running my private Facebook cancer group was when one of the valued members passed. It was a small group of a few hundred people which meant there was a certain amount of intimacy inherent with the tribe. It's truly painful when you become close to someone on the cancer journey and then they die. It's a common reality to hear of friends with cancer passing. Unfortunately, I learned to get used to the reality.

I wrote this piece when I was feeling the impact of yet another dear friend's death:

Tribute to Annelise:

Another young, beloved friend died yesterday from cancer. I refuse to say, "she lost her battle with cancer," as Annelise wasn't fighting. From my perspective, she lived her life with pure love and embraced the opportunity to grow from her guru cancer.

The last seven years of my life I've experienced numerous friends die young from cancer. The first was Morgan Fieri, whose death at thirty-nine years old shook me to my core. I knew she was sick, but I didn't think she would actually die. Her death woke me up to the reality that young people are mortal too. Morgan lived life fully and was a beacon of light to many! Her death inspired me to get a large dragonfly tattoo in between my shoulder blades. The tattoo was a reminder of Morgan, as she loved dragonflies. It was a mark for me to remember to embrace each moment, as life is precious and fleeting. With her death, I was wakened to the reality of how temporary life is.

Then there was the passing of Deb and Rowen. Sandwiched in between Rowen and Deb's tragic deaths was my own stage 3 breast cancer diagnosis. Just in case I wasn't getting a taste of my own mortality, cancer came calling to evolve my soul at a rapid rate.

As I've been in the public eye with my healing journey, I've gotten to know many cancer patients along the way. Some have healed. Some haven't. In the company of illness, death is a constant companion.

The topic of death intrigues me. I was diving into its luminous mysteries with fascination after Deb's death. Little did I know that I was going to be tapped on the shoulder by the angel of death.

In the past year, I've known many who have died from cancer. Jenny died this spring at the age of forty-two from breast cancer, leaving behind a cherished four-year-old daughter and husband. Peg Hall died a week after Jenny. Susan Smith, a beloved member of my community died this summer. Laura Williams, a dear friend and avid horse lover died a week ago (not from cancer but from a horse accident). Now Annelise has passed in the last twenty-four hours from breast cancer at the age of forty-eight. Many others have passed whom I wasn't close to.

Dawn Higgins Andrews, another dear cancer thriver, wrote this in reflection of Annelise's death:

> *When you're diagnosed with a life-threatening disease, you find your tribe and you love on each other. You can relate in a way no one else understands. It's a special bond that isn't determined by geography, that doesn't require face-to-face meetings to become dear friends. These friendships are a blessing and a curse- because, as I'm learning, loss is inevitable. The commonality that bonds us is cancer, and cancer kills people. It's a tough blow that another young one in my tribe has passed. It is a reflection of my own journey, and the reality of what I face.*

Annelise and I traveled in similar circles, though we never met. We had much in common. We were both single moms on Maui in our twenties with our young children (our kids are the same age). We were born the same year. She was diagnosed around the same time I was, with a similar diagnosis. We became immediate friends. We would speak every few months, send texts, and encourage one another. Annelise was a bright light of inspiration for many, and her loss impacts countless lives. I feel immense compassion for her daughter as she's losing her mother at a young age.

Part of me wants to proclaim, "Fuck cancer!" but I know this attitude isn't constructive to my own healing. I'm upset that it seems that many of my dear friends are dropping like flies. Yet, I know there's so much more beyond what I can see. As I face my own mortality with the death of my cherished friends, I'm incredibly grateful for the lesson of knowing how precious this life is. Cancer can be a blessing to help awaken us mortals to the beauty of what we're given.

The depth of loss I feel is equal to the love I have for each dear friend who has died.

Francis Weller, author of *The Wild Edge of Sorrow*, wrote: *"Grief is a sustained note of being alive. We're most alive at the threshold between loss and revelation; every loss ultimately opens the way for a new encounter."*

This world is certainly a crazy place. Cancer is becoming an epidemic. I won't sugar coat it. With our toxic world, we'll continue to see more and more people diagnosed with cancer. Cancer reflects the toxic nature of our society, environmental devastation, the greed, the hunger, and the unaddressed pain we all carry. There will be more sickness and illness, until there's ecological balance upon Earth. This is dependent on humans waking up as a collective to realize what a serious issue climate change is and making the changes necessary to reduce carbon emissions.

There's a powerful gift to be witnessed within the mystery of loss. It teaches me to embody my life fully while I have a body to enjoy it. I could die in a horse accident like Laura, cancer could easily snuff my life out, or I could completely heal from cancer and beat the odds of the diagnosis.

Whatever my fate is, I plan to treasure each moment. Every tear that I shed for the death of Annelise is a remembrance of how sacred each breath is.

I pray for the lives of my friends on the cancer journey. I also pray for my own life. Each prayer is a wish that we may awaken to what true healing is for each of us, even if that means embracing death. It all comes back around to love and what we choose to do with the sacred gift of our heart.

Annelise's last Instagram post read,

> *And the Ultimate Power is Love. My heart is blown open by the profound love I have experienced in the last few weeks. Totally agree with RA ~ "The purpose of incarnation in the Third density is to learn the ways of love."*

I saw Deb in the last month of her life capture this infinite truth as well. From what I've witnessed, the gift of dying is to realize what truly matters.

Love is all there is. To embrace and love those whom you cherish is the most important thing. Love heals. Love transforms.

I have seen far too much death in a short time.

Cherish your health. Fully embody your life as it's the most precious gift. Don't wait for illness to teach you this lesson.

I wish I had acknowledged this fragile reality before cancer came to knock me upside my head!

Annelise's death brings me to a deep sense of surrender. It also fuels my desire to live. None of us knows when our time will be.

I'm determined to find my way, face my shadows, find my joy, and live each day to the fullest.

The deaths of Morgan, Deb, Rowen, Jenny, Peg, Susan, Laura, and Annelise have all left indelible marks on my heart. As Leonard Cohen says, *"There is a crack in everything; that is how the light gets in."*

I strive to keep my heart open despite the sorrow and grief of these losses. In embracing this life, I surrender and accept it all, even death.

OFF TO MEXICO:

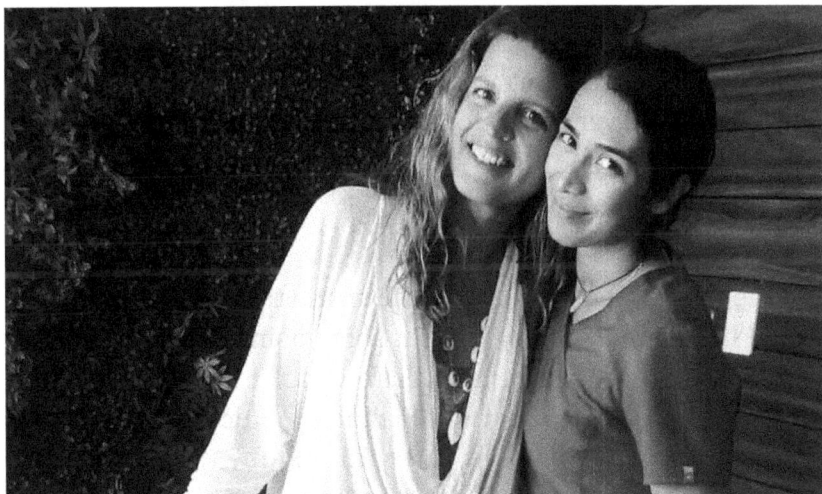

Me & Briseida (Brisy) Melchor Martínez at Hope for Cancer, Cancún, Mexico

In the fall of 2018, my health started spiraling down. Unfortunately, I started to feel the effects of cancer in my body. I had a perpetual hip & inner groin pain for months which I thought was an injury. The perplexing thing about the injury is that it never went away! I also had a painful sensation in my ribs that was a mystery. I had no idea that it was sign that the cancer had spread to my bones. It never occurred to me that the pain was indicative of the cancer spreading. If I had known, who knows what I would have done? It was definitely a stressful time in the midst of having to consolidate WHS, figure out what to do with the horse herd, and getting ready to sell the ranch.

During the cacophony, I realized I better get my butt in gear and do something to stop the spread of the cancer. I started exploring the possibility of visiting alternative cancer clinics in Germany and Mexico. I dove into deep research mode talking to a plethora of cancer clinics, comparing the crazy astronomical prices, and talking to friends who had visited various cancer clinics. I knew the need was immediate, as the scans had shown the cancer had spread to my lungs and sternum bone.

After a vast number of long-distance calls to Germany and Mexico I concluded that the Hope for Cancer clinic in Cancun, Mexico was the right place for me. There was a tiny issue though.

It was astronomically expensive.

My ranch was about to go on the market; therefore, I knew I would have money to pay for it at some point. After pouring my heart out to a very close friend, I asked him if I could borrow the money to pay for treatment at the clinic. I was desperate. I wanted to live. I would do anything to try to find my way through the quagmire of bone pain and the spiraling down health diagnosis I found myself in. I was so grateful that he generously agreed to lend me the money!

I hurriedly did what I could to get my things together in order to leave the ranch for three weeks. Syris and I boarded a plane to visit the beautiful azure sea of Cancun, Mexico for full time cancer treatment. During my time at Hope for Cancer (AKA

Hope4Cancer), I met many wonderful cancer patients who were in the same boat as me. We might have had different religious beliefs, colored skin, and ethnicity but we all had one thing in common: we wanted to stay alive.

During my time at the clinic, I was fortunate to receive the latest and greatest nontoxic treatments available. Six days a week I took a bus with the other cancer patients to the Hope for Cancer Clinic. From 7 AM to 3 PM we received vitamin infusions, laser treatments, coffee enemas, and ozone treatments; laid in the hyperbaric oxygen chamber; ate delicious, healthy food; received massages; did spiritual healing therapy; laid down in the "pizza oven" AKA hot sauna; did blood tests and ultrasounds; and tried fancy cancer treatment methods straight from Germany. (Germany is the hot bed of alternative cancer treatment clinics.)

It was definitely not a cake walk. At the end of the day, I was exhausted from the rigmarole of being shuffled from one treatment to another. While other cancer patients enjoyed time on the beach frolicking about after treatment, I was laid out comatose on the beach.

The staff at Hope4Cancer were absolutely delightful and loving, and I found it a truly nurturing atmosphere after the hell of realizing I had to give up my precious ranch. In all my world travels, I had surprisingly never spent time in Mexico. It revived my spirit and nurtured my soul. It also reminded me how the tropics were the lifeblood of my soul.

Here are some posts from that time:

11/18:

Expectations can get you into trouble! After my first week of treatment, today was my one and only day off. I had hoped I could have a stellar day exploring the beauty of Cancun. This wasn't the case!

As I have been undergoing such intense healing therapies for six days straight, the side effects of detoxification hit me hard first thing in the morning. After I ate a robust hotel breakfast Americana style, I was laid out in bed with an achy and tired body till 1:30 pm or so. I reminded myself that the intense detox symptoms mean the treatment is working.

My greatest lesson on this cancer journey is to surrender, and I had no choice but to do that! When the body aches from the inside out, the best thing to do is just ride out the experience.

After a long and satisfying nap, I kicked my butt out the door to explore the stunning beach. How fortunate am I to be undergoing such deep healing work in such a splendid location? The calming, azure blue waves soothe my soul. I'm just a tropical girl at heart!

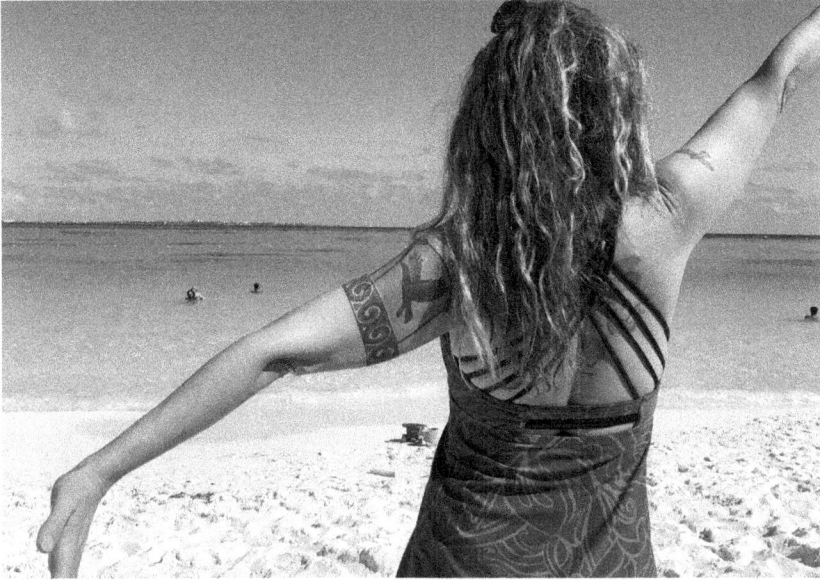

11/26:

The process of healing demands that I pick away what doesn't serve me, like pulling dead leaves off a plant one by one. Some of these dry and cracked leaves want to stay on the living, breathing body that is me, even though I know it's time the wilting leaves be composted.

I find my mind holds onto patterns and ways of being that ultimately don't serve me. These attachments to being busy, "doing," accomplishing, and worrying are all distractions from this new healed self that wishes to emerge. How to thank what doesn't serve and gracefully release the ways of being that hold firm onto illness? How to trust that I will be held, loved, cherished, and taken care of when every part of me yearns to run back into fear and the reality of the closed heart?

I'm forging new pathways to myself. I'm learning that I AM my own beloved. I'm worthwhile of the love that I choose to keep away from my armored heart.

This is tender territory, one that requires the greatest courage to face my shadows.

I feel like this creature, curled in a chrysalis, waiting to be born once again.

I'm alive, vibrant, and whole. Heart open wide and ready to embrace it all!

I see myself healed of cancer and all dis-ease that prevents me from embodying my full, radiant, and glorious self!

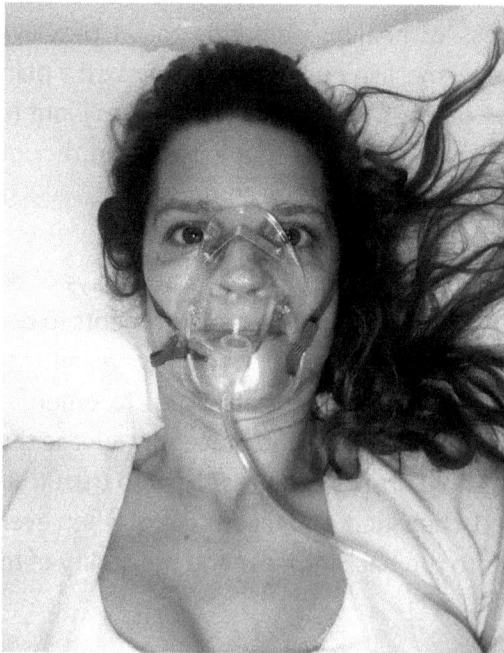

11/29:

Every day at Hope for Cancer is a packed routine of alterative cancer treatments. Each patient at the clinic goes from one practitioner and treatment to another. There's never a dull moment.

Some days are easy, some are very challenging. When the detoxification symptoms come on the inevitable side effects can range from headaches, sore body, exhaustion, and occasional nausea. Some days, I'm laid out in bed till the waves of funkiness pass. It's necessary to hold onto faith that this health protocol is working. I'm balancing on a thin line between fear and faith.

I'm super grateful for this opportunity to be here. I'm very well aware of how expensive this clinic is and that many people can't afford it. Only from selling my ranch, business, and the generous loan from a friend am I able to be here. I know I'm extremely fortunate to be receiving cancer treatments that are illegal in the U.S. or are prohibitively expensive.

One of the most healing aspects about being at the clinic is the loving atmosphere at Hope4Cancer. After the tumultuous last few months, it's extremely refreshing to be surrounded by the caring people at the clinic. I'm hearing miraculous, inspiring stories of healing and meeting many new friends. I have great respect for everyone on a serious cancer journey. It truly takes grit to get through each day and maintain a sense of positivity.

I'm nearing the end of my three-week journey and am praying for positive results soon!

11/30:

There's lots of inner work going on here. I'm processing emotions on a deep level and released elephant tears of integration today. This is a good thing!

The rainbow is emerging out of the clouds, bestowing beauty and grace, yet the clouds hold immense material and mystery to sort through.

My goal is to stay surrendered and to allow the shifting tide to move through me. It takes courage to practice the art of vulnerability. I know a pot of gold is waiting for me with all this immense physical and emotional work. My faith is strong.

12/4:

I have so much gratitude for Brisy, the special, stunning nurse at Hope4Cancer. She has cared so tenderly for me during my three weeks here. She is respectful, kind, funny, sweet, lighthearted, intelligent, and, above all, full of love!

When I arrived three weeks ago, my spirit and body were severely shaken from putting my ranch on the market, moving, and the sudden abrupt changes in my life. She and the other wonderful staff at Hope4Cancer were exceptionally caring. This helped me realize that, ultimately, everything would be okay.

The UVBI therapy was the most challenging health procedure for me.

Ultraviolet Blood Irradiation or UVBI is a treatment method that involves light. In fact, light has been used in medicine for more than 100 years to treat various conditions. UVBI or UBI or UVB is considered a non-toxic, low-cost, drug-free, safe, and intravenous method of treating a host of blood-borne viruses and other conditions like cancer.

An individual will have his or her blood drawn, and ultraviolet light is applied to the blood. The blood is then put back in the patient's body where it begins to purify the rest of the blood in the body.

The UBI process will supercharge the blood and improve the immune functions of the individual in a very effective way. The treatment has effective anti-infection and anti-inflammatory effects which are very important when treating a condition such as cancer.[8]

Due to the large needle going into a major artery, it was mentally and physically arduous. During my last UVBT procedure, the needle hit a painful vein. As tears poured out of my eyes, Bri quietly sang to me as the blood was painfully pumped out of my veins.

Thank you Brisy for your sweetness! Words cannot express how much your gentle, playful, and loving self deeply aided me in my healing.

During the end of my treatment in Mexico, I learned that there was also a small cancer spot on my liver that was there when I arrived for treatment. I wasn't aware of it till the end of my time in Mexico!

The wonderful news after my time at Hope4Cancer was that the tumor in my breast shrank by 1/3, my blood test scores improved, and two out of the five lymph nodes in my armpit vanished after treatment!

The time in Mexico was intense but very special. It was refreshing to be back in an environment surrounded by banana trees, warm humid breezes, and pearlescent water to swim in. In many ways, it felt like being home at my father's ancestral home is Kaua'i, Hawaii, another tropical location. Being in Mexico reminded me of how deeply nurtured I feel in a warm, lush environment.

When Syris and I returned home to California, we continued to jump through hoops to keep the wheels moving forward!

12/7:

I'm missing the sweet, relaxing tropical beauty of Mexico but am grateful to be back on my home ground. We're savoring the last days at WHS, as the ranch is on the market. Yup, this shit is real!

I was rocked by the waves of life before we went to Mexico, but now, I'm back on track, feeling positive and optimistic! I have a vision for how to create the optimum healing experience for this epic heroine's journey. I'm determined to manifest this reality!

While in Mexico, I realized that my ancestral homeland of Kaua'i, Hawaii was calling me back to her gentle healing shores. I believe that all the insanity of losing the ranch had unfolded because I'm meant to get my booty back on the sacred red dirt of Kaua'i again. I'M GOING BACK HOME!

ISLAND ROOTS:

I'm proud of my island roots on Kaua'i, Hawaii. My father's side of my family is from Kaua'i. We have Portuguese relatives that stretch back to 1878 originally from the Azores and Madeira Islands. In total from 1870 to 1911 nearly 16,000 Portuguese families were brought to the Hawaiian Islands to work for the booming sugar cane and pineapple agricultural industry.

I have fond memories as a child of being on the beloved small round island. The smell of the salty and tropical floral air resides deep in my DNA.

When I was in Mexico it occurred to me that there was no way I could possibly recreate the same equine retreat center setting in Northern California. I finally allowed myself to acknowledge that my body was breaking down from the cancer metastasis. Due to the mess I found myself in, it seemed to be an obvious choice to return to the sacred magic of the healing islands. I craved the ease of Kaua'i to soothe the shock of losing the ranch, and Deb's and Rowen's death.

I was blessed to have extended family and friends on Kaua'i. I felt that I could access my healing powers and leave behind the stress of the past years.

In the 1920s, my great grandfather had the intelligent foresight to buy raw land on the east side of the island. Over the years, it was passed down through the family generations. When my son was a year old, I built an off the grid, solar powered yurt on the family land. It was rented by various friends and tenants over the years when I didn't live on the island.

For my entire life, I would visit the small, round island in the middle of the ocean often for business or pleasure. Kaua'i always felt like home to me.

My life was so full at WHS with the full-time care of the ranch and four horses that I hadn't been in Kaua'i for two years. A huge lightbulb went off when I was in Mexico and remembered how much I loved the tropical island vibe. While on an exercise machine at the clinic, staring out the window at the gorgeous view of the banana trees by the bay below, I realized my heart yearned to return back to the beloved 'aina. I was so grateful to go home to the tropical paradise that was deeply embedded in my DNA.

With this wonderful realization, Syris, Xaria, and I set our sails for the lovely island of Kaua'i. There was an endless number of tasks to be done to consolidate the large retreat center and pack up our belongings so they could fit into a 30-foot yurt, but we focused on the task of getting it done!

BACK TO THE GARDEN ISLAND:

When Syris and I returned home from the tropical warmth of Mexico, it was a winter wonderland. The property had been on the market during the entire time we were in Mexico. There had been no offers. I was about to take the ranch off the market for the holiday season when, a few days before Christmas, I got a last-minute offer!

While I was waiting to see if the offer was going to go through, I finally had the courage to share my news with the world about the cancer's progression. I never shared publicly or even told my family why I had gone to Mexico for treatment. I didn't want to scare anyone by telling them the cancer had spread. My mind was already frightened, and I couldn't deal with others' fears on top of my own!

While juggling the Herculean task of selling the ranch and getting ready to move back home to Kaua'i, I had a renewed sense of self-care and a strong determination to live!

I devoted myself to a full-time healing routine, as I was aware of how serious my situation was. While I was fiercely focused on healing, I was also surrendered to what may be.

My goal was to appreciate each moment and to live as fully as I could. As my body declined, I realized how precious life was. It was a wakeup call to realize what a gift it was to be given a life-threatening diagnosis. I awoke to the beauty and joy that surrounded me in every moment.

I shared with the public on 12/23:

> I'm deeply grateful for this life even if it's much shorter than I had wished for. I plan to use all my inner fortitude, drive, vision, focus, and stamina to heal!
>
> I'm not a victim! Please don't pity me now that you know the cancer advanced to stage 4. My goal all along has been to walk this cancer healing path in the most empowered manner possible. I still believe in this vision! I'm grateful for this opportunity, and I'm doing everything in my power to heal.
>
> I have no regrets. While I might have made some slight changes to my healing protocol if I had a chance to do it over again, I fully believe in the choices I've made. I see the cancer growth as a cause and effect from the dramatic stress

my body experienced after such a traumatic jolt to my life this summer. I was doing well before that fateful letter from the planning department.

Please see me dancing healthy and whole on the beach! Visualization is a powerful thing, and you all can help me manifest this! Thank you for your help.

12/30:

The truth as I disclosed in my last beach dancing photo is that my health prognosis isn't good. My oncologist has told me there's nothing he can do for me. I don't give standard medicine a lot of credit, but this reality slaps me in the face.

The truth is that on the outside, my earthly body is almost forty-nine years old, but as I look young, most people think I'm in my 30s. At first glance, I look healthy, but the reality is there's cancer in my left breast, lungs, sternum bone, and a bit in my liver.

I sometimes experience pain and shortness of breath. It's scary and real to feel my strong body to be limited like this.

These are the hard knocks of life. I'm well aware that I will be a miracle case if I survive this. I know my prognosis isn't good. Sometimes, it feels like there's a gigantic worm crawling in my brain telling me I'm doomed to die. I'm not giving up, though!

I get up each day, take numerous pills, give myself shots, receive infusions, and pray to all that I hold dear that I will beat the odds and live to tell my tale. I believe I can heal! My love of life is strong! Despite this fucked-up world, there's still so much beauty.

My main drive is to see my gorgeous twenty-six-year-old son live his life. The boy whom I raised as a single mother deserves to have at least one parent stick around for him. It breaks my heart open into a thousand pieces to think of leaving him behind. A mother's love runs deep.

I'm moving back home to my beloved father's homeland of Kaua'i in a month. My wish is that the sacred earth will heal me. I hope my body can finally be in a parasympathetic, relaxed state so I will truly heal. Please help envision this for me. I want nothing more than to live a long life. Thank you from the depths of my heart.

2019

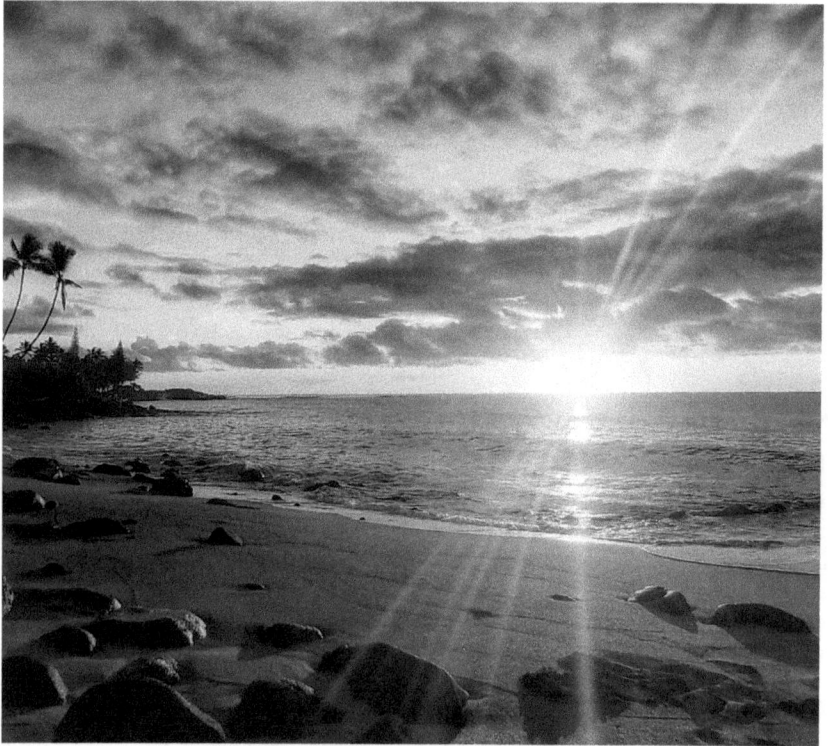
Beautiful sunrise on Kaua'i - Photo by Danny Hashimoto

1/24:

Super Blood Full Moon Eclipse Writing:

I'm fucking determined to live yet surrendered to the greater fate of what will be! While many of you call me brave and inspiring, I'm simply just showing up to the best of my ability. There are shitty days when I'm a total bitch and curse this challenging path. I've been known to hurl plates in fits of rage! There are days when I want to give up as it's been over two years of being dedicated to this path. Yet, I still keep showing up.

The choice is basically to sink or swim. I know this challenge is here to shine the diamond of my soul. I embrace every challenge that comes my way.

If the path leads me to embracing my own young death, then I'll accept that too. I will NOT give up easily, though. My tenacious, feisty, Portuguese fire is too stubborn for that!

When Syris and I arrived on Kaua'i, it wasn't the serene arrival I was hoping for. I had an idyllic vision that we would be stepping back into permanent vacation land. This wasn't the case. Unfortunately, life had more hard knocks in store.

It was a rough reality to come back to the twenty-six-year-old yurt that desperately needed some TLC. At the ranch in Northern California, I was used to living in a fancy retreat center with modern-day appliances. Moving back into a 30-foot-diameter soiled yurt in the middle of an unseasonably cold and rainy tropical winter was tough! In case you didn't know, there are no heaters in Hawaii! If the weather is 60 degrees, you can't just crank up the heat.

Upon arrival, everything that could possibly break did. If appliances were already on the brink, living off the grid in a yurt made for janky living. The stove refused to work. We were lucky to get a minute of hot water out of the water heater. Rats lived in the small kitchen.

Calgon, take me away!

My body was rapidly declining.

Adjusting to our new reality was unnerving and not the lovely slide into paradise that we thought it would be.

Sometimes, the trials keep coming to yank one into the present moment.

Not everything was rough, though. Some elements of coming back home were filled with ease and grace.

Fortunately, health-wise, things were lining up for me in a magical manner. I found an extremely knowledgeable naturopathic doctor to get vitamin IVs from. At the hospital, I met a Russian woman oncologist who was open to complimentary medicine. I even connected with someone who had a top-end hyperbaric oxygen chamber who was open to me using it. At this point, I needed to use all the tools I could to save my life!

After arriving on Kaua'i, I felt an immense amount of rib and bone pain. It felt like a backlash after pushing myself physically the month before to sell the ranch. I hoped it was just my body's way of scolding myself for not resting much. I continued to stay optimistic in the face of adversity.

ANCESTRAL ROOTS:

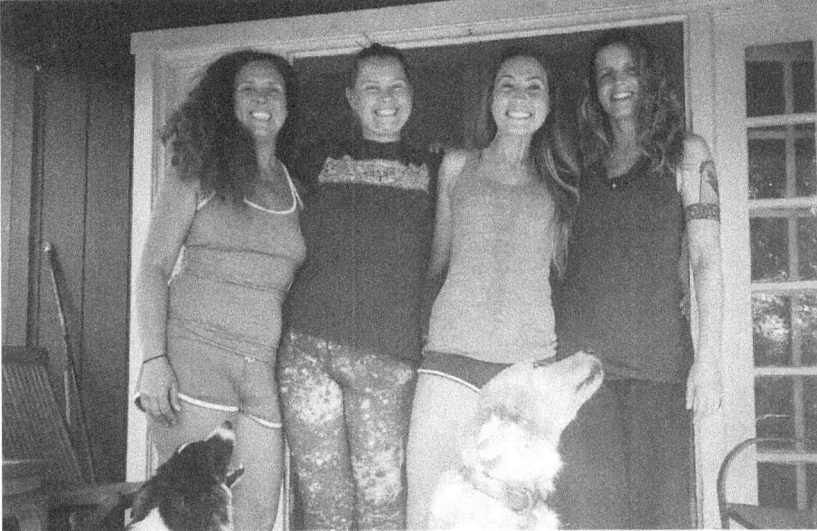

My cousins (Kaua'i ohana) - Laura, Emma, Stef, doggies & me

2/1:

In the 1870s, my adventurous sea-faring relatives arrived on the shores of Kaua'i. Due to the multilayered generational experience here, every inch of this island has a story for me.

My soul is etched upon the red clay soil of this tropical wonderland. From the time I was an infant, the years I lived on Kaua'i in my twenties and thirties, and the long history of relatives born here, this island holds my heart. I have memories of visiting my aunts as a toddler and being fed delicious opihi (limpets found on the rocky island shore) and yummy red bumpy fruit called lychee. I loved breaking apart the hard-red shell to find the soft white fruit inside.

I have countless stories of when my Uncle Eddie drove the car over the bridge in Kapa'a, the Irish officer my grandmother fell in love with in the 1940s but wasn't allowed to be with due to his religious background, and other stories.

There was a fair amount of trauma here within my family lineage, which has been my soul's responsibility to heal in my lifetime. It's fascinating how trauma gets passed down through the generations until it's finally healed.

It's no mistake that I was guided to my homeland to heal.

It's fabulous to be in a place where I randomly run into family members! We Portuguese women are a wild bunch. I love that my spirited female cousins are here! They have provided a warm welcome which I'm so grateful for.

The stories will undoubtedly continue to unfold as we create a new life here. Hopefully, this new path will be one of deep, vibrant healing, and I'll have many years to experience the rich wonder of this soil.

STORIES OF OLD HAWAII:

2/8:

Today I went to register an old beater island car at the Department of Motor Vehicles in the big city of Lihue on Kaua'i. The DMV is the same building that my dear grandmother worked at in the 1940s. However, in her time it was the sparkling new upscale Liberty House store. Liberty House was a department chain store based on the Hawaiian Islands which sold quality goods. When I first moved to Kaua'i in 1993, there was still one remaining on island in another location in Lihue. Years later the chain was bought out by Macy's department store. My grandmother would get dressed up each day in the fashion of the 1940s and sell jewelry at Liberty House. I can picture her coiffed hair, high heel shoes, long pencil skirt and sparkly jewelry.

There are ghosts on every corner.

Tales of roots and wings embalm themselves in my memory. Each building whispers secrets of the past.

Such a rich legacy to inherit in my genes.

TESTS:

2/10:

Kaua'i has the uncanny ability to test new arrivals on the island. It's common for visitors and people moving onto island to be continually challenged till they pass the test and find their peace with the island. Many don't make it over this hurdle and end up leaving the island in frustration. It's common for tourists to have an epic healing vacation on Kaua'i, decide to move here, and then leave the island soon after, as they're not able to endure the trials the island delivers. Many people end up spending six months to a year here and then flee back to the mainland!

Since we returned, every appliance except the refrigerator was on the blink. The hot water kept going off, the stove was pumping out major toxic propane fumes and the washing machine broke. Due to the vicious storm, fallen trees were scattered all over the property and we had no hot water for days, as the wind kept blowing out the flame on the hot water heater. High wind of 50-60 MPH is no joke!

We were clearly being tested!

I know this is Kaua'i's way of making sure we can endure the tests she delivers. I'm hanging in there and holding gratitude for what's working out and breathing deep into the challenges that come our way.

2/14:

The storms continue to rage endlessly, turning our driveway into an impenetrable mud puddle only accessible by 4-wheel-drive vehicles. Kaua'i is indeed the "wettest spot on Earth", with the 5,148-foot-tall Mount Waialeae receiving more than 400 inches of rain annually. Hanalei averages 78 inches per year.

I know, in time, eventually everything will be ironed out. The island is challenging us to see if we're able to ride the turbulent waves of change.

Isn't it interesting how the human ego craves solidity and stability? I believe these confrontations keep pouring in so I can truly learn to let go and surrender.

As the rain pounds on the yurt roof, I release again what I cannot control.

A VISIT FROM THE BOY:

My son Willow knew my health was in jeopardy and managed to pull some major strings to visit me. Willow and his girlfriend Mia visited for eleven days. As they were leaving the freezing winter of Minneapolis, they were understandably looking forward to being in sunny Hawaii. Unfortunately, their time on Kaua'i was marred by constant tropical storms and chilling weather. Locals said they hadn't experienced such a cold winter for years with the temperature dropping into the high 50s and low 60s. Remember, there are no heaters on an island!

2/16:

Willow, Mia, Syris, and I took a break from the endless fixing of broken things, treatments, clearing up storm debris, and unpacking to escape the rain for a moment only to find more rain on the South Side of the island. (Usually on Kaua'i you can go from one side of the island to another to find the sunshine. If it's raining on one side, just drive to the other.) After one turbulent downpour after another the sun eventually came out! We were overjoyed to see the sun, and have it dry out our wet sopping jeans.

We journeyed to the otherworldly splendorous rainforest of Kokee, overlooking the foggy Kalalau viewpoint. Soaked to the bone, in the freezing rain and wind, we hobbled about on the slippery red soil, trying not to fall on our asses in the mud.

As we drove down the mountain, we pulled off on the side of the road and laid our wet garments and towels out on the car to dry. We were like happy cats soaking in the glorious hot sun. We hadn't seen the sun for days!

On the long winding drive back, we were blessed with about ten different rainbows! I've never seen so many rainbows in my life. This felt like a gift for all the hardships we had endured after our arrival on the island.

It was such a treat to spend time with my son and Mia, who are both such intelligent, wonderful, and playful young adults. It's always good to take a break and gain perspective on what truly matters in the big picture. I'm incredibly grateful for family and the blessings it brings. Despite the challenges, I'm surrounded with beauty and abundance!

PARASYMPATHETIC/SYMPATHETIC NERVOUS SYSTEM:

I was grateful to have a handful of astute practitioners following my progress, issuing out blood tests, and helping me navigate the wacky path of stage 4 breast cancer. I was completely dedicated to my healing protocol.

As I had guests, I pushed myself physically and didn't get the down time I needed between treatments. I was starting to feel an active strain in my lungs and ribs.

Moderation is key to finding the balance for healing. I was striving to enjoy my life but also to have chill time for the healing to occur. Finding this balance is tricky for me, as I tend to never stop moving. This was a continual lesson in this lifetime. Hawaii was good for me, as the pace was so slow.

The sweet home island of my father's lineage was working its magic into my bones and slowly bringing me to a place of calm, rest, and healing.

As the past year had been incredibly stressful, I realized that I was primarily dwelling in the sympathetic nervous system (a state of fight, flight, or freeze). I was desperately yearning for my body to return to a parasympathetic, tranquil state of being.

When the body is in a parasympathetic state, the breath slows down enough to create relaxation within the body. This allows cellular repair to occur on a deep level, which, in turn, creates a perfect level of homeostasis. The body naturally brings itself back to equilibrium again and healing occurs.

Then there's the sympathetic nervous system which allowed the human species to survive. This fight or flight response helped our cave man predecessors quickly learn how to navigate danger! When a saber-toothed tiger was drooling outside the cave door and your Pleistocene relative learned how to avoid yet another casualty, you can thank the sympathetic nervous system for doing its job well!

Unfortunately, the reality in our modern-day civilization is that our reptilian brain is hard wired to react in the same manner as when that saber tooth tiger was looming at our cave man relative's door. This same panic response is triggered when an incident of a smaller magnitude occurs. Events such as when a battery dies in the car, an argument happens with a friend, or anything that jolts the nervous system can easily trigger the basal ganglia (also referred to as the reptilian or primal part of the brain) into thinking your life is in danger. The solution is to find the calm within the center of the storm and realize that your life isn't in danger just because there was a disagreement with a friend. This is why the parasympathetic nervous system is so necessary and important!

We're a civilization of people running fast, balancing Starbucks cups full of highly caffeinated, sugary drinks to keep our productivity level high. Being constantly busy has become the norm. How often do you find yourself quickly inhaling your food to get where you need to go?

We've learned as a civilization to constantly dwell in our sympathetic nervous system state. No wonder with each passing year, cancer and other illnesses are becoming more prevalent! As society speeds up, so do our nervous systems which makes it increasingly more difficult to heal. Stress kills, this is no joke!

The more time I spent in Kaua'i, I found myself transitioning from the sympathetic state of being to the parasympathetic state. This was a wonderful thing and I know it helped to contribute to my healing.

Even though the hurdles kept coming, my goal was to embody each moment the best I could. After the major storm, we had to deal with no hot water for five days, no water at all for two days, multiple trees scattered all over the property, and a slew of flaky workers who never arrived to work when they said they would. Island life is idyllic but the downside to a relaxed lifestyle is that it can be hard to get anything done. Tasks took three times longer to complete on the island than on the mainland!

We were finding our way. An immense amount of patience was necessary. As we didn't have hot water for five days, a hot shower was a simple and joyous celebration!

After being on Kaua'i for a month the plan was to go back to CA for scans, Mexico for treatment, then back to CA to figure out what to do with the two horses and try to sell the Tiny House. The adventure continued!

FACING DEATH:

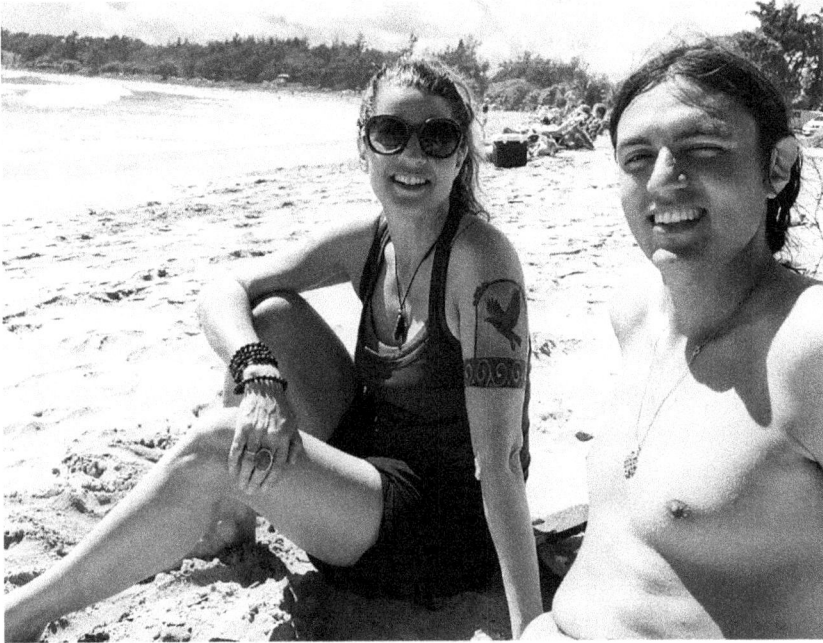

A powerful talk on the beach with Willow

As I was going quickly downhill physically, it was important to address the issue of my possible death with Willow. I wrote:

> Today, I had a teary, difficult conversation with my son about what might happen in the event I don't heal from cancer. All my focus is going toward healing, but as my ex-husband says, "Trust in Allah and tie your camel." Believe me this is a tough conversation to have with a twenty-six-year-old! I'd much rather he not endure the loss of his only present parent dying. It fucking breaks my heart to think of my possible death and how that might impact his life.
>
> After witnessing so many young friends pass from cancer and witnessing the immense amount of work it takes to sort out the logistical details of finances and material items after

death, I feel like it's a gesture of kindness to sort it out, so my beloveds don't have to. Figuring out the logistics needed before one's eventual death is a wise thing to do whether you have cancer or not.

I'm getting my will and practical details together; meanwhile, I'm living life as FULL as I can. I plan on living a nice LONG LIFE! I want to see my brilliant son live into his 30s and beyond!

ON THE ROAD AGAIN:

As we got ready to leave for our brief mainland trip, I found myself experiencing moments of peace of mind and serenity creeping into my consciousness. Kaua'i was starting to touch me with her healing magic.

I was aware that the island liked to challenge naïve new arrivals upon arrival on its dreamlike shores. I feel like I passed a massive test to make it through the first few weeks of challenges!

One reason I was going back to CA was that I still had medical care there and hadn't gotten insurance coverage on Kaua'i yet. The day after arrival in Grass Valley, I was going to get a PET scan. PET scans work by injecting the body with a sugar substance though the veins. The body is then scanned with nuclear medicine to detect where the cancer cells are. As cancer loves sugar, the cancer cells light up like a Christmas tree!

I was a bit nervous about the process. Ultimately though, I would rather know the reality if there was progression of cancer in my body.

One of the reasons why I refused to do any PET scans, MRIs, or CT scans for a year and a half was due to past trauma around Deb's experience with leukemia. In fact, much of my resistance to standard medicine was due to the PTSD around being with her for twenty-two months as she received treatment.

It took a huge amount of courage to do the PET scan. To say I was resistant to the experience was to put it mildly.

The evening before the PET scan, I woke up at 1 am with the disturbing memory of being with Deb when she almost died after receiving a CT scan. The uncanny part of my experience of being by Deb's side during treatment was that for some reason I was the main one there when difficult experiences unfolded. In this particular incident Deb didn't wake up after receiving the CT scan. At this point of her treatment, she was going downhill. She had been staying in the hospital for weeks. When she went in for her CT scan, she was already mentally and physically taxed.

After her scan, the nurses told me that something was wrong with Deb. She was lying flat out on the scan table, and no one could wake her up. I tried to rouse her, but Deb was out stone cold with no oxygen pumping through her lungs. We hurriedly rode the elevator up to the floor where her hospital room was to find fifteen nurses and doctors frantically wanting to know what happened to her. Utter pandemonium erupted. In the background, I heard the words "Code Blue" announced on the hospital loudspeakers. (The translation for "Code Blue" is "What the fuck? Something really terrible has just occurred; get your butt here ASAP!")

Deb's mom, Mary Lou, came out of Deb's room with nervous concerned eyes wondering what the fuss was all about. She immediately realized the commotion was focused on the issue that her beloved daughter wouldn't wake up. I had to explain to

Mary Lou and countless nurses what had happened after the CT scan.

As Deb wasn't breathing, the nurses needed to know immediately if Deb should be resuscitated. I stood dumbfounded with my feet trying desperately to root into the linoleum hospital floor. I deferred this immense decision to Deb's mother. A moment after this, a priest arrived and asked if we wanted the "last rites" to be performed on Deb.

As my head spun with total confusion, my goal was to hold solid ground for Mary Lou and Andy (Deb's husband who arrived soon after) as they absorbed the shock that our beloved Deb might be dying.

Deb was wheeled away to the ICU to be hooked up to a machine that would bring her back to life. She ended up having a tube inserted down her throat for three days (intubation) while she slowly came back to consciousness.

When she woke up in the ICU days later, she was pissed that she wasn't allowed to die. At this point, she had already been through innumerable hurdles.

This was just one of the many traumas that played out during my time of being a caretaker to Deb.

This PTSD of being with Deb when she almost died scared the shit out of me. The horrid memory crept up to greet me each time I had to do a scan. I saw Deb lying motionless on the bed, nurses swarming around us, "Code Blue" booming on the loudspeaker, and a frantic mother and husband coming to terms with Deb's possible death.

It took years of separating out Deb's cancer experience and mine to understand that I could write my own story. I didn't have to relive Deb's experience. I had my own version to tell.

When we were in California, it was such a wonderful treat to visit with Comanche and Blue! It had been a month since I'd seen them. It was a heartwarming homecoming to see them again; I felt like a part of me had been missing, as I hadn't seen them for so long.

My horses were an integral part of my soul. Just a short time of being near helped to bring my feet back to the sacred Earth again.

TO MEXICO:

When I received the results from the PET scan, I wasn't surprised to find out that the cancer had spread. The last eight months had been incredibly stressful with consolidating the ranch, moving to Kaua'i, and dealing with endless repairs on the island.

I wasn't giving up, though! My oncologist reminded me I'm a tough cookie and not to dig my grave yet. He recommended I try some hormone blocking medicine to stop the estrogen fueling the cancer growth.

After a necessary emotional release, I mentally jumped back into action mode once again. As Syris and I were on our way to Cancun for a week of treatment at Hope for Cancer, I was optimistic I could find help with the knowledgeable doctors there!

I was confident that I could create a lifestyle in which I could heal. I knew it might take a while to get there, but I was determined to find that balance!

INSIGHTS FROM THE JOURNEY:

In this period of dangling at the edge of death, there was a lot of wisdom and awareness that was bestowed upon me. I wrote the following while undergoing cancer treatment in Mexico:

Living with a life-threatening diagnosis is walking on the razor's edge of life and death. I'm actively choosing life yet surrendered to death.

The past two and a half years have been a deep dive. It has stretched me to the far reaches of my soul. It's been challenging, beautiful, terrible, enlightening, life gratifying, and full of wisdom. I thought I'd been through tough times before, but living with the knowledge that my life is dangling by a thread makes me aware of what's truly important!

There's so much beauty in the everyday sacred. It's really a gift to be staring your mortality in the face as you recognize how damn precious it all is.

There's no time to fret that my thighs are too big, I have too much belly fat or issues that might have weighed on me before. The fact that I'm alive today is enough. Life in a body is indeed a gift that I wish I had appreciated pre-diagnosis. To live in a functional, healthy body is all I wish for now. For those reading this, please take a moment to appreciate your healthy, pain-free body. Once you lose it, you realize how valuable it is!

THE LAYERS OF GRIEF:

During this time, I also was processing another layer of loss around Deb's death. Even after releasing immense grief in the three and a half years after her death, there was still many more layers to release. For years after her death, I facilitated grief rituals that created safe space for others to feel grief. This also allowed me to be present with my grief. When I was honest with myself, I realized that part of me was still holding onto her. Even though I knew her spirit was free, I still dearly missed her.

As I had recently realized there was cancer in my lungs, I energetically explored what that meant for me. When you look at various body parts and what each area represents, the lungs symbolize grief. Deb was my rock. She was my best friend for nineteen years. It made sense her death would have a dramatic effect on me. Her death was a major loss. There was no one quite like Deb.

The recall healer named Leslie at Hope for Cancer helped me tune into this deep-set grief. She guided me to see the emotional/ energetic element of my story beyond just the physical appearance of cancer. I realized that I had experienced many major losses including Deb's and Rowen's death, divorce, death of a dog, and letting go of the ranch and two horses.

I wrote:

> It's time to let go of the shadows that linger after experiencing so much loss. It's time to call in the light and free myself from this emotional bondage!

In this action I'm choosing to let go of the stories around my friends' deaths. I'm separating myself from their story, actively rewriting and choosing my story!

In this awareness I choose joy!

I let go, one tear at a time.

GOODBYE GRASS VALLEY/ NEVADA CITY:

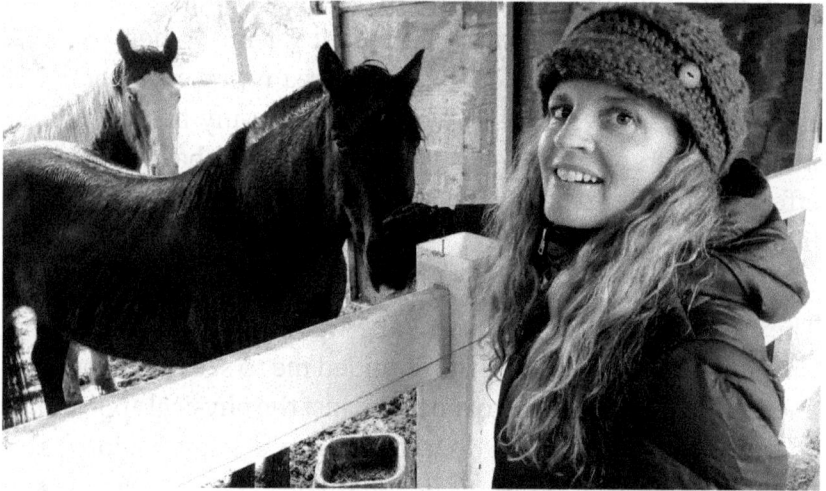

Blue, Comanche & me

Before we knew it, we were back in Nevada City for one week tying up loose ends. I loved spending time with my mustang Comanche. Spending time with him was like coming home to my heart.

The big decision was to figure out if I was going to bring both horses, Comanche and Blue back to Kaua'i. For them to get back to the Hawaiian Islands it required that they undergo an immense journey which would take about three weeks.

My hesitation to go forth with bringing them home wasn't so much about the financial expense, though it definitely was expensive! I questioned if such an arduous journey would be too much for them. I was afraid that being on an ocean liner with no sunshine for days would be torturous for these wild and beautiful beasts to endure. Horses are skittish creatures and don't like to be contained in small spaces. My horses always had large areas to roam around in; therefore, being enclosed in a Matson shipping container sounded like a horse nightmare. It was a big decision to make.

During my time with Leslie, she brought up a relevant point. She reflected that my profession is to help others heal with horses. She asked me, "Tara, why are you not utilizing the horse's restorative powers for your own healing when you dearly need it now?" This was an excellent observation that I took seriously!

Before Syris and I left the area, we had a goodbye party at my favorite vegan restaurant, Café Tara in Grass Valley. I liked to joke that it was my restaurant! About fifteen to twenty friends came to say goodbye to us for our final hurrah before we left town. As my body was increasingly feeling more pain daily, I tried to disguise the discomfort I felt from sitting for a few hours at a time. I was also coughing quite frequently from the cancer in my lungs. I shoved one cough drop after another into my mouth to avoid have a raucous coughing fit in front of my beloved friends. I didn't want anyone to know the serious state I was in.

It was a festive event where it was delightful to see everyone! I felt deeply loved by the beautiful friends who showed up to formally see us off to the islands. I dearly loved my time living in Grass Valley and Nevada City. The seven years spent in the community was an incredible healing, jubilant, and productive time after splitting up with my husband Tom and leaving Marin. It was a vital, creative, and vibrant community that I knew I would miss.

With all the physical challenges I had been through, the love, devotion, and care of dear friends makes the struggle worthwhile. To realize I'm truly loved is a profound healing force.

We had one more drive past WHS, the place that had been my sacred home, business, retreat center and the cumulation of eight years of hard work. I didn't know when I would see it again. It was an emotional, bittersweet day of saying goodbye to the ranch, the Grass Valley/Nevada City area, and my past life.

There was also a joy in letting go as I knew that releasing the past ties ultimately freed me to have the financial room to fund my healing journey. It had been years of endless, exhausting fundraising to raise enough money to keep my head financially above water. The monetary freedom gave me space to tap into my parasympathetic nervous system and truly heal on my beloved ancestral island of Kaua'i. There were no mistakes!

I celebrated all the workshops taught at the ranch and every guest who visited its pristine ground. I celebrated every dollar spent to keep the wild, verdant beauty of the ten acres stunning. I'm thankful for every worker who helped to keep it picturesque.

I embraced my new wild and precious life on the Hawaiian Islands. My hope was that the 'aina would heal my body, mind, and soul.

After leaving Nevada City, we stopped by to see Spirit and Daisy (the two horses I had given up when I let go of the ranch) who were thriving in their new home with their new family. It was a thrill to see them!

BACK HOME AGAIN:

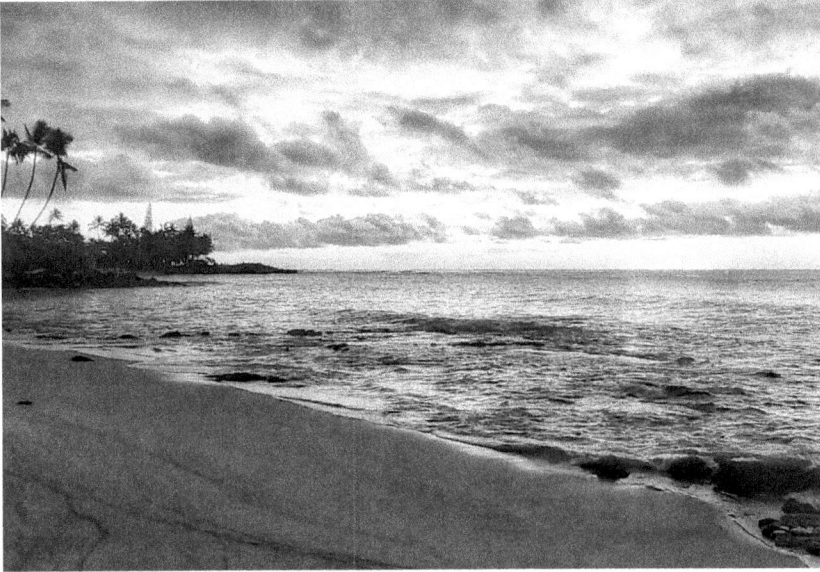

After arriving back home, Syris and I were worn ragged from our mainland and Mexico travels. We were definitely needing to slow down and were very happy to be back. I was aware that I needed to drop into a deeper state of being to allow my body to do the healing work it needed to do.

Kaua'i had always been a potent place of healing for me since I was a child and visited the islands. I had always thought of it as home. Due to having such deep roots on the island, I also felt like the mana of the island was extra strong for me.

As my body broke down, I literally was faced with tearing apart all my past perceptions and limiting belief systems that didn't serve me anymore. Not only was I looking at my own personal false beliefs, but I was also aware of the layers of family trauma from my father's Portuguese side of the family on the island.

As my Portuguese ancestors had lived on Kaua'i for 150+ years there was serious family history layered in the iron-rich dirt. Ancestral ghosts of yesteryear plus my own childhood and adult memories lurked around every corner.

I knew it wasn't a mistake that I was drawn to the island during the most accelerated healing adventure of my life. I was aware that I would either find a way to heal this prognosis or die on Kaua'i.

I was 300% committed to doing the work, showing up and exploring all the avenues that might restore my health. I realized that facing unhealthy karmic family patterns were a big part of my necessary inner process.

SELF-PITY:

It's easy to let the mind worms of self-pity creep in while on a cancer healing path. Since my diagnosis, it definitely has been a daily check-in for me to acknowledge my fears and move forward with a positive stride. I felt that, overall, I did quite well with my state of mind.

During this time, my body had been pretty slammed with new painful symptoms that were pushing me to the edge of my comfort zone. I was also experiencing an abysmal exhaustion from a full month of traveling. I was forced to practice faith in my body's ability to heal. It was a new thing to be experiencing such profound discomfort within my body. In the past, I was a powerhouse amazon superwoman and prided myself on my limitless strength and ability to do things others couldn't do.

I found myself in a frequent inner dialogue with the limiting demons of self-pity and voices of doubt that wanted to stop me from rising above these new healing opportunities.

One day I went to the ocean. It was divine to remember the majestic grace I was surrounded by on the island. Nature brought me back to myself every time I touched her.

I was on a profound healing journey that was growing me by leaps and bounds. I kept reminding myself that whether I died from the prognosis or miraculously healed, the diamond of my soul was being brilliantly polished. The growth I was receiving from the experience was all that truly mattered.

I chose daily to stay in gratitude despite the stinky mind worms!

THE BREATH OF LIFE 1:

My body continued to take a rapid downward spiral. As part of my healing routine, I was fortunate to find someone on Kaua'i with a hyperbaric oxygen chamber which saturates the blood with oxygen. This helps fight bacteria and stimulates the release of growth factors and stem cells, which promote healing.

After one particular session, I felt an acute sense of irritation in my lungs. For three days straight, I had trouble breathing. I believe that the cancer nodules in my lungs became extremely irritated with the huge blasts of oxygen I was receiving. It was too much for my body to handle.

When I wheezed like someone with serious asthma, I was struggling to get enough oxygen into my lungs. It was impossible to sleep at night as I ended up choking in my sleep. For about a month, Syris stayed up with me at night, as he was concerned I would choke and die in my sleep. Hour after hour in the dead of night I was constantly sucking on cough drops, chugging cough syrup, and trying every trick I could to breathe with no avail. This was scary! It was so severe; I almost went to the emergency room several times.

I was grateful for another dear friend who had an ozone machine. I inhaled the ozone into my lungs, which brought a sense of relief.

I had to be in a state of constant awareness to make sure my body stayed calm when I had a coughing fit. It was easy for the sympathetic system to take hold and fall into a fight/flight/freeze mode when a coughing fit came on. This only made the coughing fit worse.

This experience helped me become aware of what a gift it was to breathe normally. I vowed to never take for granted the wonder of oxygen pumping freely in and out of my lungs.

THE GODDESS INANNA

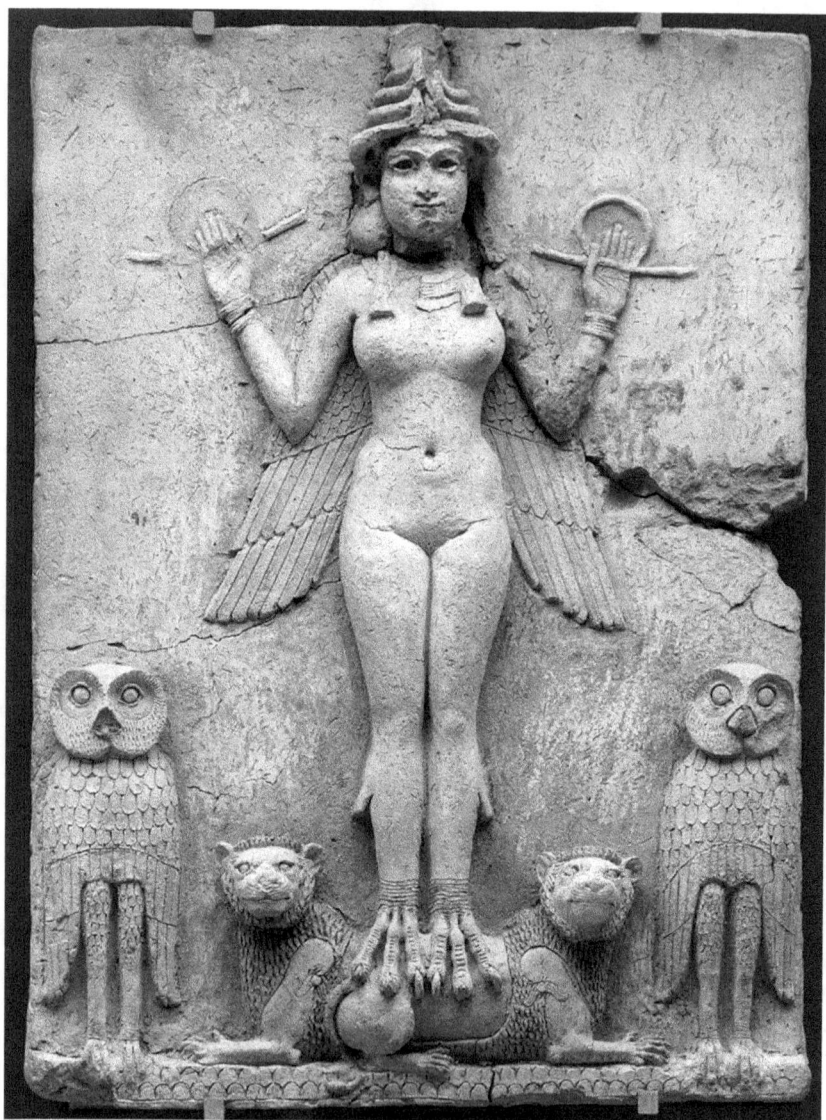

Inanna - Burney Relief 'Queen of the Night' - from Southern Mesopotamia between 1800 and 1750 BCE

I have followed Inanna to the depths of the shadows and back again.

Inanna is a 5,000-year-old goddess of ancient Mesopotamia. Her stories were recorded on stone tablets between 1900 and 1600 BC and are some of the earliest extant myths that we have. Inanna is related to the goddesses Ishtar, Isis, and Aphrodite. She is a goddess of sex, but not of marriage. Inanna is also known as "Queen of Heaven and Earth."

In this ageless tale, Inanna travels through the seven gates to the underworld. The "Descent of Inanna" tells of the eponymous heroine's journey to the Underworld to visit / challenge the power of her recently widowed sister, Ereshkigal who is the queen of the realm. *"One explanation for Inanna's interest in the Underworld is that she hopes to extend her power into that realm."*[9]

Before her departure, she outfits herself in all her jewels and raiment. She had seven sacred pieces that included a crown, jewels, scepter, and robes. She begins to descend into the netherworld, only to be stopped at each of the seven gates during the journey. At each gate, she is required to give up another symbol of her status, from her crown and scepter to, at the last gate, her robes. She arrives at her sister Ereshkigal's domain stripped of everything that she had and is completely naked. Once she appears before her sister, Ereshkigal kills her, and hangs her body on a meat hook in a corner of her throne room.

Prior to entering the Underworld, Inanna had instructed her servant Ninshubur on how to come to her aid should she fail to return at the expected time. Thus, Ninshubur went to the god Enki, Inanna's father, for help. Whilst Inanna was successfully revived by the servants sent by her father, she is unable to leave the Underworld as easily as she entered it.

A substitute had to be found, and Enki's servants tried to take several of Inanna's followers, though the goddess stops them from doing so, as they were all mourning for her supposed death. In the end, Inanna encounters Dumuzi, her husband, who is clearly not in mourning, as he was "clothed in a magnificent garment and seated magnificently on a throne." This infuriated Inanna, who ordered him to be seized.

Dumuzi prays to Utu, the sun god, to save him, and is transformed into a snake. Nevertheless, he is captured in his attempt to escape, and is brought to the Underworld. Geshtinanna, Dumuzi's sister, volunteers to be her brother's substitute, and in the end, it was decided that Dumuzi and his sister would each spend half the year in the Underworld. Like the Greek myth of Persephone and Demeter, this event is used to explain the changing of the seasons."[10]

Inanna travels back to the upper world, and as she does so, she gathers her regalia at each gate.

This is a tale of death and rebirth.

During this time, in the spring of 2019, I was fully initiated into the realm of Inanna. I had been through hardship before, but nowhere to the extent of this time.

Jean Shinoda Bolen, in her book *Close to the Bone*, talks about Inanna as the mythical equivalent of someone with a life-threatening diagnosis. On page 21 of her book, she writes,

"Over and over, at each gate, symbols of power, prestige, wealth and office were taken from her. Over and over, at each gate, the removal of something else that covered her, was unexpected. Over and over, she would say, "What is this?" and be told, "Quiet, Inanna. The rules of the underworld are perfect. They may not be questioned."

In this time, I was forced to face my fears of standard medicine. I basically had to eat a huge slice of humble pie as I had boasted through all my social media channels, blog pages, videos, & interviews that I was healing cancer naturally. I was forced to face my stringent belief systems around any sort of medicine that wasn't "natural."

This took great courage for me to share with others. I did a huge amount of self-reflection with my dear friend, author of *My Cancer Guru*, and cancer thriver Bethany Webb with "The Work of Byron Katie," questioning my belief systems.

In the next posts I gingerly make my announcement to the world about trying standard medicine:

Here's a little Tara update for your Instagram ears only! Those who have been following me for years now with the cancer healing journey know I've been 100% Miss Natural! I've been questioning my beliefs big time around this lately as my health has become in such a serious state.

I'll cut to the chase: I started taking Tamoxifen last week! Shocking right? Tamoxifen is a hormone blocker to help stop the flow of estrogen that's feeding the cancer in my body. My doctors tell me it's the best chance I have of healing now.

My love of life is strong! Lately, tears freely flow down my cheeks when I feel how dearly I love life and want to be in this body for many more years.

In the past, I thought of Tamoxifen as poison. I've shifted my thinking to see it as the medicine that will heal me.

I'm faced with staying within my old belief system of only doing "natural" medicine and dying as a result OR embracing new ideas that could literally save my life!

I choose life!

I'm facing my own inner judgment and shame that comes with taking mainstream medicine.

The side effects after a week of taking Tamoxifen are moodiness, highly emotional at times, hot flashes, and night sweats. This sounds like menopause, doesn't it? I'm riding the waves.

So, I go forward, pink unicorn bag in arm and a supreme willingness to grow despite the challenges and repugnant side effects that come my way. Onward and upward! Shazam!

***

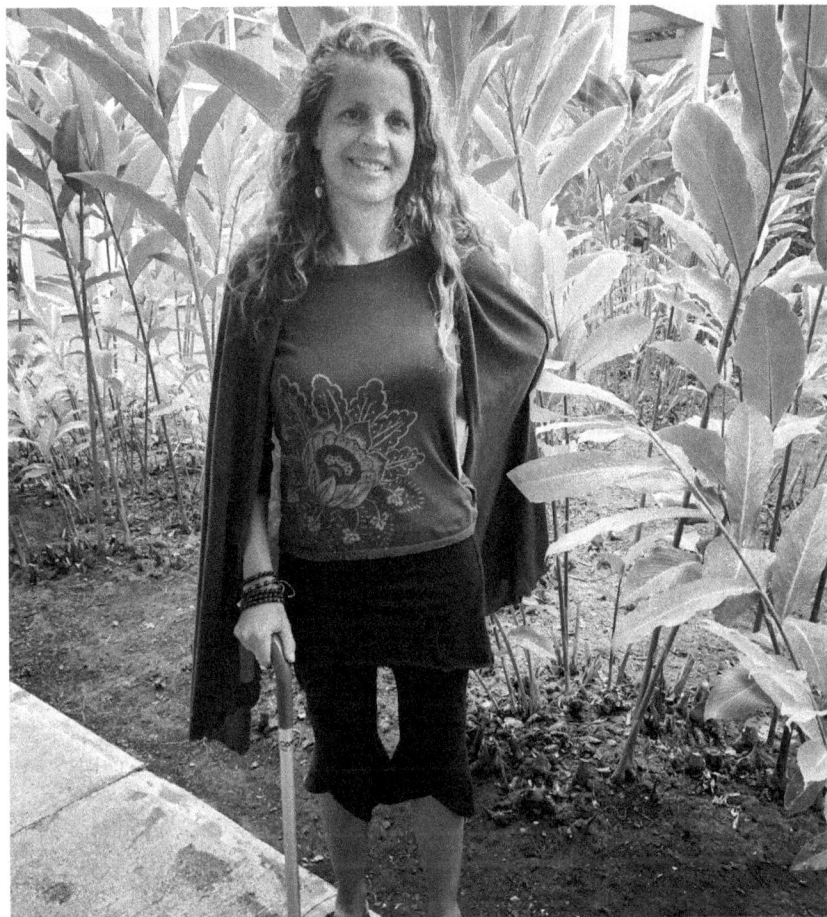
My benevolent cane Frida

This time was one of great decline where I was navigating a body that was becoming consumed with cancer. I tried my best to hide it from the outside world, but I was suffering in my daily life. I was walking with a cane due to the cancer metastasis in my bones, having a hard time breathing due to the cancer in my lungs and I couldn't sleep lying down for two months, as I was gagging too much in my sleep. It was frightening.

One of the lessons during this time was how to practice impeccable self-care. As my body was increasingly becoming more limited, I couldn't push myself the way I usually did. This was actually a gift to slow down and take care of myself, as I had no other choice.

Despite the agony, my goal was to remain as positive as possible. Finding light in the shadows made everything much better.

Sharing my journey on Instagram was a huge help during this time, as not only did I receive the love and support of thousands of people in an extended community from all over the globe, but it was also a cathartic release from the intensity of my daily life.

April:

Today, I feel the beautiful expansive nature of the universe and choose to say yes to life!

Yes, there are many challenges, and for all I know, this could be the last year of my life.

Despite the odds, I'm choosing to believe I'm healing! I believe this metastatic breast cancer experience came to me to grow my soul to a place of unimaginable depth. I'm choosing to be thankful for the pain, struggle, and fear of what this path might bring. I know if I'm brave enough to accept it, I'll transcend it!

Each challenge I face is an opportunity to embrace it and grow or not.

It's very simple.

Sink or swim.

In many ways having a serious diagnosis is a blessing, as it teaches me how damn precious each moment is!

Today, I will dance and celebrate life to the best of my ability. Life is short, and, despite the rough spots, I choose gratitude, life, love, and beauty!

THE JOURNEY BEGINS:

The horses were soon to arrive! My heart was eagerly anticipating the arrival of the two boys, Comanche & Blue. Before they touched ground on Kaua'i, they had a long journey ahead of them.

4/10:

Tomorrow morning, these two gorgeous horses, Blue and Comanche, start a two-week journey that will take them from Grass Valley to Sonoma, then on a 2,500-mile journey across the Pacific Ocean to Kaua'i. They will leave the Port of Oakland next week, be put in a shipping container with other horses, and then travel for four days from Oakland to Honolulu. They will then spend the night in Oahu and take another boat to Kaua'i.

Although they both are wonderful, easygoing horses, they've lived a life on large, green pastures. They aren't the type of horses that have lived their lives in small stalls. I'm a bit nervous for them to be enclosed with no sunlight for four days in the shipping container, though I know they'll be okay.

EATING HUMBLE PIE:

As I waited for the arrival of my blessed horses, I wasn't getting the results I wished for with Tamoxifen. Because I was experiencing dramatic pain in my ribs and my left hip, a kind radiologist told me that it would be helpful for me to try five rounds of focused radiation on these tender areas.

Announcing to the public that I was going to do radiation was deeply humbling. I previously had held the proud flag of "Tara Coyote, the natural healing Cancer Warrioress"! It was time to get real in the face of my crumbling body.

There were often humorous occurrences that would unfold when dealing with others about my serious diagnosis. I learned to just laugh at the perceptions and trust that everyone had good intentions.

For example, at a physical therapy appointment, my PT asked me if my diagnosis was terminal. I almost broke out laughing in response and felt like saying, "Isn't life a terminal condition?"

I forged ahead with what I felt would give me a good quality of life. I was learning to embrace certain aspects of the allopathic world that I had shunned before. Along with the Tamoxifen I was taking for three weeks, I decided to do five rounds of radiation. The acute bone metastasis pain in my hip and sternum area was becoming more severe. The radiation hopefully would minimize the pain and stop the cancer growth.

This was a huge shift for me, as two years before, I was blogging about the dangers of radiation. For me to publicly change my route of treatment took a lot of inner courage. I was definitely eating some humble pie! My will to live dominated any old dogma that kept me in limited belief systems.

At this time, I apologized publicly through my social media posts to anyone I placed judgment on for their choice to use standard medicine for cancer treatment.

I was a headstrong woman and was learning big lessons through this epic process! I learned that every individual has their own journey, and each person must choose what their own ideal path for treatment is at any given time.

I planned to use the best medicines of the allopathic world and combine it with the stellar alternative therapies I was doing to forge my path ahead. One moment at a time, one foot in front of the other.

The first day of radiation was rather anticlimactic. As I laid in the mold made for my body with the large machine whirling around me, I focused deeply on the procedure successfully healing me. When thoughts of fear crept in as I felt my body restricted, I would gently let them go and remind myself of the light technology freeing my body of cancer. The deeper I breathed, the more of a surrendered Zen space I entered into. I think I may have fallen asleep near the end of the process.

The whole experience was rather surreal! I released into surrender as I allowed the allopathic medicine in.

Robot Dream:

I had a dream of being attacked by machines after doing four days of radiation. I lay in bed surrounded by the chirping and croaking of tropical sounds. My body feels pummeled by the new medicines I've chosen to embrace on this heroine's journey. Tamoxifen, Tramadol, low dose Naltrexone, and radiation run through my veins. This creates an entirely new story for this self-prescribed "all-natural girl." Self-doubt and faith roll into one as I bow to what is.

Where's the edge of your outdated belief system? Would you sacrifice your life to hold onto that belief? Is there a cost for choosing life over death? How far would you go to claim your life? When does one gracefully choose to surrender to the reality at hand and allow the tide to seize your soul? When is enough Tamoxifen? How far would you go to preserve your one short and precious life?

I'm facing the hardest question I've encountered on this two-and-a-half-year cancer healing journey. Thoughts of mortality and what I truly embrace to be my truth ripple through and cause me to question everything. I won't be imprisoned by my past belief systems, yet I need to honor what my heart says. This tale is yet to be told.

I humorously tossed and turned last night as I dreamed of machines attacking me. Between the radiation, X-rays, CT scans, and ultrasounds of the past week, I'm being asked to accept the modern technology that will possibly save my life.

I will keep going forward the best I can till it's clear I can't, robot nightmares and all!

I sampled one new allopathic medicine after another in the effort to save my life. The saving grace of the experience was being back home on Kaua'i. The tranquility of the island was deeply nurturing when I most needed comfort and peace. It was exactly where I need to be.

I was starting to see that there were no mistakes. Sometimes, what might be seen as a cataclysmic event can serve as a transformative reawakening. Being forcefully uprooted from my beloved horse ranch was the best solution for my healing. I saw that all was perfect, and I was actually being guided all along! Never doubt the mysterious power of the universe.

GIVING UP MY REGALIA:

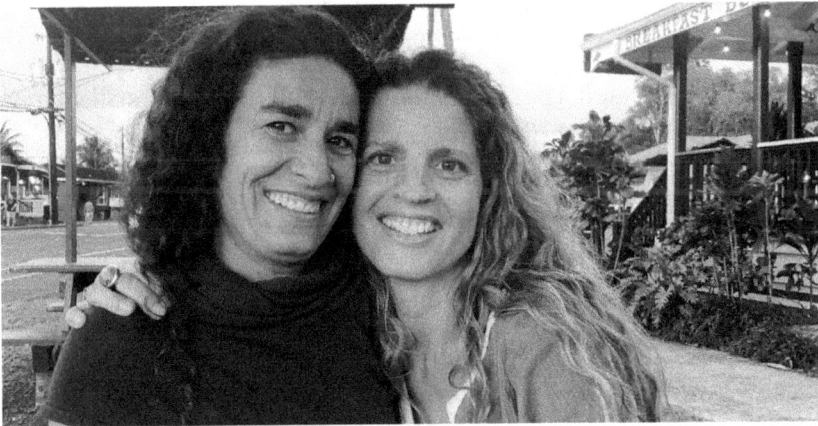

Michelle & me

The bone metastasis pain kept getting worse. The throbbing nature of bone pain was beyond anything I had experienced in my life.

I could feel my bones eroding. It was starting to affect my quality of life. I was limping and walking regularly with a cane. My bestie Michelle, playfully named my cane Frida (after the artist Frida Kahlo who dealt with a considerable amount of pain in her lifetime) to make light of the dire situation I found myself in. It was like I had a camera watching me from afar and I was witnessing my athletic, invincible body breaking down. In slow motion I saw myself losing the physical prowess that was my natural state of being. I felt stupefied and honestly didn't know how to cope with it.

It was extra challenging, as I always prided myself on my Amazonian strength. My body and mind were both equally pushed due to the hellacious circumstance.

I dreamt of waking up in the morning feeling normal. I yearned to do something as simple as riding a bike and not having to worry about my bones breaking due to falling off the bike. I fantasized about the day when I didn't have coughing fits every hour.

I reminded myself that I was still alive. There was still beauty to be found. Even though my body was in grappling pain, I still had the ability to appreciate the luminous clouds, flowers, ocean, blessed animals, and humans surrounding me.

I chose to focus on the gifts surrounding me.

I chose gratitude.

I chose to continue on with the faith that the hard moments would eventually pass. And if they didn't, I vowed to enjoy the ride the best I could.

If I survived, I would never take my functional body for granted again.

RETURN OF THE HORSES:

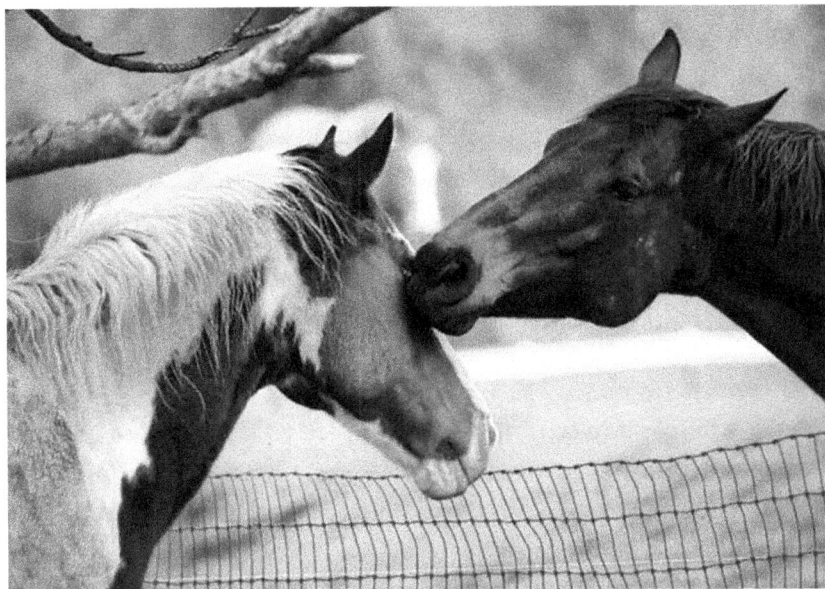

Blue & Comanche - Photo by Melinda Vienna Saari

All wasn't lost, though. Comanche and Blue were soon to arrive! After a three-week trip from Grass Valley to Kaua'i, I was eagerly anticipating their arrival.

My dear friend Michelle was visiting to help me through the fear of receiving radiation. We went to a feed store to gather goodies for the horses' arrival. Just the smell of horse feed, hay, and the sight of horsey items lifted my spirits. You can take the horse away from the girl, but you can't take the horse out of the girl!

The horses were an intrinsic part of my heart. They fueled my drive to live. My seven-year relationship with Comanche and the rest of the herd had already seen me through the toughest of times. I was elated to have them by my side to help me face the biggest challenge of my life.

Thank goodness for horse medicine. Bless the beasts!

***

When the horses arrived, I felt an immense sense of relief. Even though I was deep in the throes of the underworld on my Inanna journey, there was an immediate comfort to feel their presence on the island.

I wrote:

> The horses arrived, bringing with them a blast of joy to my tender heart! What a tedious three-week 2,500-mile journey they've been on. I wish they could talk and tell me of their adventure from Grass Valley to Kaua'i! They both lost some weight but, overall, are doing great.

> Of course, my paint horse Blue, with his white and brown coat, was impeccably clean when he arrived. Can you guess the first thing they did when they stepped upon the red dirt soil? They happily rolled their ocean weary coats on the ground! Their hooves hadn't been on the earth for three weeks. So much for a clean horse!

> My outcome was unknown, and my destiny was unclear. All that was certain was that I was present in the infinite eye of grace.

GRAVEYARD INSIGHTS:

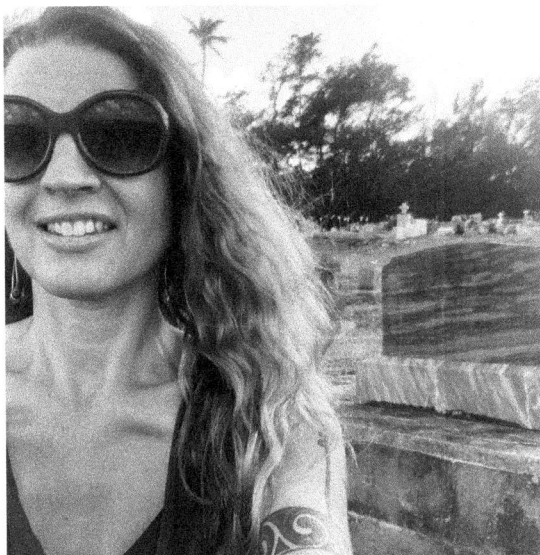

Whenever I felt lost, Kaua'i would shine some of her healing magic upon me. The yurt was cradled under the magnificent Makaleha mountains. Seeing this mountain range while driving home and while on the land brought a constant sense of awe.

I have a clear fascination with death. I love hanging out in graveyards. A particular favorite of mine is St. Catherine graveyard where all my Portuguese ancestors from Kaua'i were buried. Several generations of my homies dwelled here! This special spot overlooking Kealia beach was a constant source of peace and comfort for me throughout my whole life.

Great-Grandma Rosie, Great-Grandpa Joe and Great-Uncle Eddie raised my father throughout his fragmented childhood and were buried here. I had been coming here since I was a baby to honor these beloved ancestors. My dad would plop me on the side of their grave and share fantastical stories about them. We would place tropical flowers in the permanent glass vases that laid deep in the sand over their decaying bones. Even as a child, I felt incredibly held by my ancestors when I visited this graveyard. Their presence was tangibly felt.

Surrounding Rosie, Joe, and Eddie were my great-great-grandparents on both sides of the family line going back to 1878 when they arrived from the Azores and Medeiros islands off the coast of Portugal. After we spent time with Rosie, Joe, and Eddie, we would make our rounds around the graveyard and visit Rosie's parents Ernest and Maria Mladinich and Joe's parents, Joe and Maria Bettencourt. I reveled in the fact that they had been in the ground far beyond my young life. Besides all the great-great-grandparents, there were over a hundred cousins, aunts, uncles, and distant relatives in the graveyard with names such as Carvalho, Fernandes, Rapozo, Freitas, Aguilar and Lizama. Portuguese families were all related on an island as small as Kaua'i through one descendant or another. There were some serious roots here.

I especially loved visiting the Jesus who was embalmed in a cave built of stones on the hill of the graveyard. When I was a child, a lifelike prone image of Jesus laid in this cave. I remember his piercing blue eyes staring at mine and wondering as a child if he were real? It was surreal. In the 1980s, this iconic Jesus was stolen and a smaller version that wasn't as fascinating was put in his place. Who would steal Jesus? The fake Jesus still lives in the stone cave.

Although I was baptized Catholic on Kaua'i and felt a great affinity for the graveyard, I wasn't religious. As a young lad, my dad served as an altar boy for two years from the age of nine to eleven at St. Catherine's Church in Kapa'a. He came from a strict Catholic family on a small island; therefore, he had strict Catholicism shoved down his throat. When he moved away to college at the age of eighteen to immerse himself in the study of biology, he became increasingly more affiliated with the magic of the DNA strand than the holy wafer that symbolized the body of Jesus. He vowed to never make his children walk a religious path. (I was grateful for this!) My younger brother and I were baptized on Kaua'i to appease Great-Grandma Rosie, who was highly religious. Overall, I probably attended church two times in my life. The fact that I was baptized on Kaua'i was proof to me of my devotional bond to the island; it had nothing to do with religion for me. The island was an integral part of my soul.

I was rooted to source in the graveyard. I would visit Rosie, Joe, and Eddie, sit on the side of their cement grave wall and stare at the pounding waves of the ocean below. I came here in times of great need to pray and ask for guidance. I would feel them whispering in my ear, sharing words of guidance to help me find my way.

As I was facing my own possible death it was time to take Frida, the cane to the graveyard. It was time to consult with my relatives, as I had a colossal decision to make.

On a trip to the graveyard in May 2019, I wrote the following:

What if you were told you had just a year or two to live?

Would you have the courage to change the toxic relationships and circumstances in your life?

Would you choose to transform your life, live large, and dare to do the things you always dreamt of?

Given the fact that life is temporary, and anyone's life could be snuffed out in a moment, why not do it now?

I'm immersed in the reality of my own mortality. I'm questioning everything.

One thing I know for sure:

Life is far too precious to be wasted in anger, regret, and hatred.

I'm learning to embody my own needs, even if it means saying NO to those closest to me. Boundaries are vitally important when it comes to healing!

If spending time in a graveyard doesn't remind you how short life is then I don't know what will!

JUST KEEP DANCING!

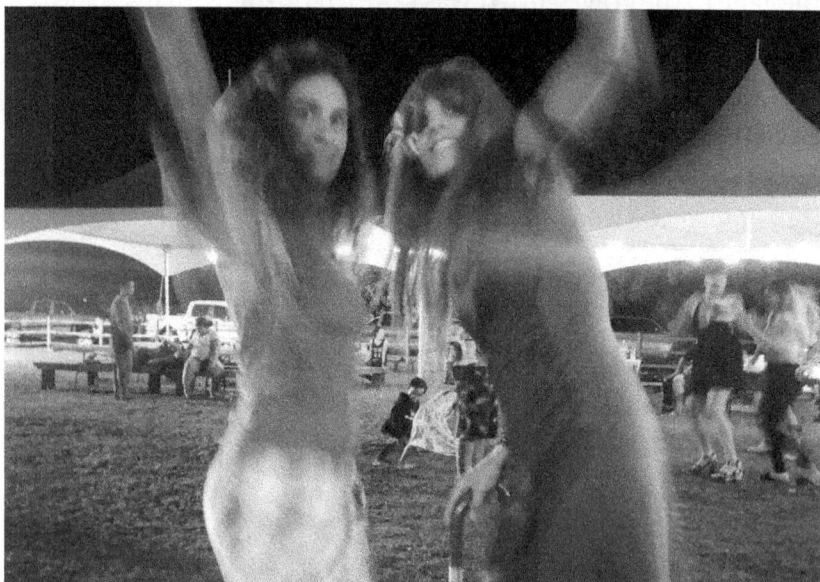

Michelle, Frida & me

Even though my body was having a rough go at practically everything, I was determined to get out and have some fun every now and then. I was well aware that if I stopped pushing myself to go out then I would perish in a cloud of depression. Therefore, cane or not, I made myself get out to dance if the opportunity presented itself. I didn't care if others looked at me or judged me; I wasn't going to let my deteriorating body prevent me from enjoying my life!

I wrote:

> Good ol' Jerry Garcia! Frida, my cane is such a brilliant dancing partner! Last night there was a Grateful Dead dance where friends replayed a 1989 DVD Philadelphia show. Deadheads, do you remember those days?
>
> There was young Brent, the keyboard player with his raspy, unique voice. Bobby had the sporty clean look and Mickey Hart looked suspiciously like Spock. Then there was Phil who I'll always love for the song "Box of Rain" and Billy banging on the drums. Then, of course there was iconic Jerry!
>
> Yes, I was a Deadhead! The New Year's Eve show going into 1989 was the first Grateful Dead event I attended. I didn't go physically into the show but fell in love with the fellow misfits in the parking lot. There was an immediate affinity with the tousled bohemians dancing in the drum circles. I loved the sight of women in long flowing Indian dresses, guys in tie dye shirts with the smell of patchouli wafting through. There were people of all ages selling grilled cheese sandwiches, burritos, and hand-made jewelry with the sound of pounding drums in the background.

After feeling like a stranger in a strange land in high school, finding the Grateful Dead community was an invitation into an exciting world where I felt like I could be myself. The Dead and their followers showed me there was a world far beyond the linear box I felt limited by in high school. I experienced a joyful liberation of sorts in the parking lot jubilee!

Thirty years later it was a delight to stumble upon a Grateful Dead replay of a show on tiny Kaua'i and connect with my Deadhead roots. I was proud of myself for not letting my fear of being seen with a cane limit me.

My advice to you: Don't worry about your limitations. Keep striving to live large no matter what your limitations might be! It felt SO GOOD to dance! Frida and I had a damn good time!

ACCEPTANCE & SURRENDER:

As I shared my healing journey vulnerably on social media, the announcements to the public about me embracing new forms of standard medicine (Tamoxifen and radiation) was a perpetual reality. These announcements took great courage. I was eroding the posterchild natural healing "Cancer Warrioress" façade with every new announcement.

This next particular announcement was the hardest one to make. I knew I would lose some of my "natural healing" cancer followers after they heard my decision. I felt like hiding from the world with this dramatic decision, but I knew it was important to share it with the world:

5/14:

Cracked open, raw, and vulnerable.

Today, I'm going to have a port put in me. I'm nervous. I'm having a foreign entity put just above my heart, so infusions and blood draws are easier.

Why am I getting a port? My big confession is that I'm going to start chemotherapy soon. This may come as a shock to many of you who have been following my story for years now. Miss Natural is changing her tune!

I've tried almost every natural healing possibility, spent an absurd amount of money (if you have donated to one of my fundraisers, thank you!), yet my quality of life is rapidly declining. Walking and breathing are becoming increasingly more difficult. Even my natural doctors are urging me to do chemotherapy! I dearly want to live, and this is my only chance left.

I have decided to fight fire with fire.

It's taking all my inner power and strength to go forward with this radical change of plans. I'm facing my worst fear: putting a medicine in my body that could kill me!

Remember I was the girl who boldly shared in posts, videos, and interviews that chemo killed? Well, now this girl is doing the medicine she feared most! Stay tuned friends!

It became increasingly clear that I would either stay stuck in my past belief system or die.

I had seen numerous other friends refuse to try standard medicine and sadly die. Who knows what might have happened if they had opened their mind up to allopathic medicine? Was I going to be another casualty like them?

Would I be willing to let go of my stuck belief system, try something new, and possibly live?

I dearly wanted to live!

THE BREATH OF LIFE 2:

I had a condition called "pleural effusion" which is caused by cancer cells in the lungs.

Cancer cells that inflame the pleura and this makes fluid. The fluid builds up in the pleural space and is called a pleural effusion. The fluid stops your lungs from expanding fully. So, you have to take shallower breaths and make more effort to breathe.[11]

The fluid buildup had increasingly caused more difficulty in breathing and created endless coughing fits. I was having uncomfortable side effects such as sore muscles and lack of sleep due to trying not to cough. It was necessary to get my lungs drained.

One month before, I had tried to have my lungs drained, but I was told there wasn't enough fluid to take out. This was very disappointing to know I had to continue in this uncomfortable state.

Another side effect of the liquid in my lungs was that my heart was overworking and beating dangerously fast to try to pump enough oxygen throughout my body.

My prayer was that the lung drainage would stabilize my body, which would create more oxygen in my body. A body that's deprived of oxygen easily can be overcome by disease and creates a breeding ground for cancer to proliferate. Having enough air to breathe is vital to healing.

I was told it was a simple, quick procedure to drain my lungs and would create immediate relief. Other friends reported a miraculous change within their bodies after getting it done. I hoped to have the same story!

I had an order for oxygen tanks from the island lung doctor that was taking forever for the insurance to approve. I had been waiting for six weeks, which, considering my situation having trouble breathing, felt like an eternity!

This was a time of being pushed to an extreme level and surrendering into trust. I tried to believe that I was exactly where I needed to be.

I knew my soul chose a path of rapid acceleration in this lifetime. I prayed for a bit more ease.

It was an extremely busy period full of endless doctors' appointments, scans, and preparation for port surgery. The big goal was to get my body and mind ready to start chemotherapy.

I had been to the hospital every day of the week for random spontaneous scans in preparation for port surgery. All week long, I had received phone calls unexpectedly saying, "Tara, can you make it down in the next two hours for an X-ray?" The following day I was called down for an ultrasound. I would grab my basket full of whatever necessary items I would need and off I went!

Now the level of importance for having my lungs drained was on the doctor's radar. As I couldn't physically lie down due to the fluid in my lungs and the violent coughing fits that would erupt, it was necessary to drain my lungs so I could get surgery. The doctors were afraid I would start choking during surgery, which was a realistic fear, considering I hadn't been able to lay down to sleep for six weeks!

The lung procedure was successful. It was a tremendous relief to be free of the one liter of nasty pond scum liquid that was drained out of my lungs!

After my lung was drained, the fact that I hadn't coughed for seven hours in a row was a total miracle! My brain and body were slowly becoming accustomed to having enough oxygen to properly saturate my body. My lungs had become accustomed to constantly fighting for air due the gelatinous pond gunk that took my breath away. During this adjustment period, I was a little loopy, dizzy, and out of breath, but I felt better!! Hallelujah! At this point, every small victory was a tremendous milestone.

I was grateful. Never would I take for granted how important breathe and lung function is again. When you're struggling to breathe, it puts everything into perspective!

The day after I had my lung drained, I had another hurdle in front of me: port surgery. In this marathon week full of endless procedures, I was definitely drawing on a Herculean source of strength.

I was told not to eat after midnight the night before. The surgery was scheduled for 12:30 pm but typical to island time it didn't begin till 3 pm. I tend to get dramatic blood sugar dips if I don't eat. My mind was starting to go a bit haywire from not eating for over eighteen hours! Anticipating surgery on an empty stomach in a hospital bed made me bat shit crazy. Sitting still was never easy for me. Due to low blood sugar and being stuck in a hospital setting, it stirred up the trauma of being with Deb for months in the hospital. My mind was having to do some serious work to stay calm while my belly screamed for food and water!

Surgery seemed to go okay, though when done, I was told I was only getting 70% of the oxygen my body needed. Hello lungs! The staff wanted to keep me overnight hooked up to an oxygen machine. Fortunately, the unfulfilled oxygen tank order from six weeks ago finally went through so Syris was able to pick up the oxygen equipment needed. I could now breathe safely at home.

After these frantic few days, I was resting and sleeping a lot. My body was banged up from having my lungs drained on Thursday followed by the port operation and another breast biopsy on Friday.

It was strange to have a port under my skin. It felt like I was implanted with an alien probe!

My body was in a hard place. I tried to rest when I needed to, was active when I could be, and tried to stretch my aching body in between it all. I attempted to find that fine line of pushing myself and fierce self-care.

It was extremely therapeutic to finally have an oxygen machine to help me breathe. I realized I hadn't been getting enough oxygen to my brain in the previous six weeks due to the constant cough.

My body was starting to calm down from the constant fight or flight trigger of needing more oxygen.

It was a bizarre situation to have my right lung drained and then transition to breathing air again. My lung felt like it had been waterlogged and stretched out and was learning to breathe oxygen again.

The plan was to do two months of A/C with four doses with two weeks in between each other. Then after that I would do twelve weekly doses of Taxol for three months straight. A/C is a combination of two chemotherapy drugs used to treat breast cancer. It takes its name from the initials of these drugs:

- Doxorubicin (also known as Adriamycin)
- Cyclophosphamide

FACING DEATH:

This poem was written when I was referred to hospice and facing death. I had just started chemotherapy. Chemo was my last hope to hold onto the thread of life that I held so dear. I had only told those closest to me what a decaying physical state I was in. I didn't want to scare those outside my inner circle.

After birthing this poem, I only showed a few of my most beloved friends that I knew could handle hearing it.

> Who will walk into the deep end with me,
> The place where the shadows lie,
> Where few dare to go?
> Who will face their fear of death?
> Who will hold my hand as I face my own?

Who is not afraid to see that death and life are
interconnected as one?
Who is brave to see that to embrace life, it's
necessary to accept death?

Who will witness my body breaking down, muscles
atrophying, and the once gorgeous athletic body I
had turning to dust?
Who will stand by my side when the mental demons
visit and, I face my deadliest fears?
Who is not afraid to dance in the darkness with me?
Who can bear the hollow skeleton of Kali embracing
our bodies, her bony, clawed fingernails running over
crackling bones?

I'm seeing the edge so clearly.
I could vanish in an instant if I chose to.
Life and death, the great fork lies before me;
It's a choice I must make.

Who is brave enough to cross the abyss with me?
We will cover our naked bodies with garlands of
roses as we step beyond the beyond.
We will celebrate our timeless souls.

A GLANCE OF THE HORSES:

Two days after the first surreal chemotherapy infusion I was
riding some big emotional and physical waves and missing the
horses something crazy. I yearned to see them again. Comanche
and Blue were adjusting well to their new life on over 80 acres.
As they were on such a huge chunk of land, and I couldn't walk
far due to the bone metastasis and hip pain, we were seeing them
only once every few days.

I wrote:

> Syris, Xaria, and Kismet the cat, who liked to go on walks with us, joined me on an adventure to find them. Lo and behold, they were waiting on top of the hill closest to us!
>
> It was such a joy to see them again! Unfortunately, my accident-prone Blue had a big cut on his leg. We decided to contain them in the small space near the yurt where I could care for his injury before they were put out in the great wilderness of Kapa'a once again. I was grateful to have them temporarily close by during the hard stretch of getting used to chemotherapy. They are a great source of power for me.
>
> Living with horses is pretty sweet. I'm so thankful for these gorgeous beasts that help keep my wahine feet tethered to the earth!

DIVING INTO THE DARKNESS:

It took me a few days after the first A/C chemotherapy infusion to return to my body again. What a strange, dreamlike trip it was. It was unlike anything I've done before!

In the past, through various mind-expanding substances (light hallucinogenic drugs), I learned how to wield the power of my mind and find clarity on whatever psychedelic journey I embarked upon. The dive into mainstream medicine and the turbulent physical and mental side-effects of chemotherapy took all my inner strength to stay centered. The medicine evoked dark energy such as fear, doubt, and anger. I had to be present with the process or it would consume me. A/C carried a heavier energy than any of the other substances I had tried before. It took all my power to stay on the razor's edge of clarity. Even though my body was being pummeled, I was losing my hair and rapidly losing weight, it was imperative for me to remember that my inner light was still vital and alive. This process brought up emotions that pushed me to another level of healing. It was necessary to face repressed shadows and be honest with myself about the level of self-care that was necessary to truly heal. This was a beautiful thing!

Usually, it's fairly easy for me to transcend the shadows and find my inner light, but this medicine was definitely challenging! Being a purist (in the past, I hardly ever took aspirin) the big guns of the cancer killing medicine sent me for a serious loop! One moment I was fine and the next I was emoting big tears of self-doubt, wondering if I could get through the heavy gauntlet. It makes sense that a substance used to kill cancer would have this extreme reaction.

I made it through the first round and was intact. My friends who had experienced a similar heroine's journey with chemo were a great help. They reassured me, telling me that everything I was feeling was normal. The love and support of my social media friends and community truly made a difference as well. The lessons that I was worthy of love kept coming through!

I don't know what I would have done without my partner, Syris. To be totally broken down and needing help with the simplest things (getting food, feeding the animals, driving to appointments) was utterly humbling. Words cannot express how grateful I was for his profound patience and holding my hand through the nightmares. I truly was blessed.

I had a week and a half to integrate till the next round of A/C. I knew I was soon to lose my curly long locks. I intended to enjoy every moment and every strand of hair I had before then!

My attitude was, *Take that, cancer! Life is meant to be lived and I intended to live it fully!*

***

Bolen writes in page 23 of her book, *Close to the Bone:*

> *This stripping away makes it possible for us to reach depths within ourselves that we otherwise might not reach, where whatever we consigned there or abandoned or forgot about ourselves, suffers the pain of not being remembered or of not being integrated into our conscious personality or allowed expression. In remembering, we find ourselves connecting with soul. What is actively sought in a depth analysis may be inadvertently revealed as a result of having a disabling physical illness or entering a hospital with a condition that will take a patient through a difficult and uncertain course, through making a descent into the underworld. Psychological depth is the realm of Ereshkigal, as is death. When death takes on a reality and becomes close, soul questions arise.*

This next post illustrated my attempt to see chemo as an alchemical mystery. It was a definite turning point of transforming my fear into faith. There were formidable soul questions stirred up within this medicine experience.

5/26:

Making peace in the belly of the beast: here I am this past week getting ready to drink the first infusion of chemo medicine, the nectar that shall heal me.

I'm realizing how it's all about a state of mind! I can make this reality whatever the heck I want. Chemotherapy was my worst fear (dragons and demons and all) for years, ever since my dear friend Deb died. I vowed I would never do it! I did countless interviews, podcasts, and articles sharing how chemo completely annihilates the immune system. Now I'm consenting to allow this toxic medicine in my body? What peculiar change of mind occurred to welcome in the medicine I abhorred?

It's called life, folks! You see, I have this amazing son who is twenty-six. He's accomplishing brilliant deeds in the world. I want to see his life unfold more than anything! When push comes to shove, my belief in life far exceeds any attachment to fear about chemo. I know I can get through this hurdle!

This past week, doing the first round of A/C was extremely challenging. I found myself dancing with the mind worms of the toxic medicine.

Darkness be gone! I'm calling in all my angels to make it through this five-month gauntlet.

There's something highly alchemical about drinking in this heavy medicine to call in the light. I'm starting to think of chemotherapy like a homeopathic treatment. The definition of homeopathy is: "A system of medical practice that treats a disease especially by the administration of minute doses of a remedy that would in larger amounts produce in healthy persons symptoms similar to those of the disease."[12]

Is it possible to ingest the medicine that I feared would kill me and, instead, ask it to transform me? How absolutely awesome would that be?

It's like one of those reoccurring nightmares where a scary big purple monster is chasing you. One evening, you eventually build up your courage, stop running, and ask the putrid creature what it wants? Lo and behold, you discover the monster just wants to give you a hug!

Could chemo be equivalent to a prickly purple monster for me? I think there's a potent transformational force here if I'm courageous enough to face my shadows.

Facing my fears.

Transforming the darkness into light.

I'm calling on my highest power for this healing dance.

Watch me fly, like the Phoenix from the flames!

I shall not shrink from the fear that calls me to witness my greatest truth. Each of us is a powerful magician of the soul!

***

Despite the challenges, there was still so much beauty to behold. I would occasionally wake up in tremendous discomfort from the pain in my spine and the side effects of chemo and cancer. I would hear the soft pounding of rain on the yurt roof and realize I had a choice what to focus on. I could pay attention to either the gentle tapping of rain or the pain. If I tried to ignore the physical sensation, it would persist and most likely become more irritating until it was completely consuming. My goal was to say hello to the pain, feel it, acknowledge and welcome it in, then kindly let it go.

No thank you, pain; I would rather hear the tapping of the rain now!

Linda Kohanov, whom I was fortunate to train with at Eponaquest, teaches how to use emotions as information:

Horses use emotion as information to engage surprisingly agile responses to environmental stimuli and relationship challenges.

1. Feel the emotion in its purest from.

2. Get the message behind the emotion.

3. Change something in response to that message.

4. Go back to grazing. Let go of the emotion and return to living in the present moment.

The horses were valuable teachers, and I chose to listen.

EUGENE:

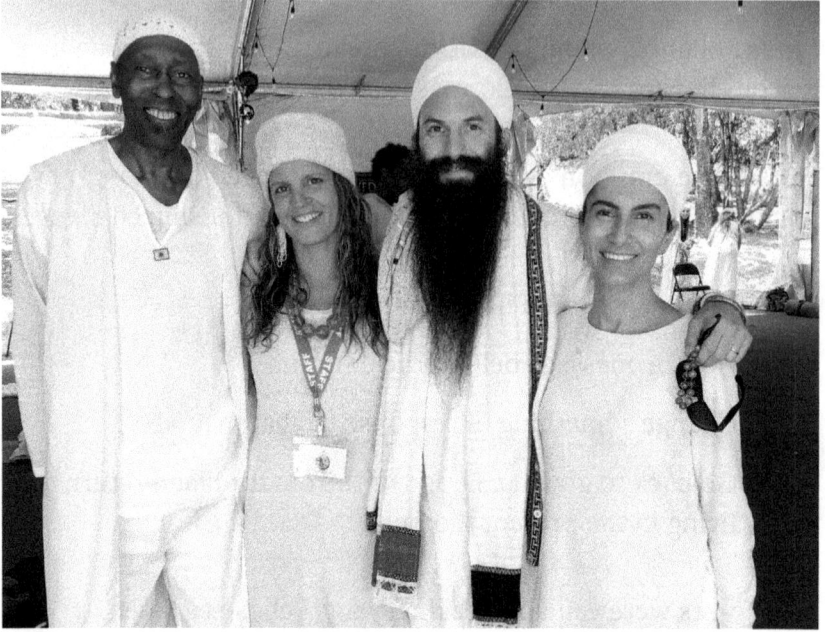

Eugene Turner, me, Jai Dev Singh, Simrit Kaur

When the demons of chemotherapy started playing havoc with my mind, my beloved friend, Eugene stepped in to be a big brother ally for the hardest part of my journey.

Eugene is also a cancer thriver who has defied the odds and is a miracle case. He was diagnosed with a rare blood cancer, Waldenstrom Macroglobulinemia, twenty-five years ago. For five years, his life was hanging by a thread as he received acute medical treatment and was in and out of the hospital. He came close to dying several times. His life was precariously held in the balance till he made a conscious choice: he wanted to be here. Through his tenacity of spirit and his mission to share his light and wisdom upon Earth, he decided to stick around.

I met Eugene through Jai Dev, my kundalini yoga teacher. Eugene would regularly come to the summer immersion programs that

Jai Dev and Simrit would offer. At one of the events, I raised my hand to ask Jai Dev for guidance in front of 150 people as my cherished friend Rowen was close to dying at that time. With a shaky voice and trembling hand, I asked a question about death as my heart was hurting to be alienated by Rowen during her decline. Jai Dev suggested in front of the group that I talk to Eugene at some point during the immersion.

Dressed in our white Kundalini yoga clothing, Eugene and I sat at a table, sharing a meal and surrounded by a few new friends. Eugene kindly shared his story with me of journeying with cancer. Immediately, I realized we had very similar paths and understood why Jai Dev wanted us to meet. We both had an affinity with death. We both were walking with cancer. We both spent time with others when they crossed over to the death realm through working/volunteering at hospice. We immediately bonded.

This man is very familiar with dancing with lady death. He has spent the last fifteen years being present with hospice patients and midwifing them through the death process.

When we met, I had stage 3 breast cancer, had volunteered recently at hospice, and was trained as a death midwife/doula. I had already seen my fair share of death too after the death of my best friend and the approaching death of another dear friend.

As the years went on, we got to know each other a bit more although I was constantly busy with my ranch work. When my health started rapidly declining, Eugene's presence in my life became more prominent. When I thought I might be dying, he coached me about what I might expect when my soul would leave my body. I was reluctant to hear his words of wisdom, as my tenacious spirit refused to believe I would die!

When I was in the hell of chemotherapy, Eugene was my guiding light. With his wise, angelic grace, he was the one I would reach out to when the dark shadows of the medicine threatened to take over my soul. I would send him a text and he would remind me that the light was stronger than the darkness. He knew the depths of darkness and shadows I was dancing through and reminded me that the moment would pass.

This is an experience that someone can only understand if they've walked through the gates of death and decided to return to this earthly plane. When one has held hands with the dying and shared their last breath, a vast knowledge is given in exchange. Eugene holds this wisdom, and I'm so honored to be in his close circle of friends.

If it hadn't been for Eugene constantly reminding me that my soul had a divine purpose upon Earth, I wouldn't be writing my story right now.

LETTING GO:

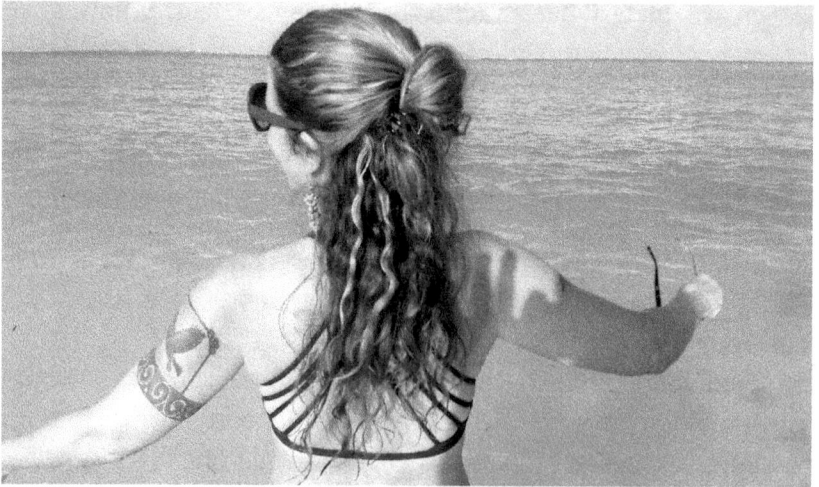

On this metaphorical journey with Inanna, I was asked to sacrifice my precious, curly hair that I loved so much. Twice in my twenties, I had cut my extremely long hair into a pixie cut. Letting go of my hair this time around was more difficult, as it wasn't my choice to cut my hair. I had to ask myself, "Would I rather die to keep my lovely hair or lose it and be given a chance to live?" When I thought of my son, Willow, that choice was crystal clear. I wanted to be here for him.

This was a journey of releasing ego attachment. Inanna was journeying farther into the underworld with every ritual of release. Little by little, I was being stripped till all that would remain would be the essence of my soul. I hoped to still be physically in my body then!

Bolen writes on page 24 of *Close to the Bone* about chemotherapy treatment:

> *Chemotherapy and radiation patients make an Inanna descent. Each treatment is another gate. After the second or third chemotherapy treatment, hair often falls out in clumps. On the descent at this gate, you surrender your head of hair, and even if you were expecting it, this is a shock. For a woman especially, it is a loss that strikes at identity and femininity. It is often a low point, a depressing time. The face in the mirror is unfamiliar. "Who is this?"*

SISTERS OF THE SHAVED HEAD:

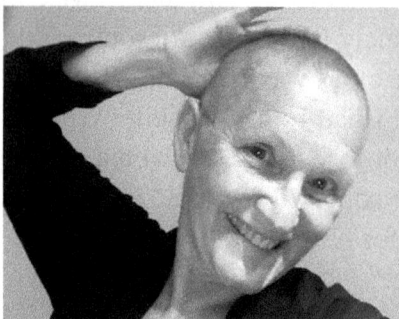

Photo by David Steinberg   Photo by Bradyhouse Photographers

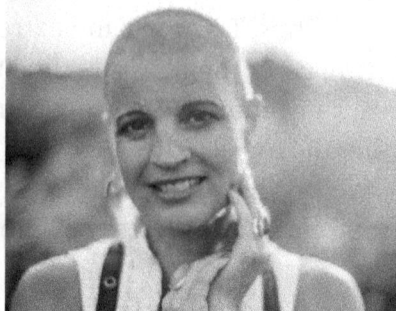

Kim Mears & me

It was finally time to say farewell to my hair, which was now in a bob form. Many cherished friends stepped up to help me magnanimously. My benevolent friend Kim Mears from Santa Cruz, California turned out to be a solid ally who walked through fire for me. I had met Kim when she had attended one of my horse workshops at WHS two years before. This particular act of kindness truly meant a world of difference for me.

Kim chose to shave her head with me, as she knew it was challenging for me to let go of my hair. Words cannot express how much this meant to me. The fact that she would bravely let go of her hair with me gave me tremendous courage to do it myself. My hair was falling out from the chemo and I had no choice, but she did!

Sometimes, this cancer journey can feel very lonely. With Kim doing this brave act, I felt like I had a buddy by my side who was courageous enough to walk in the shadows with me.

On a Zoom call 2,500 miles apart from California to Hawaii, our heads were shaved in tandem. On the rickety, faded green deck of the yurt, my son Willow shaved my head. With Jasmine, Syris, and my mother physically in attendance, I watched as my hair fell out in dark brown globs onto the deck.

My scalp felt super sensitive to the touch right after my hair was shaved off, so I kept my head wrapped in a scarf for a few days, as the sensation was so peculiar. It felt like I had a vulnerable, newborn baby head!

DEEP IN THE CAVE:

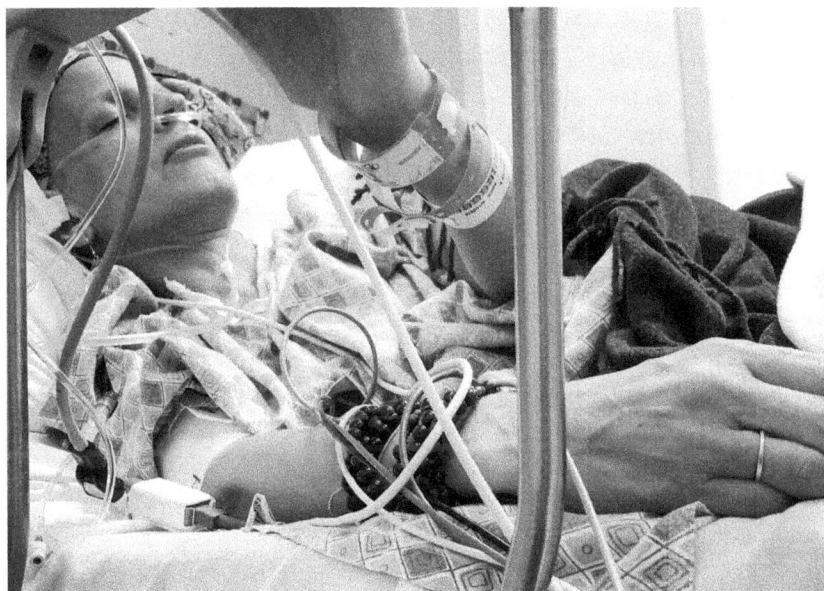

Days after shaving my head I was plunged into the depths of mental and physical shadows. This coincided with running out of painkillers and the intense chemo making its way through my body. Perhaps letting go of my hair provoked a huge emotional release for me.

My inner guidance said, *Keep going through the pain, discomfort, trials, and tribulations; there's a greater purpose to the suffering! I promise you this.*

The shadows kept growing till I ended up in the hospital. This was an extremely low point of my healing journey.

Bolen writes in *Close to the Bone* on page 29:

> *There are many good reasons for an immediate admission to the hospital, such as traumatic injuries from accidents or violence, severe burns, a likely myocardial infarct, hemorrhaging, being unconscious, having a raging fever – any state in which immediate care could make the difference between life and death. At Los Angeles General County Hospital, where I interned, anyone who arrived in a critical condition was called a "red blanket." The patient was immediately put on a gurney, a red blanket (in actuality, a bright red sheet) was thrown over him, and an attendant wheeled the gurney on a nonstop elevator to an admitting ward. When a red blanket arrived on the floor, that patient was seen immediately.*

> *This is a critical moment. The decision to be immediately admitted to the hospital may be the right one, and you may be relieved that this is happening, because you have had a feeling that something quite serious was not being attended to, and now it is. You may intuitively trust the doctor and the decision. Or, as is sometimes the case, there may be an inner resistance, an intuition or feeling that you need more information, or need to sort out the situation, or need to take care of other matters before you can go in. For the soul, and quite possibly for the body, it matters whether you are ready or not. For you are not just being admitted to the hospital, you are on a soul journey that will take you into the underworld.*

I was in a critical position health wise. One of the side effects of A/C is called thrush or mucositis which is very similar to canker sores:

My tongue hurt so much, I couldn't talk, eat, or drink due to the sores on it. I had a severe case of mucositis and hadn't been able to eat for days. The sores were in my throat, mouth, tongue and on my lips. Due to the lack of food and extreme immune reaction response, I was getting increasingly weak and had a burning fever.

I had been warned that the mouth sores were a possible side effect of the chemo. Due to my immune system being severely compromised, it was hard for my body to fight off simple things like mouth bacteria.

My entire family had been visiting for the last month. Willow was leaving that day after a lovely three-week visit. As I was in such a broken-down state, he called Wilcox Hospital to talk to the on-call physician to ask for advice. It was decided I would go to the emergency room for serious chemo complications. In retrospect, it must have been very scary for my son to say goodbye to me, knowing I was soon to be admitted to the hospital!

When it was time to go to the hospital, I was so weak that Syris had to carry me to the car!

As soon as I arrived at the hospital I was hooked up to endless wires, antibiotics, hydration fluids, and painkillers. As I hadn't been able to eat or drink for days, I was severely malnourished and dehydrated and resembled a limp noodle.

When I arrived, I found out my white blood cell count was dangerously low, so I received a blood infusion. I was grateful to get a bit more energy from it. It's common while going through chemotherapy for either the red or white blood cell counts and/ or platelet levels to go down. While the medicine eradicates the cancer, it also is rough on the immune system.

I kept the faith that my Wilcox hospital detour was an important part of the path. I was grateful to receive excellent care with every doctor and loving nurse I encountered. This made the process much easier and allowed my body to heal faster. The aloha spirit was alive and well in Kaua'i!

My body felt like it had been hit by a train from the last chemo round. I was frustrated and exhausted by the relentless effort it took to keep going in the face of such physical adversity, lack of sleep (Syris and I only slept three hours one night due to the nurses constantly coming in), explosive nosebleeds, barfing, etc. It was rough!

One night in the hospital, I was determined to get more sleep so my body could heal. I ended up asking for a bigger dose of painkillers to knock me out, and it worked! I started feeling a bit better after that due to the hydration and blood infusions I received. I slowly recovered and was able to eat small amounts of very bland food. After not being able to eat or drink for three days, even hospital food was delicious!

After five days in the hospital, I realized it was the closest I had ever been to death besides the time I almost drowned in Maui in my twenties. I was a pretty strong wahine, but this experience had pushed me far past the edge of my comfort zone!

Surviving the hospital adventure was a major milestone. I had lost a fair amount of weight, my muscles had atrophied from lying in bed for five days, and it was hard to walk after leaving the hospital. I was determined to keep going through hell or high water. I figured if I had faced my death and made it through, I could get through anything. My goal was to not just survive but to thrive!

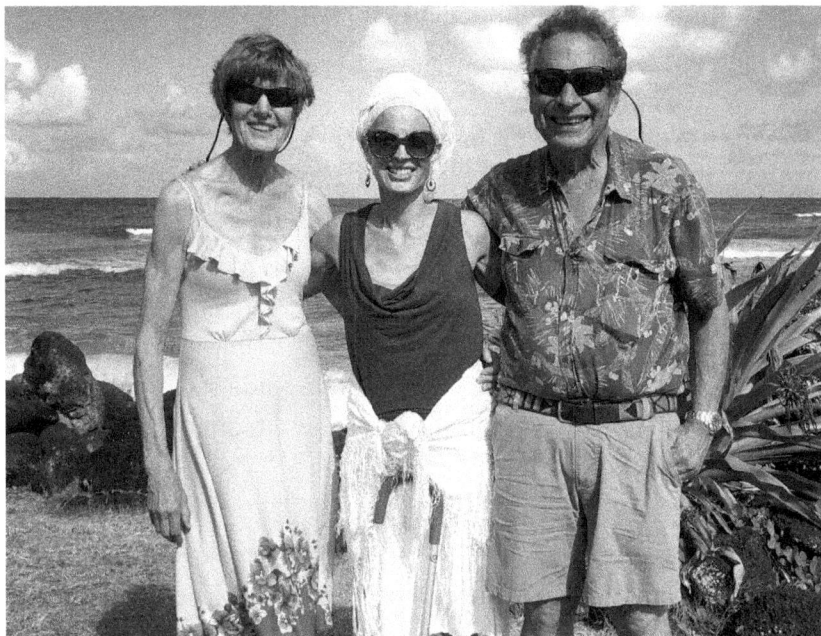

My mother, me, Frida & my father

6/16:

I was deliriously happy to be out of the hospital! After five days in a tiny room with hardly any sunshine, I was going a bit batty. After I returned home, I appreciated smelling the air, seeing the birds, the verdant, green jungle of Kaua'i, listening to music, being home, sleeping in my bed, and of course, seeing my precious animals I missed so much.

I was slowly coming to appreciate the wonders of modern medicine in a new way. If it hadn't been for the care I had received at Wilcox, I would have died.

Anyone who has spent time in the hospital knows that it's not the easiest place to rest with nurses and doctors coming in constantly to monitor you, take your temperature or get a blood sample. I was grateful to not be poked by a kind nurse taking my blood at 5:30 am.

The gift of the hospital visit was to remember the incredible beauty that surrounded me daily. I recognized clearly that it was a gift to be alive and I vowed to never forget this truth.

I was aware that my life was dangling on a thin thread. I had just barely escaped death. As I hobbled about with Frida the cane, lady death walked so close to my side that I felt her warm breath on my skinny arms. I knew I might not make it to my next birthday.

This close brush with death caused me to make a choice. I decided that no matter what the future held, I would enjoy every moment of my life to the best of my ability. I realized that even though my body was broken down by cancer, I was incredibly fortunate to be alive. There was always something to be grateful for even in the darkest moments!

HEALING IS A CHOICE:

I was starting to realize how healing is a choice. I saw that my perspective could color the fabric of every experience I had if I chose to let it.

I asked myself, "Did I truly want to live?"

Bolen write in *Close to the Bone* on page 63:

Siegal described three types of patients. He characterized about 15 or 20 percent as unconsciously or consciously wishing to die. These were people who on some level welcomed cancer or another serious illness as a way out of their problems. As the doctor is struggling to get them well, they are resisting and trying to die. If you ask them how they are or what is troubling them, they say, "Fine" and "Nothing."

6/17:

My feet are dangling perilously over the canyon of death. I'm fully aware that I possess the choice in this moment to live or die.

With such a severe diagnosis, it's primarily my sheer willpower that's dictating if my feet stay upon Earth or not.

I have witnessed others with a physically widespread cancer diagnosis like me give up. Sadly, they usually are dead within the year. The chemo I'm being given is termed "palliative care." This basically means I'm doomed to die. I was told the medicine is extending my life by hopefully two to five years.

I directly asked my oncologist and radiologist how much time I had left if I chose not to do chemotherapy. Their answer was around six months.

Usually, I would doubt a prediction like this, but due to the side effects of the cancer rapidly breaking down my body, I knew they were right, and the cancer was killing me. That's why I chose to do the thing I said I would never do: chemotherapy. This was a choice of seeing my death and actively CHOOSING to LIVE!

Chemo is kicking my ass! This near-death experience in the hospital this week and the last month has pushed me mentally and physically beyond anything I've ever experienced before. There have been times I've wondered why the hell I consented to this torture, but then I remember that this is the potent medicine I need now to save my life. The potion is in the poison. Chemo is dramatically healing my lungs. My left hip is less painful. I'm visualizing the chemo dissolving the tumors in the same powerful way it created the mouth, throat, and lips this past week in the hospital. I know it's working on all levels, and I have great faith in that!

I'm aware that my stubborn, strong demeanor is keeping me going. It would be so easy to give up. I often feel like absolute shit and curse this path. Then I move on and strive to continually find the beauty.

When I'm having a difficult time, I have faith that there's sunshine around the corner. It's true that it's always darkest before the dawn.

The exultant relief I felt after leaving the hospital is proof that the sun will always come out. I'm grabbing onto this nugget of truth to pull me through the challenges.

I choose to dig my heels into the ground. Even though it sometimes physically hurts to walk, I will keep going! There's no other choice. I will continue to choose LOVE over FEAR!

I started visualizing life beyond my confined health journey. Beyond the veil, lay a dazzling view of life that I was deeply grateful to be a part of! To think that the week before I was in the hospital close to death brought appreciation for the simplest things. Even going to the ding dang DMV was its own special version of joy. I was still alive after all!

ZAHRAH:

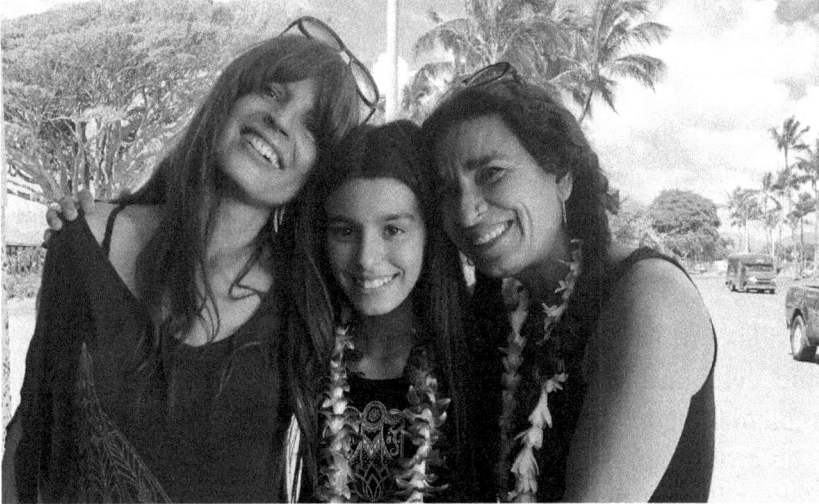

Me with my Zahrah wig, Zenobia & Michelle

Now that I had a baby bald head, I gave myself full permission to have fun with the process. I started playing with different identities with wigs.

When I was in my late twenties, I did a lot of performance art mixing dance, visual art, and poetry together. I had a fantasy about shaving my head, wearing different wigs, and taking on different personas to see how believable it was. It was time to play with that unfulfilled fantasy. Life is art!

My first and favorite character was Zahrah. This wig had long dark red hair and straight cut bangs. Zahrah was named after an actual real-life friend of mine who's hair looked remarkably the same as the wig.

Zahrah's character was spunky, tons of fun, vibrant, and the life of the party. I was told I looked like a rock star. I got a kick seeing how unsuspecting strangers responded to my Zahrah persona! When I noticed a man at the grocery story stealing a sideways glance at me, it made me laugh. If he only knew the reality of what lay under the wig!

My darling friend Michelle and her daughter Zenobia came out to Kaua'i to help me through the rigors of chemotherapy. Michelle had already visited months earlier and was well aware of the gauntlet I was in. Michelle gave me the gift of being authentically real.

Besides fun wigs, dressing up, going dancing, Michelle's arrival, and celebrating being out of the hospital, I was focused on replenishing my body to get ready for the next round of chemo. The mouth sores and the hospital stay had slammed party girl Zahrah like a freight train!

My mission was to eat! I hit an all-time low weight of 110, which was a twenty-two-pound drop from my usual weight. I was pounding the vitamins and trying to gain the flexibility back I lost in the hospital. Michelle did a great job of feeding me carbohydrate-rich pasta smothered with olive oil and butter to get my weight back on me. Mangia Italiana!

I loved having a joyous week-long break from the crazy roller coaster effects of chemo. Experiencing a temporary vacation in the hospital certainly put it all into perspective. It was a detour I would prefer not to do in the future!

SACRIFICE & SURRENDER:

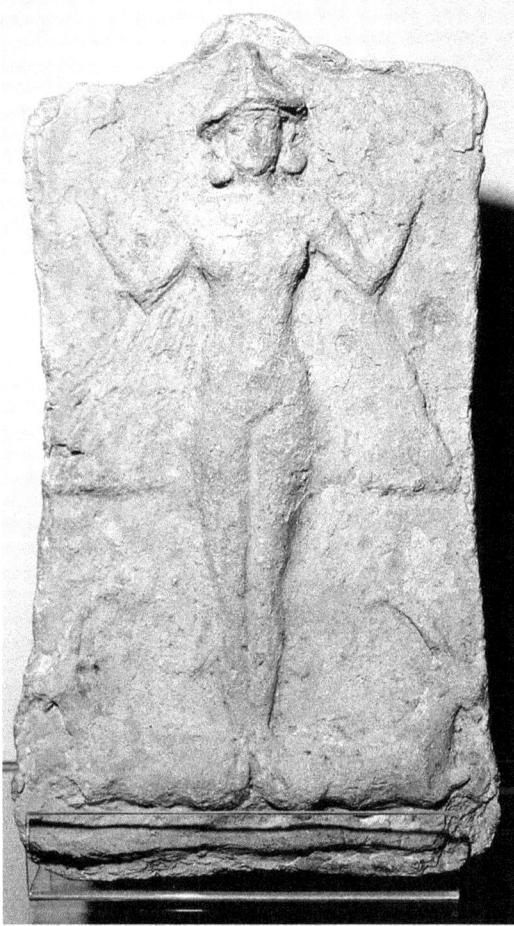

Terracotta relief of the Goddess Inanna standing on two animals

It was time to dive deeper into the cave of Inanna as the time for the third round of A/C was approaching.

Bolen writes in *Close to the Bone* on page 47:

> *When Inanna went down through the seven gates into the Great Below, the proud and powerful goddess entered naked and bowed low, looked into the baleful eyes of death, and*

was struck down. Her body was hung on a hook to rot. She became a slab of green meat. This is a picture of how it feels to be reduced and humbled, powerless and without illusions, to be vulnerable and rejected, to feel putrid. There are phrases of being ill in which people feel like Inanna on the hook, when the infected, dysfunctional, or malignant cellular level of their being permeates the soul, and they feel as if they were dead and rotting. This is what suffering can feel like as well to those who make a psychological descent to uncover sources of chronic depression and anxiety in the depth work I do as a Jungian analyst.

I was nervous. The last round of chemo almost killed me. I figured it was normal to feel trepidation after such a harrowing experience.

I allowed myself to break down. A wall of exhaustion, depression, and fear hit me as my mind prepared for yet another dance with the healing nectar. I was letting go of all the things precious to me on the quest for life!

My long golden locks were gone. In my body's sacrifice to annihilate the cancer, another loss was my voluptuous curves. I watched my body become skinnier and observed my muscles slowly lose their tone. My butt practically disappeared! My friend Bethany playfully called this stick-figure look "the model runway look." I decided to playfully embrace this idea, even though seeing myself the skinniest I had been my entire life was frightening!

I was balancing precariously on the razor's edge.

I was literally putting poison (AKA healing nectar) into my body so I might live. I had faith and trust that this was the right choice, but mamma mia, there were some heavy sacrifices that were being made! I was like Inanna traveling to the underworld, having to give up all her worldly possessions and sacred attributes in order to become truly free.

The gift was life, and I yearned to gobble it up with all the power within me! Yet, I had to accept that I was walking with a cane. I was skin and bones. I was bald. Where did this leave me?

Societies' viewpoint of what a cancer patient looked like is due to the gross side effects of chemo. After so many years of people exclaiming that I looked too healthy to have cancer, I finally looked like a "cancer patient."

I wrote:

> Closer to source?
> In the center of the spiral?
> Stripped of all my earthly attachments?
> Am I ultimately free?
>
> Death looks on from her pearly place and laughs as I do.
> I know I'm beyond description, form, or definition of self.
>
> This is all just a surrealistic dance; therefore, there's nothing
> to fear.

***

After I allowed myself to feel and release the terror of doing another round of chemo, I was back to my fearless self again.

LOOK LIKE A QUEEN:

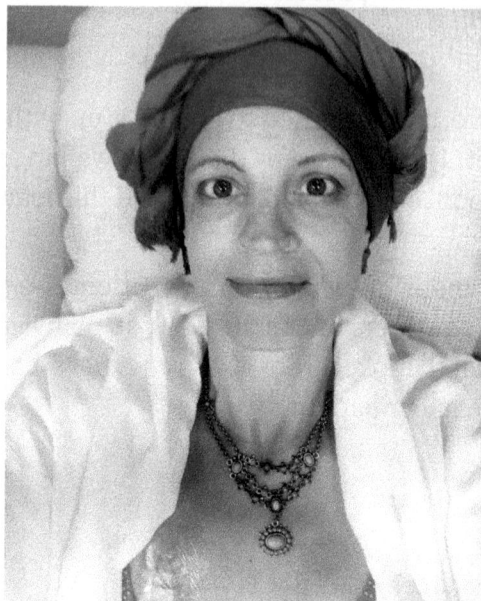

My goal was to look like a queen when I went to the infusion center. I figured if I looked like a goddess during treatment, I would enjoy the process and the medicine would be easier to physically integrate within my body.

On my first day back post hospital visit, I wore my favorite color: a vibrant teal/turquoise hue. This color reminded me of the immense power I possessed to transcend whatever obstacle came my way. It helped me shine even in the darkest hour.

I realized that if I could survive horrendous mouth sores and escape death, I could bravely face another round of treatment. Looking like a queen and wearing flagrant clothes with colors that I loved helped to lift my spirit.

During treatment, a delightful Tutu was in the chair beside me. With her lauhala hat perched upon her dark, curly hair and her brown wrinkled skin, I could tell she was deeply loved by her daughter who lovingly cared for her. It warmed my heart as I watched her daughter, with a sing-song voice, care for her elderly mother who was clearly hard of hearing.

Tutu and I were connected by experience. She was a reflection of my ancient aunties and relatives I dearly loved as a child on Kaua'i. A reminder of my treasured island home was everywhere I looked.

The sacred is everywhere, even in the oncology ward in the hospital. You just have to open your eyes to see the magic!

As I mentally prepped myself for another tumble down the rabbit hole of my third A/C treatment, I prayed for more ease this time around. My goal was to find grace in the storm that threatened to capsize the fragile boat of my soul.

Despite the turbulence in my treatment, my love for the horses was a constant source of strength. Since I rekindled my passion for the equine world nine years before, their mere presence had carried me through turbulent times.

And as I faced my darkest demons, I returned to the heart of horse wisdom to guide me through the shadows.

I was close to the last (fourth) round of A/C. The plan after that was to transition to doing Taxol (a lighter and easier form of chemotherapy) once a week for three months. Being a natural medicine girl, it was comforting to know that Taxol was derived from the yew tree.

NEVER GIVE UP:

On 7/9 I had exciting news to share:

> I'm KICKING this cancer, friends! Yes, my dearies, I got stellar test results back today! I just saw my sweet Russian oncologist, and my breast tumor markers (CA 27-29 test) have dropped by half! In May, it was over 900; now it's around 400. My liver markers have dropped too. We both are very happy with the results! My lungs are clearing up and my hip pain is better too! Half the time I'm forgetting to take Frida the cane with me. My weight seems to have stabilized at 110 pounds and I haven't lost more weight in two weeks, which is great! This is fabulous news all the way around!!
>
> Who would have thought with my fierce resistance to chemo, that it would actually be helping me so much?! It took having my spark of life almost snuffed out from cancer to make me examine and question my stubborn belief system! It's about time, girl. Mahalo modern medicine for this extension of my life!

****

Even though I was elated by the positive news, it still was hard work. I was pushed to the edge, but I was determined to keep going!

I wrote on 7/11 after receiving my last A/C infusion:

> Today I'm broken down to bare bones. I must surrender to the epic wave that rages through my body. I'm surfing and

surrendering. I'm grateful to the spirit medicine (chemo) as it's helping me to reclaim my body again.

I'm thankful for the ability to let go and allow others to help me. How ironic that I usually am the one in the caregiver role, but now, in order to make it through the gauntlet of healing, there's no choice but to learn to receive help.

This is like a shamanic journey. To find the most valuable pearl, it's necessary to courageously dive through the depths of darkness. While descending, you see strange globular creatures with sharp pointed teeth shining brightly in your direction. As you hold your breath, trusting your lungs won't burst from the pressure of the water, you bravely search the ocean floor for the cherished pearl. You spot the shiny gem hiding within a clam's shell! Treasure in hand, lungs yearning for oxygen, you rise to the surface where air meets water and gracefully rejoin the world.

The message here is before you can find your own gem of knowledge, it's necessary to face your shadows first. The pearl represents your inner wisdom and tenacity to face any challenge you might encounter.

This is also the story of Inanna. This ancient goddess had to let go of all creature comforts and face her shadow to ultimately be reborn again. This is the hero/heroine's story that has been enacted for thousands of years through multiple cultures. It's a timeless tale, eloquently described by Joseph Campbell in *The Hero with a Thousand Faces*.

It is a reoccurring theme on the hero's journey that the main character has to lose something sacred in order to claim their life. For example, Luke Skywalker in Star Wars loses his arm, the Lion King loses his father and home, and Harry Potter loses his life. One of my favorite movies is the Star Wars movie: 'The Rise of Skywalker'. The bold heroine, Rey sacrificed her connection to her royal blood family (the 'Palpatines') who were the dark forces of the universe to take on her new role of being a 'Skywalker'. In embracing the light, she also sacrificed her twin soul 'Kylo Ren' AKA 'Ben' when Ben gave up his life to save Rey. This altruistic, valiant act ultimately helped to bring balance to the universe and defeated the dark forces.

Another similar example of this is the mythological story of the 'Twin Horses'. I first learned about this from my teacher Linda Kohanov in the Eponaquest training. You can see this story throughout various cultures around the globe. Usually when twin horses are born, one dies. This is a great metaphorical symbol that can be applied to the story of Rey and Ben. I also strongly related to this symbolic story after Deb's death. It was through Deb's death I realized the preciousness of life. It was through the tragedy of her illness and death that I came to life.

The thread through all these stories is that the loss is necessary for the heroes/heroines to find themselves again. Patients on a cancer journey lose their hair, vitality, weight, relationships, jobs and more. Some die and come back like Anita Moorjani in her book *Dying to Be Me*. Perhaps resisting these losses and not accepting the brilliant pearls of wisdom the path offers may be why some people don't survive their cancer journey?

My wise friend Eugene shared this nugget of truth that echoes the symbology of Rey in Star Wars:

> *Yes, you must face your shadows, your fears. But you know what? When you find your strength and when your light of confidence grows brighter within you, the shadows disappear. The demons shrink away from the light that*

you illuminate. You become the candle in the night. Your spiritual presence WILL be felt. It will protect you, as do I.

***

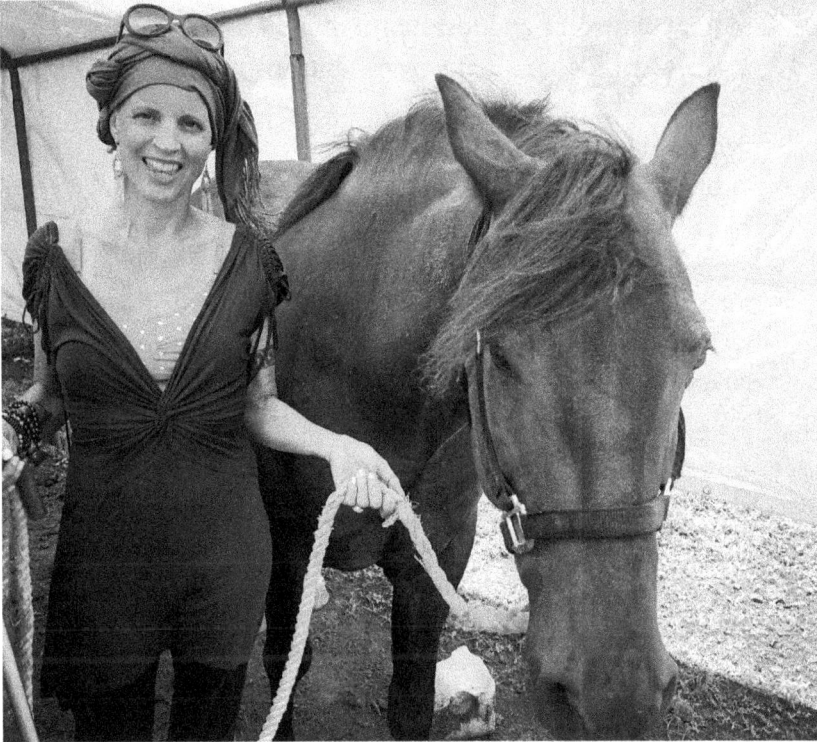

It was apparent to me that the horses, Xaria, and Kismet the cat were holding a huge amount of space for me and my healing. I could actively feel them balancing my energy as I went through the harrowing depths of treatment. They were silent sentinels of the soul, helping me by just being present.

I wrote:

> I have such love for these vibrant horse spirits that give endlessly of their gigantic, loving hearts. Their presence is

an immense gift. They truly emanate a depth of peaceful awareness through the channel of love and wisdom.

There certainly are no mistakes about how circumstances have unfolded. As the horses helped me through the tragedy of divorce and lost motherhood years ago, they're now present for me during my healing crisis.
Facing death,
Claiming life,
Through the dark crevasses and shadows of the soul,
I'm calling on the light that sustains me.

Horses, spirit guides, and treasured friends by my side,
I will feed the flame that illuminates my way through the darkest moments.

LIFE AS A TECHNICOLOR DREAM:

The twists and turns kept coming. The diamond of my soul was definitely being polished!

My beloved mother was in the hospital. We didn't know what was wrong with her. I was praying that it wasn't anything too terrible. It was bizarre that I was recently in and out of the hospital, and a month later, my mother was going through a similar experience.

At this point, I knew way too much about all thing's related to cancer. I was trying my best to keep my mind quiet and trust that everything would be okay. In a bizarre twist of fate, she also was getting her right lung drained and having heart issues. I had seen how in my body, the heart speeded up due to the lungs being overworked. This was completely bizarre to me, as it was exactly what I'd gone through in the last months.

I had observed both humans and animals taking on the same symptoms and maladies as their beloved family members and human owners. I manifested a serious cancer diagnosis one year after my friend Deb died from leukemia. I witnessed my animals, countless times, manifest the same physical issues I was going through. Due to this knowledge, I asked my mother to please not take on my physical symptoms. They were mine and mine alone. I wanted her to stay healthy.

I was also requesting a change in my relationship with Syris. I asked him to move out of the yurt, but with the goal for us to still stay together. It was time to create a bit more space between us. I was called to foster a deeper sense of clarity within my soul. I realized that if I only had a year to live, it was necessary to live each moment with embodied intention! I hoped that the transition would unfold in a way that would serve us both. It wasn't a breakup but a need for breathing room. Overall, I viewed it as a healthy shift.

Bolen writes in *Close to the Bone* on page 58:

> *Sometimes I wonder if a life-threatening illness or condition is a last-ditch opportunity to pay attention to soul needs for authentic expression, for creativity, for intimacy, for solitude, for retreat inward, for something significant to happen. Perhaps when all else has failed to call attention to pain at the soul level, disease not only may result but may become the means through which we go inward to find buried feelings and cut-off or dismembered aspects of ourselves.*

Bolen captured it perfectly here. I was understanding that there were parts of myself that were yearning for expression. When I felt my mind and body being pulled to pieces within the chemo gauntlet, it presented a mirror into everything in my life that wasn't congruent.

I was realizing that I deserved to shine, no matter what. Regardless of what car I drove, clothes I wore, relationship I was or wasn't in, what job I had, or how I looked, I was worthy just as I was. Chemo helped me find the gem of self-love. I was worthless to anyone else if I didn't take time to love myself. I was inherently deserving of happiness and I aimed to find it!

***

It was a huge turning point for me when I finished the heavy doses of A/C. It took all my strength to get through this time, but I had made it! I felt like a heroine on a journey who, after defeating great odds, realizes she might possibly *survive* the horrible death-defying escapade she's been on. I was starting to see the light peeking through the clouds.

While I was finding a newfound sense of levity for myself, the heaviness of what was happening with my mom started creeping in. It took all my effort to keep my mind calm. This was definitely the greatest Jedi training of my life!

My mom had been in and out of the hospital getting tested to try and diagnose what was out of balance with her body. It was hard to be 2,500 miles away and not be present to help.

All I could do was to keep the faith that all would be okay. I showed up the best I could from a distance.

TAXOL TIME:

It was time to start the next chemotherapy drug, Taxol. I was scheduled to do three months of weekly treatments. As the treatment schedule was so intense, I chose to find joy when I could. I found it was important to celebrate the milestones, as you never knew when the next rough wave would hit. My blissful choice for this particular day was gluten free pizza!

7/31:

My joyful moment today was eating gluten free pizza! I've been craving pizza for days! Due to treatment, my stomach is often supersensitive, which means I can only eat the blandest foods. Today was the day to celebrate all that I've come through in the past two and a half months of intense A/C chemo treatment!

We thoroughly enjoyed our pizzas! My body is so happy to have experienced a hedonistic moment of pure food enjoyment. The best thing after that is I have leftovers!!

Due to my weight loss (AKA runway model look), I'm now trying to eat as much as I can to maintain my weight and try to put on pounds. It's liberating to eat more calories instead of curbing my enjoyment of food. Is this an excuse to eat more Italian food? Sure, why not? As they say in Italy: Mangia tutto! (This is loosely translated as "Eat a lot!")

THE BEAUTY TRAP:

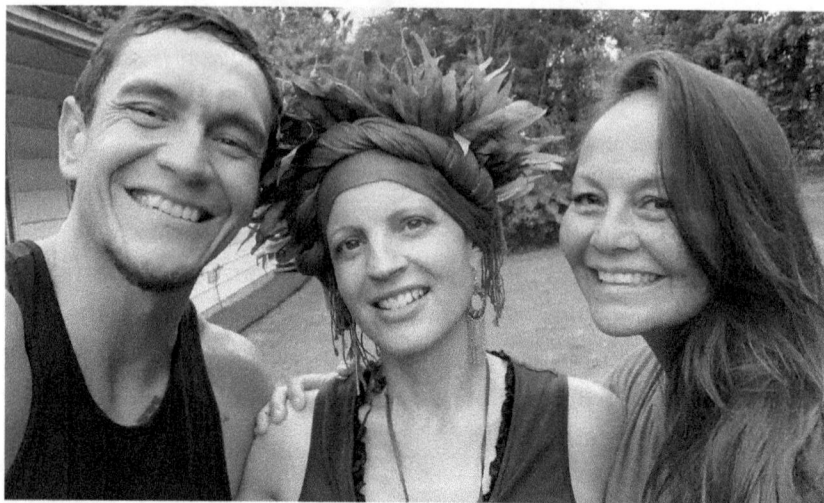

Ke'oni Hanalei, me & Marni Sue Reynolds

Although I would not have consciously chosen this cancer path, I'm deeply grateful for the lessons I've learned. This path has been a rapid evolution of growth. When I think back to before Deb was diagnosed, I see myself as an innocent woman who had no idea how precious life was.

When Inanna bravely travels to the depths, shedding her regalia for the sake of her important mission to be reborn, she learns what's real and worthy of her time.

For many women, losing the identities we worked so hard to create, whether it be our career, what we've physically manifested in our lifetime, or the way we physically look, can be extremely challenged during rigorous cancer treatment. Quite often, long, flowing tresses are sacrificed to the chemotherapy chemicals. A fit body can easily be whittled down to skin and bones due the toxic side effects. Other side effects emerge such as body sores and unpleasant maladies. Often, while undergoing chemotherapy, it's necessary to step outside of your predictable life and take a break for healing.

When I did chemo, I went from being 125 pounds (which was already on the light side for me) to 110 pounds. My ultra-skinny, super model body was shocking to behold as my usual curves and big bum were reduced to mere bumps. Friends reassured me that I would regain my curves again and possibly even miss my light-as-a-feather body.

The gift of losing the physical form your ego clings to is a great opportunity to redefine yourself by how you truly are separate from your physical identity! It's a hard lesson but one that's important to examine. After all, aging is inevitable when you dwell in a body. Even the most gorgeous super model is eventually going to have wrinkles and saggy skin somewhere on her body, even with the most technological surgical and medical devices. You can't run away from time. Cancer treatment tends to speed up the aging process, but the benefit is your life quite often is extended beyond your prognosis. This was my case at least!

In our Western society, women are taught to value themselves by how others, particularly men, see them. Seeing beyond the illusion of defining ourselves beyond what we physically look like is a valuable lesson of self-love. We're so much more than what our physical appearance is. As I dove deeper into the healing process during the hard months of chemotherapy, I realized that true healing comes from self-love.

In the spring of 2019, I was fortunate to meet a Native Hawaiian man who works with traditional fern medicines. Ke'oni Hanalei was born from a long line of Hawaiian healers on the island of Maui and has a fascinating history of being of Scottish & Native Hawaiian descent. His Scottish ancestors dated back to 1831 after arriving on the ship New Englander on Maui. I had no idea before meeting him that there were Scottish people on the islands!

Ke'oni has a business called "Pohala Botanicals" and makes rare fern botanical medicines. He has a prominent following on Instagram, and one of my other cancer thriver friends told me about him. When I heard his story, I was stunned!

At the age of twenty-eight, he was diagnosed with Stage 4 Embryonal Carcinoma. This incredible being was recommended to go into hospice. He did some deep soul searching and, in six-months, experienced spontaneous radical remission! The medical world ended up studying him, as they couldn't comprehend how he had accomplished such a feat!

Years later, he manifested an incredible line of fern and plant medicines. He's intelligent, hilarious, wise, kind, fiercely strong, unique, and has the heart of a pure warrior. It's a true honor to know him.

I reached out to him when I was recommended to go into Hospice to find out how he healed from a dire stage 4 cancer diagnosis. Since then, our friendship has grown, and I'm proud to call him a close friend. He's truly a shining brilliant light during a transformative time in human his-story!

I was fortunate to get to know him well on his many visits to Kaua'i. I hosted him at my family's house, attended his workshops, and did some private mentoring sessions with him when I needed guidance. He gifted me with wisdom, levity, and many of his precious herbal concoctions.

Ke'oni's vast message to me was to practice "Aloha Mā" which translates to "self-reflective love." In the deep dive of my Inanna experience, I sacrificed my curly crazy locks for something that was far more precious, an insightful sense of self love/Aloha Mā. This was a gift beyond what I had experienced in my lifetime.

With my body broken down by the effects of chemo, I took the opportunity to examine who I was beyond my physical appealing self. I learned that when I chose to cultivate my own sense of self-reflective love (Aloha Mā), I was happier.

MOTHER:

In July, we found out the startling news about my mother:

> My heart hurts and my head is spinning. We got news of my mom's diagnosis; it's a doozy! She has stage 4 peripheral T cell lymphoma, cancer of the lymph nodes. We were dreading this diagnosis.
>
> I'm always one to look on the bright side, but really? Hasn't there been enough cancer in our family? Rowen, the mother of my beautiful niece died two years ago from colon cancer at the age of forty-seven, there was my diagnosis, and now my beloved mother. This morning, when I got the news, I hit the ground crying with the mantra, "FUCK NO!" going around my head. The day was spent in shock while texting and calling family members.
>
> Here we go. She's getting a port put in and most likely will start chemo next week. I keep hearing that lymphoma is actually much easier to treat than what I've gone through. This is a relief. Apparently, it's 80% curable, depending on the severity and how she handles treatment.

I know that my parents are both unbelievably bright, optimistic, powerhouse people. I was so proud of how both handled the roller coaster of the past weeks. Attitude is everything, and that speaks volumes when dealing with cancer!

I'm digging my roots in the ground to find the strength to face this. Four years ago, when I got the raven tattoo on my left arm, which symbolized wanting to learn the mysteries of death, I had NO idea what I was signing up for. I've learned enough of this lesson, thank you very much!

I'm envisioning my mother and I riding these magnificent waves with grace.

Life is sure fragile and precious.

My soul signed up for some huge lessons in the past seven years. It's been one transformative lesson after another. The consistent theme revolves around death, dis-ease, and letting go of the unnecessary shards that hold me back from true expansion. Like the Phoenix from the flames, I'm asked to let go of any sense of comfort, step fully into the flames, and transmute the experience.

Turning the sorrow, pain, and grief into gold,
Precious lessons of impermanence,
I will embrace the adversity,
Use it as material to shine my soul,
Turn the darkness into light,
And rise again!

SELF-CARE:

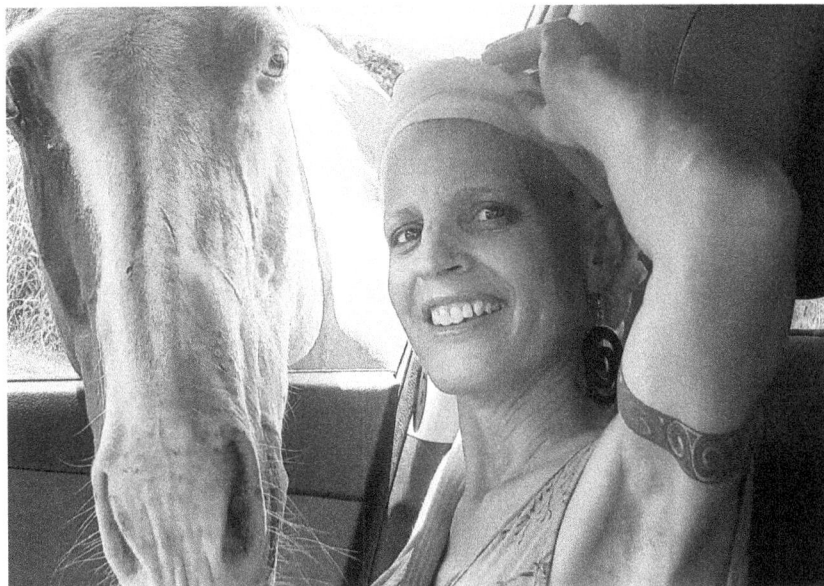

One of the biggest lessons of the cancer journey was how to put myself first. This lesson kept repeating itself during my healing journey at different levels of intensity. In many ways, cancer was a blessing to get me to truly care for myself!

With the relentless routine of receiving chemo, I was starting to take a hard look at my nurturer/caregiver pattern. I was examining that fine line of what it meant to give to another, yet still maintain my own personal boundaries. How much is too much when it comes to giving to another? Where do I stop and you begin? It's an act of kindness to give to others, but if I overextend myself, then I'll become depleted. Resentment invariably follows depletion.

In my years of witnessing many women with breast cancer, I saw how it tended to affect those who are givers. After caring for my best friend Deb through her twenty-two-month journey with leukemia, I was diagnosed with stage 3 breast cancer exactly one year after she died. I was definitely overextended during the time of caring for her during her illness. I would often drive seven hours in one day to spend the afternoon with her while also trying to care for two horses, start a business, and run a ranch. She never asked me to go the extra mile for her. She always encouraged me to take care of myself. It was my responsibility to find the fine line of self-care. When my own life was on the line, I finally understood this important lesson of self-care!

It was also a valuable lesson to learn how to receive. Being knocked down by chemotherapy taught me the necessity of asking for help. I had no choice.

With my mother's recent diagnosis, I had to take a hard look at a pattern of codependency I possessed. In trying to help my mother, a part of me wanted to maintain control in the guise of loving care. I struggled with my need/desire to help my mother, which was coupled with a vast feeling of helplessness.

I was aware that my caregiver pattern was one of the causes of the cancer diagnosis. I knew my health was fragile and while I was doing relatively well, the reality was that I had been close to death mere months before. I wasn't out of the woods. I reminded myself that if I became consumed with the care of another, I would stop the dynamic process of healing within my body. I would be putting my life at risk.

I was scared. My mom wasn't doing well. I knew my parents weren't going to live forever, but couldn't this have happened at another time? I dearly loved my mom. I had experienced a shit load of death in a short period of time. I knew I had signed up for rapid transformation and growth in this lifetime, but, heck, this was over the top!

I knew I was strong. I kept the faith that there was a way to find balance and heal despite another obstacle in my path. I was determined to walk the razor's edge of self-care while still being present with what was real.

The saving grace was that I had been connecting quite a bit with Blue and Comanche. The horses truly fed my spirit. They were the holders of such beauty and profound peace. Truly, my love of horses had gotten me through the rough times. I knew I'd be okay because of them.

HEAD WRAPS:

My goal was to try to enjoy the ride! I made the best of my baby bald head look by playing with wigs and head wraps. My egoic self was severely stripped bare by the side effects of chemo. My goal was to counteract the loss by having fun with my identity.

I found my mind rebelling against my new physical identity. With no hair or eyebrows, I really did look like an alien. Having no eyebrows was actually more challenging than being bald. It was surreal to look in the mirror and not have eyebrows framing my eyes. I was like a stranger in a strange land.

A friend wisely reminded me that I was in a new reality. To expect my life to be the same as it was before I started treatment was holding onto a past false perception and expectation of myself. I was a different person than I was before. The reality was that the side effects of cancer and cancer treatment were severely affecting my body. I looked vastly different with my slim frame and bald head.

I realized I needed to allow room to grieve what I had given up. It was difficult to travel down into Inanna's realm and let go of what was precious to me. I had let go of identifying with my ranch, two of my horses, career, hair, voluptuous body, and the free, independent image I clung to. Once the grieving was done, I could move forward to appreciate life and the beauty that surrounded me.

I WAS ALIVE! Wasn't it enough that I had just skirted through hell barely escaping death?

It took great courage and a willingness to see a different perspective. I kept dropping into gratitude amidst the occasional hissy fits that were necessary to release.

I aimed to be like the horses: Feel the feeling, express it, and then go back to grazing.

I was an occasional fireball on the roughest days:

Today the frustration of my situation got to me. I said, "Fuck it!" and went to the beach. As I dove into the turbulent waves, I allowed my anger to sizzle off into the water. I listened to the pounding of the waves, sunk my feet into the sand, and everything was okay again.

Sometimes, it's necessary to shift your perspective. I went to get another chemotherapy infusion of Taxol today. After sitting for ninety minutes, waiting patiently, I was told my white blood cell count was too low to receive chemo. I had been feeling pretty crappy the last few days and wasn't surprised.

What did I do? I got frustrated from the insanity of the roller coaster, the up moments of feeling great, then the down moments of feeling like total crap. It's completely unpredictable! Compounding the reality is that my treasured mother is now on this path.

I turned into a fiery Portuguese cyclone. Watch out!

I had a good laugh with Syris today about how I should start a Portuguese women anger management group on the island as there are so many of us flamboyant, temperamental creatures on the island. We could release our fury by exclaiming loudly about what bothers us. After we would cathartically release our emotions, we would jump in the ocean and watch the steam rise!

***

I felt pulled between California and Kaua'i with my mother's new diagnosis. I decided to go back home to see my family. My oncologist said it was fine to travel, as I was doing so well. My goal was to be present and help, while still staying on track with my own healing regimen. I felt fairly confident about this plan of action. It was important for me to visit. My cherished mother was my root to the world.

Such uncertainty sure put everything into perspective. There was no time to waste.

LOOKING UP!

I was on my third round of Taxol and doing great! I had gained back 10 pounds in the past weeks. I even noticed that my muscles were returning! I was thrilled to go out dancing for two hours and attended a yoga class.

The other happy proof that I was healing was that my lung doctor said my lungs were improving. Also, my tumor cell count was 135 with the CA 27-29 test. When I started receiving treatment, it was in the 900s. The normal amount is under 40.

I was taking it one day at a time. I continued to take each moment as it arrived, putting one foot in front of the other. Breath by breath, I was determined to heal.

MOTHERING THE MOTHER:

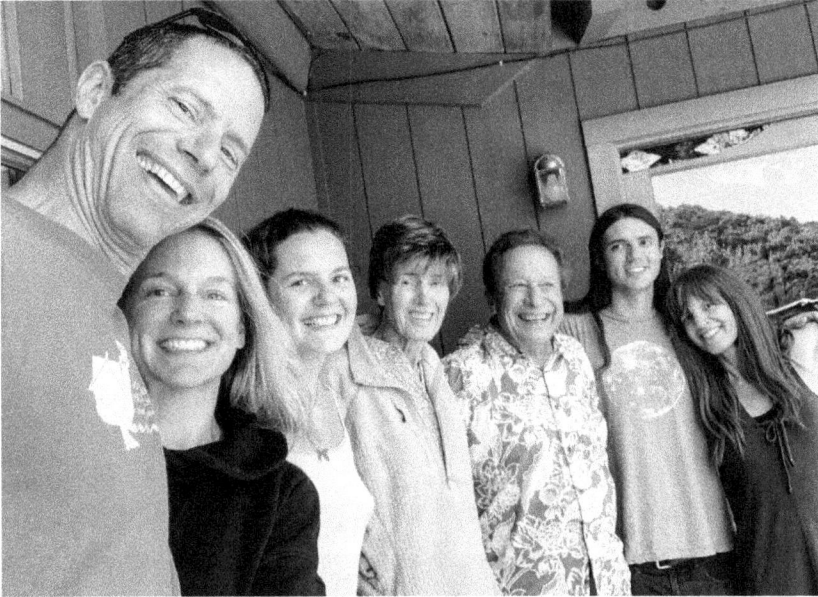

My family: Ted, Renee, Jasmine, my mother, father, Willow & me

I decide to take a break in treatment to visit my family in the Bay Area, Northern California. On the flight over, I was suitably masked up to protect my sensitive immune system from germs. For a sense of fun, I donned my red Zahrah wig. It was truly amusing to be a shapeshifter with long red hair for the flight over!

When I first arrived in California, it was hard to see my mother with a stage 4 cancer diagnosis. I was at peace with my own cancer journey. As a natural caregiver, it was always hardest to see those I love suffer. My codependent tendency was to try to take away their pain and save them from suffering. I kept reminding myself that each person must go through their own experience; it's not my job to save anyone except for myself. This is a lesson I need to be reminded of frequently.

It's quite the experience to see your parents age and witness the roles of caregiving reversed. Every inch of me wanted to take my parents in my arms and protect them. They took such good care of me as a child; it was only natural that I would want to reciprocate, mothering the mother as it were.

Inanna traveled down another layer into the underworld. I hit another layer of grief with the realization that my mother had stage 4 cancer. My parents had always been a solid rock of support for me. Even though I possessed a fearless attitude with the "stage 4 cancer" label, the concept that my mother might be facing her death soon hit like another anvil upon my tender head.

LADY GRIEF VISITS AGAIN:

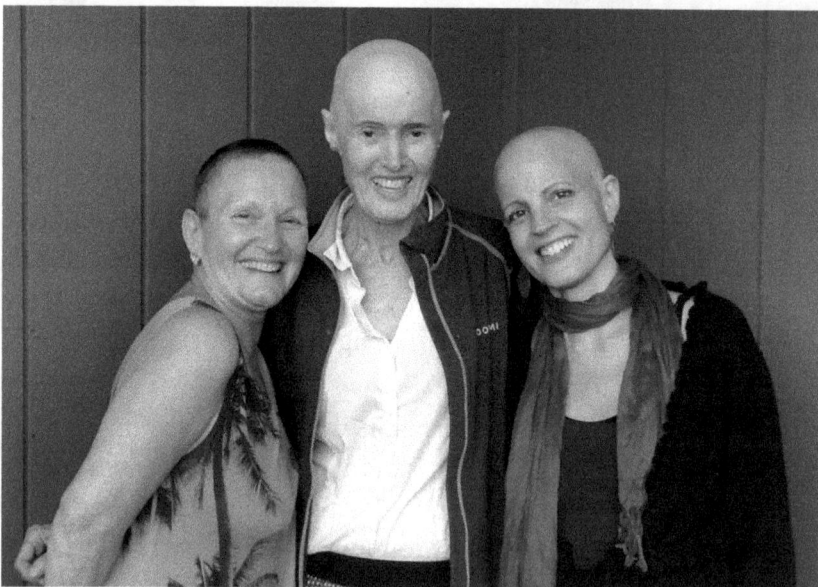

Photo by David Steinberg
Kim Mears, mother & me

I spent years leading "Grief Rituals with Horses" at my retreat center. After Deb's death, I was guided to create these sacred rituals, as I realized that grief was a suppressed emotion in our society. It was a powerful journey and an honor to hold safe space for others as they released a lifetime of grief. Rivers of suppressed tears would flood out, which would allow for a miraculous transformation within their healing process.

Once past traumas were released, it allowed for a new sense of vibrancy to emerge. I witnessed my clients claiming their own empowerment as they released the baggage of grief that held them as prisoners of the past. They were finding their own sovereign selves. This was an incredible transformation to witness.

Grief would still visit me occasionally, though not as intensely as the first year after Deb's death. When lady grief would visit, I would do what the horses taught me to do: I would welcome her, express my sorrows, and let it go to the best of my ability. I knew that this was the key to my healing. If I didn't release the past trauma, the stuck energy would hold me back from embracing my vibrant healthy self!

I allowed myself to cry when I needed to while I was in California. In the process of feeling the grief about my mother's diagnosis, I could return to JOY once more. The sacred tears were a gift to bring me back to wholeness.

The truth sunk in a bit more when I accompanied my mom to get her head shaved. My mood swung from shock to acceptance to disbelief and back again.

My mother and I now shared the same experience: shaved heads, chemotherapy, and all that treatment entailed. I wished she didn't have to experience all the twisted gifts of cancer, yet I had no choice but to accept that this was her path. I had to trust that her soul chose it for her growth. I was reminded yet again that it was much easier to go through a health journey than to witness your loved one's face difficulties.

Surrender, girl.
The idea of being in control is just an illusion.
Keep the faith that all is perfect and in divine order.

There were some tender, powerful family moments of witnessing my mother drop into a layer of vulnerability I had never seen before. I observed her be open in a new manner after her diagnosis.

The weather we endure daily definitely shapes our personalities. My mother was born and raised in New Hampshire. New Englanders possess a hardworking, frugal, solid mannerism. They must endure frigid, freezing winters, which, in turn, roots their feet solidly to the ground. In contrast, people from the sunny West Coast of the USA tend to be more on the flighty, flaky side of things. I've noticed that folks who live in warm locations are more relaxed and not as productive as the cold weather hardy types. When I've traveled across the United States from New York to Hawaii, I've seen this gradual demeanor shift in the general population from east to west. After living in Hawaii for a good portion of my life, I can say that getting a project done that requires assistance from other islanders requires incredible patience and fortitude. This is due to the lackadaisical, warm tropical air that so lovingly infuses its inhabitants. It's lovely to live in paradise, but it's lacking the productivity of the bustling East Coast! In my opinion, this is a good thing.

Due to her New England upbringing, my mother always tended to have more of a reserved, quiet nature. When my mother was diagnosed with cancer, I observed her loosen up and spend more time talking with her loved ones on the phone and relaxing after dinner. It was refreshing to witness the positive transformation that unfolded with her.

I was grateful to see my family in California, but it was lovely to go back home again.

COURAGE:

When I got back home to Kaua'i it took a bit to integrate after the deep dive into family dynamics. The time with my family led me to take a hard look at the health of all my relationships, particularly, the love relationship with my partner. When your head is on the grindstone and you're faced off with the demons of hell, it's natural to examine the fine line between a healthy and toxic relationship. My goal was to foster healthy relationships with everyone I spent time with. It became clear to me that if I wasn't in right relation with those close to me, then it would directly impact my body's ability to heal. Toxicity in relationships can creep into mental balance, which, in turn, can affect your body's health.

It required immense courage to make a change in the relationship with my partner. It asked me to shift out of old, familiar patterns and see beyond the limited realm of what was comfortable.

I love this definition of courage which connects the concept of true vulnerability with having your heart open:

> *The root of the word courage is cor – the Latin word for heart. In one of its earliest forms, the word courage had a very different definition than it does today. Courage originally meant 'To speak one's mind by telling all one's heart.' Over time, this definition has changed, and, today, courage is more synonymous with being heroic. Heroics is important and we*

certainly need heroes, but I think we've lost touch with the idea that speaking honestly and openly about who we are, about what we're feeling, and about our experiences (good and bad) is the definition of courage. Heroics is often about putting our life on the line. Ordinary courage is about putting our vulnerability on the line. In today's world, that's pretty extraordinary.

–Brené Brown, *I Thought It Was Just Me: Women Reclaiming Power and Courage in a Culture of Shame*

As I was examining the sustainability of my personal relationships, I was increasingly feeling more physical bone pain in my body. This Mahina poem describes it perfectly:

Waking up in the wee hours of the morning with the glorious full moon rays streaming in through the yurt window, I toss and turn releasing all that doesn't serve. Sometimes, bone metastasis brings incredible pain in my left hip and lower back, along with the physical pain from chemotherapy side effects. I allowed the waves of discomfort to move through me. I matched the pain with the expression of grief that begged to be released.

Sound escapes in the form of primal cries, my furry friends cuddle by my side to bring comfort and relief. The previous week of seeing family stirred up unresolved emotions and evoked great sadness in me. I allow these emotions to pour on through as the pain shoots through my breast, sternum, hip, and leg.

The animal is awakened!
The wild full moon shakes and cries with her intensity and grace!

Resolution is found as the waves slowly return to a calm state. Sleep creeps in, bringing a sense of surrender to my soul. I'm released to the wonder of her mercurial depths, Mahina, mother Moon, holding me close.

Whatever mysteries this path holds for me:I'm held.
I'm loved.
I'm adored.

I know not of the future; all I know is now.

All is perfect, pain resolved, peace returned, Mahina's white glowing arms surrounding me with grace.

Mahalo, Mahina for returning me to your bosom repeatedly.

This Pisces girl is so very grateful.

MOLD BE GONE!

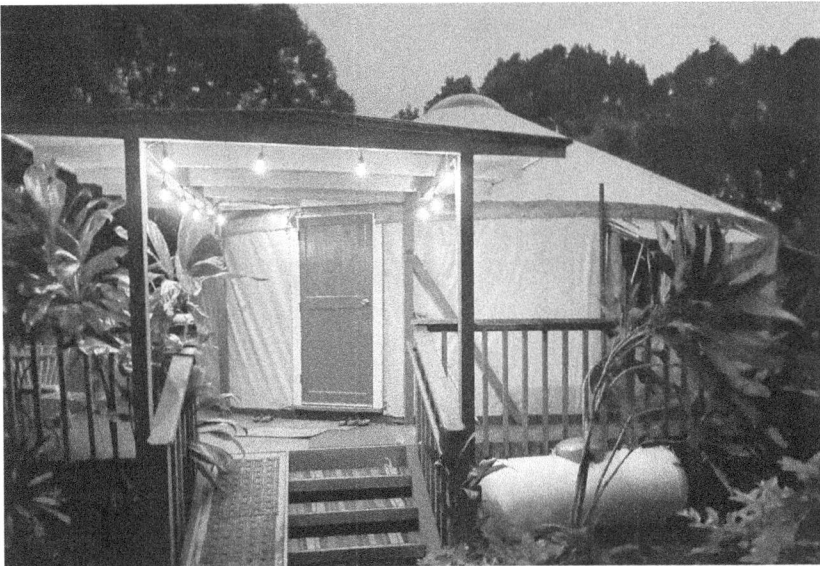

The waves kept coming. Within a few weeks of returning from my trip, while undergoing treatment, I realized my beloved yurt home had a terrible mold infestation. I woke up one day and noticed the mold creeping up the furniture, eating away my most beloved leather items, growing on the wooden kitchen utensils, and swallowing my clothes alive!

It was necessary to completely renovate my home. Living in a vinyl tent on the wettest spot on Earth was a bold invitation for mold growth. I dove into research about what was necessary to eradicate the mold.

I wrote:

> This earthly plane has continuous learning opportunities for growth. Life never seems to stop. I'm determined to find the beauty in the rough spots!

> Due to a dangerous mold situation, I have to temporarily move out of my home. It's necessary to gut the yurt and remove all traces of the toxic mold. My health is already so precarious, I cannot take a chance of backtracking with all the progress I've made. I'm incredibly grateful that I have another place to stay.

> These past years have been rough! I feel like Julie Andrews in *The Sound of Music*, optimistically singing, "These are a few of my favorite things" to stay focused on what keeps me smiling and laughing through the absurdity of it all.

> Despite it all, I fiercely love this island and welcome the growth she has to offer!

KUMU:

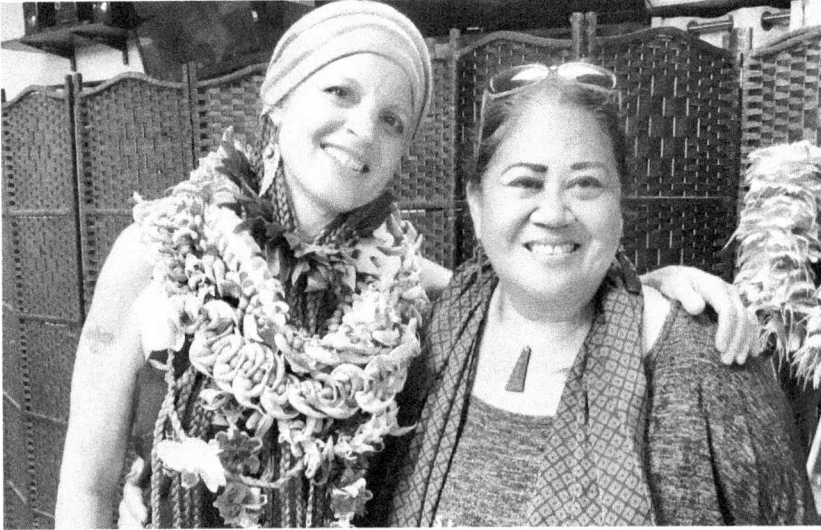

Me & Kehaulani Kekua

I was taking a Hawaiian spirituality class with a beautiful Hawaiian woman named Kehaulani Kekua whose native wisdom had been passed down through several generations of spiritual elders. She is a life-long practitioner, disciple and scholar of traditional hula and Hawaiian culture. She taught a weekly class which shared the teachings of Hawaiian spirituality. I had reached out to her, sharing about my health situation, and asked her if I could join her class. I was so overjoyed when she allowed me to join! This was a rejuvenating experience to be able to partake in a "normal" activity after being so close to death in the last year. Learning from Kumu (Kehaulani) was fulfilling a long time wish about wanting to learn more about Native Hawaiians on the islands. I was grateful she saw beyond my physical limitations and allowed me to join her class.

Grateful for the light, beauty and depth surrounding me! Life is so rich. I'm currently taking a Hawaiian spirituality class and just was steeped in two hours of learning the language and sacred chants. So much power, grace, and wisdom to behold.

It's a blessing to be learning it while I'm on such an intense health journey. It helps to provide context for the deep waters I'm in! Tonight, we spoke about the Kumulipo, and learned Hiki Mai Ka La E & Ka'i Kukulu. (These are the names of specific Hawaiian chants.) I'm thankful to have access to this sacred knowledge, being of European ancestry (even though my Portuguese ancestors have been here on Kaua'i since the 1870s). I'm well aware that these teachings are only recently accessible to those outside of Hawaiian ancestry. The world is united. Many tribes are coming together to find peace and balance.

INANNA ENCOUNTERS MOLD:

Inanna might possibly have never dealt with mold. We'll never know, as the toxic black matter was never mentioned on the 3,500-year-old tablets pulled from the earth that told her story. The fungus called mold did exist then, so it's entirely possible she dealt with it!

My experience of dealing with mold meant I had to throw away many of my precious "treasures," like Inanna had to forsake her adored regalia. This was a physical and emotional Herculean task to undertake. Goodbye favorite iconic cowgirl hat! I tried to save what I could but was advised that if I kept things that were moldy, most likely, they would reinfect everything else again. So out they went!

Dealing with a terrible mold problem in the midst of chemo treatment, while experiencing body pain, wasn't a walk in the park.

I ended up throwing away a massive number of items like priceless pillows my son got me in India, wood sculptures, canvas paintings, a buffalo leather bag made by a dear friend, backpacks, leather boots, clothes, and kitchen utensils. I had to wash all my clothes that weren't already ruined in Borax. I ended up doing fifty to sixty laundry loads. The washer and drier were constantly running for weeks!

While gutting the yurt and tearing out the twenty-six-year-old kitchen and bathroom cabinets, rats' nests were found under two of the decrepit old cabinets. Gross!

Everything I owned needed to be either thrown away or cleaned with chemicals in order to kill the mold. I had no choice but to hire a professional mold remediator to do the job. I knew my health and my life were at stake.

Just when I was at my wits end, I remembered I had countless friends who had repeatedly offered their help to me. Duh! It was time for me to practice one of the greatest and most difficult acts of vulnerability: asking for and learning to receive help! Six loyal friends agreed to come help me dispose of moldy items and help me pack and move my belongings.

I started using Frida the cane again after enduring the extreme stress of traveling and dealing with mold. My body was reacting with violent spasms of pain. My hope was to get back on track when all the craziness settled down.

Just in time, my superstar friend Michelle came out to help me through the mold and chemo escapade. She was a bright light during a very intense time. It was the third time she had visited me in the past year. I was incredibly blessed to have such an altruistic friend helping me through the rough patches. It was truly the love of my generous friends and family that made a difference repeatedly.

It was time for my three-month CT scan! Before receiving the scan results, I was a bit nervous due to the stress of traveling, sudden mold problem, and having to move. My acute hip/back pain had returned, which brought up fears about the cancer's possible spread.

Despite the crazy twists and turns, my health continued to improve, and I received positive CT scan results! The tumors continued to shrink throughout my entire body. The tumor cell count for the CA 27-29 blood test was down to 70!

I celebrated my great news and tried my best to deal with the daily body discomfort.

Little did I know what waited around the bend.

SPREADING MY WINGS:

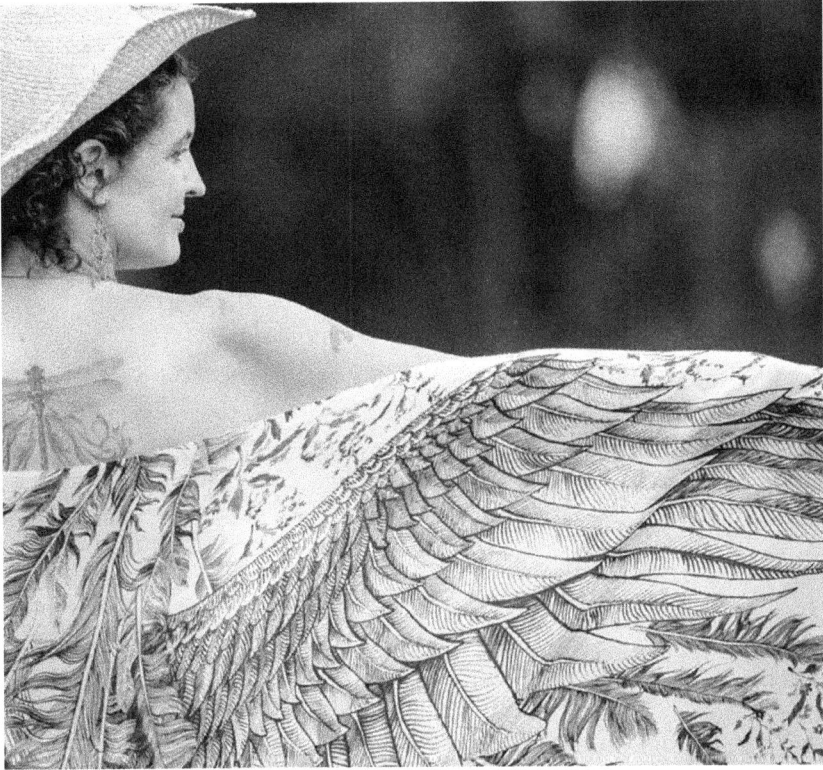

Photo by Kalalea Photography

Bolen writes in *Close to the Bone* on page 6:

> *Illness, especially when death is a possibility, makes us acutely aware of how precious life is and how precious a particular life is. Priorities shift. We may see the truth of what matters, who matters, and what we have been doing with our lives and have to decide what to do–now that we know. Significant relationships are tested and either come through strengthened or fail. Pain and fear bring us to our knees in prayer. Our spiritual and religious convictions or the lack of them are called into question. Illness is an ordeal*

for both body and soul and a time when healing of either or both can result.

I hadn't announced it publicly, but in August 2019, Syris moved out. I shared the news on social media a few months after he found another home:

> Syris is a stellar being who has stood by my side through the gauntlet of the past three and a half years. I have TREMENDOUS respect for anyone who stands by their beloved through a cancer journey. It's like watching death dance on the outskirts of their love. Syris has done this and much more! He is a magnanimous being who bravely held my hand through the darkest moments, and I dearly love him for this.
>
> About two months ago I asked him to move out so we both could find our own story separate from the cohesion that comes from such an intense health journey. It felt important for both of us. The reality is that being a caretaker can be all-consuming. (I know, as I was a caretaker for my best friend for twenty-two months.) We didn't "break up" but made a mutual decision for breathing room. This has been healthy for both of us! It's good now and then to have space to assess what works and what doesn't.
>
> I'm proud of both of us for finding our way through the quagmire of this path with love leading the way. It's so easy to fall into hatred and blame. With all my heart, I want to see him shine and embrace his beautiful life. I know he wants me to live and thrive! We're doing what we need to do to make that happen on our own individual paths, while still staying connected.

Thank you, Syris, for staying by my side through thick and thin. Words cannot express the love, gratitude, and respect I hold for your ability to love me through this shadow dance.

METAMORPHOSIS:

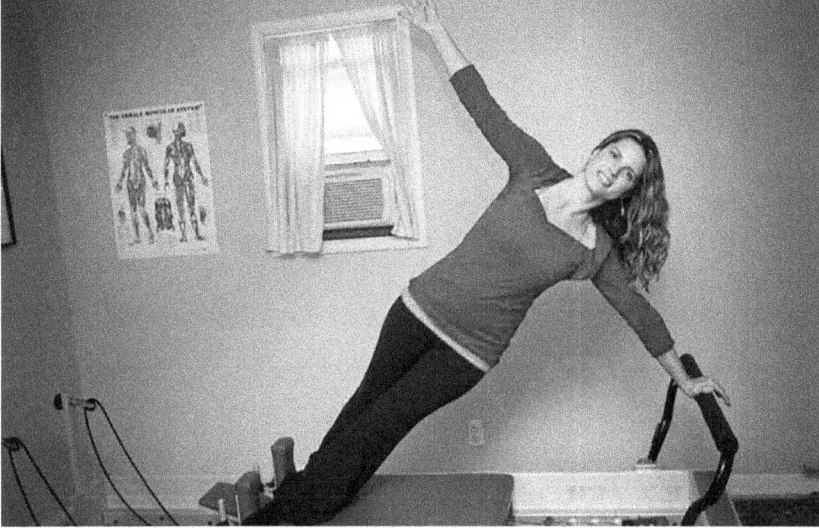

Photo of me at my Pilates Studio: Studio Equilibria

Part of the Inanna's allegorical journey to the underworld is to sacrifice ways of being, relationships, objects, job titles, and limited perceptions that have been part of the ego's identification. This may also mean letting go of a sense of security with what roles we play in the world.

I was born into a superstar fit family; therefore, a big part of my identity was my athletic prowess. I grew up with my parents challenging me to speed down advanced ski runs when I was almost learning to walk. Both my brother and I were soccer stars at a young age. My mother and brother were/are avid rock climbers who performed death-defying climbs to the tops of random mountains around the globe. Being so high off the ground like that would most likely make me chuck out my stomach contents! My courageous brother has climbed El Capitan and other challenging climbs in Yosemite. Spending the night 1,800 feet up on the side of a cliff and taking a shit in a poop bag was a normal reality for my brother. I decided at a young age, when he took me climbing, that my feet preferred being on the ground!

Being in my body and being physical was something I was proud of. Academic life was challenging for me; being a sporty, artistic girl was naturally easy. When I was eleven, I identified so much with being a tomboy that for a year, I refused to wear a skirt or dress and actually wanted to be a boy! I saw boys getting the natural respect that girls had to earn. I wanted it to be easy for me too.

To release my identity of being a super star athlete when my body was battered by cancer and treatment wasn't only physically challenging but also deeply mentally perturbing. It was the identity my mind had clung to my entire life. As I didn't feel comfortable with my own vulnerability as a child, I heavily identified with the athletic part of me that easily excelled in sports. I grew up in a science-oriented family but never identified with academia. Science was foreign to my own naturally inclined artistic orientation. I naturally excelled at sports, dance, art, writing, and outlets of a more physical nature. Letting go of my physically inclined identity was like tearing off one of my appendages. It was a huge adjustment to still perceive myself as valuable without my naturally robust, adept body.

9/29:

Today, I'm grieving my athletic body that could easily tackle advance level athletics. This is a photo of me from nine years ago *see notes above* in my Pilates studio where I used to teach rehabilitation to advanced level classes and private sessions in Pilates, the Gyrotonic Exercise Method, and Yamuna Body Rolling.

When I was a kid, I was a total tomboy and could beat most of the girls and many of the boys with my nimble body. In my twenties, I choreographed dance shows and would perform in them. My body loved the challenge and could easily do whatever I asked it to.

My current reality is that due to cancer bone degeneration, walking can be incredibly painful at times. I've been stripped down to basics. Just like I'm throwing away half of the precious items in my yurt due to mold, I have to let go of the concept of being the vigorously able Tara. It's a huge letting go for me that's requiring tons of surrender. It's not easy.

When I go out now and witness others dancing with wild abandon, I occasionally experience a mental blow as that was a vibrant slice of my past. Dancing like a crazy banshee was my prior identity. Now when I go dancing, I strive to be aware of the acute line of pain versus pleasure. If I overdo it and I'm not careful, it can throw me off for days. As my treasured friend Eugene says, I'm in a new cancer baby body and I need to tune into what it needs in every moment. It creates layers of frustration, grief, and anger in me as I can't depend on my predictable strength anymore! I'm not superwoman anymore. This is real.

Practicing surrender and acceptance in every dragon's breath.

Along with having a hard time adjusting to the physical prowess I possessed before treatment and cancer, my mind was having a hard time in general adjusting to my new "normal" reality. The shock of all the changes that my body had gone through was starting to hit me. One day, I looked in the mirror and realized my physical appearance had been possibly forever altered. Due to chemotherapy, I had no eyebrows, was stick thin, bald, and my once sturdy frame had been severely slammed.

It was helpful to process the experience by writing about it and sharing on social media, primarily Instagram. Being witnessed through my writing helped me come to peace with the new alien landscape I found myself in. Though my mind was spinning from all the changes, I knew one thing; I was very fortunate to be alive.

I knew I had to give up what was safe in order to survive, adapt to this new identity, and, hopefully, one day thrive.

BOUNDARIES:

Boundaries help create a safe container to operate within ALL of our relationships: friends, family, coworkers, and acquaintances in the everyday world. Having clear boundaries with others can help us flourish within our relationships, as we're clear what our needs are and how to get them met.

Once we learn where our boundaries are and how to set them, we can operate in the world in a healthier manner as we're clear where we stand with ourselves and others. The world becomes a safer place and we're empowered to stand strong yet aware within ourselves in a whole new manner.

-Tara Coyote, Learning Healthy
Boundaries: Tools for Healing &
Self-Discovery

Being aware about the concept of boundaries was a huge part of my learning experience since the creation of WHS. It was also a strong focus of the Equine Facilitated Learning work I taught with the horses. I was so enthusiastic about the concept of "Healthy Boundaries" that I even created a free E-book about the topic.

In my need for fierce self-care on the healing journey, I was submerged into another layer of learning about boundaries.

Bolen writes in *Close to the Bone* on page 39:

When we are seriously ill or recovering from surgery, radiation, chemotherapy, or any life-threatening or health-threatening condition, we are on Psyche's journey. If we are accompanying someone we love through the underworld, we will need all the resources we have for both of us. The need to conserve our strength, to not extend ourselves at such times, is advice we need to heed. The Psyche myth may make the point in a deeper way than a rational explanation, especially when-as is often the case-people who drain and deplete us have held us in the relationship through guilt and the assumption we are responsible for them.

When we are going through an underworld phase, there is the possibility that we will not return if we do not hold on to what we need. When this part of the Psyche myth strikes a chord, we know that the difference between making our way back to physical, psychological, or spiritual health may hinge upon very little. Like Psyche, we may be asked to do something that seems on the surface a small expenditure of time and energy, and we may be drawn to help out of compassion and because we feel mean-spirited and selfish (guilty) if we say no. It is not a small thing: it is a moment of truth. To hold on to the message of the myth when we know it is true (and yet have trouble justifying it to others) may be possible if we imagine we are Psyche making a descent into the underworld and our return depends on whether we can harden our heart to pity and guilt and say no to whatever and whomever we know will drag our spirit down and take energy and optimism from us that we cannot afford to lose.

As the yurt was being completely gutted due to the mold damage, there was close to a dozen workers I was juggling to do the different tasks necessary to clean up the space.

This is the yurt work that was completed:

- Changing the inner roof liner of the yurt. This entailed tearing the entire huge roof off, taking off the moldy liner and then replacing it with the new liner.

- Tearing out the old cabinets out in the kitchen and bathroom and putting in new ones.

- Installing new tile for the kitchen and bathroom.

- Finding new kitchen and bathroom fixtures, etc.

- Painting the entire roof and wooden window slats with anti-mold substance to stop the future proliferation of mold.

- Putting in a new wood floor

- Repainting the walls of the yurt

- Installed ceiling fans to prevent future mold growth, which required doing a complete overhaul with the yurts electrical wiring to install them.

- Refurbishing three large pieces of furniture covered by mold: sanding down and repainting them with mold-resistant paint.

I need a nap after reading the list! It's hard to capture in a list the work it took to complete each of these tasks. Each step took innumerable hours. Ordering cabinets and tiles and the complications of getting them shipped 2,500 miles away to Kaua'i was a logistical nightmare. Everything in general moves much slower in Hawaii where the concept of island time and flaky workers are plentiful!

9/30:

In the last few days, I've had my boundaries seriously challenged by four different workers during the yurt overhaul project! Of these four men: two of them were men I'm in close personal relationships with and are near and dear to my heart. It's very clear that the universe is testing me to see if I can hold my ground with kindness and strength.

Sometimes these tests arrive on a sparkling platter to challenge us to stand firm in our truth. If these growth opportunities can be met with compassion for others and fierce self-care and respect for ourselves, then that's even better!

Along with throwing away massive amounts of items affected by mold, I'm also letting go of patterns that don't serve me anymore. Why hold onto dysfunctional ways of behavior that are outdated and ultimately don't serve anyone? If I don't respect my own boundaries, then who else will?

BLOOD COUNT ROLLER-COASTER:

It's normal for cancer patients receiving chemotherapy treatment to experience the roller-coaster of blood count cell levels. Chemo and the other drugs used to treat cancer are a whopper on the immune system. While it's simultaneously working to annihilate cancer cells, it's also weakening the immune system that keeps the body healthy. It's a fine line of keeping the body healthy enough to function but also actively kicking the cancer back.

It's common for cancer patients to have a challenging time keeping their blood counts high enough while undergoing treatment. If blood count levels are not high enough for the necessary chemotherapy treatment, the infusion will most likely be delayed for a week or two till it's at a stable level. While I was receiving Taxol treatment, my white blood count level was frequently plummeting. My mother also experienced constant challenges with her platelet levels, which also delayed her treatment.

10/1:

No chemo today. I was supposed to be getting weekly Taxol treatments, but my body is typically taking a while to recover from each infusion. The bone marrow which stimulates and creates white blood cells has been worn out by the intense chemotherapy treatment.

I'm coming to peace with the fact that my body seems to be needing more time to integrate the treatment. The nurses say this is fairly normal, so I'm not too worried. I do know I tend to be more on the sensitive side compared to most people, and medicine typically impacts me more than others.

The way I look at it, it means I have more time to enjoy my week and allow my body time to recover. At the rate I'm going with seven more Taxol treatments, it means I won't be finished till January or so. Originally, I was told I'd be done with treatments in November.

I tell myself that it's not about the destination, but about the journey. My goal is to enjoy life and be grateful for what I have. I'm just happy to be alive and I trust my body is doing exactly what it needs to do to heal. Slow and steady wins the race, even if it's at a slug's pace!

SHELL BELL BELL:

You definitely find out who your true friends are when you're on a life-threatening health journey! Having a serious illness is a litmus test for who is brave enough to walk in the dark with you.

I was fortunate that Michelle, AKA Shell Bell Bell (when you've had a cherished friend for over twenty-five years, funny nicknames come with the territory), was visiting again. Michelle possesses a natural mothering nature, which allowed me the rare gift of relaxation, knowing I was being cared for. She's one of the few people I've allowed into the barred chambers of my heart in full vulnerability.

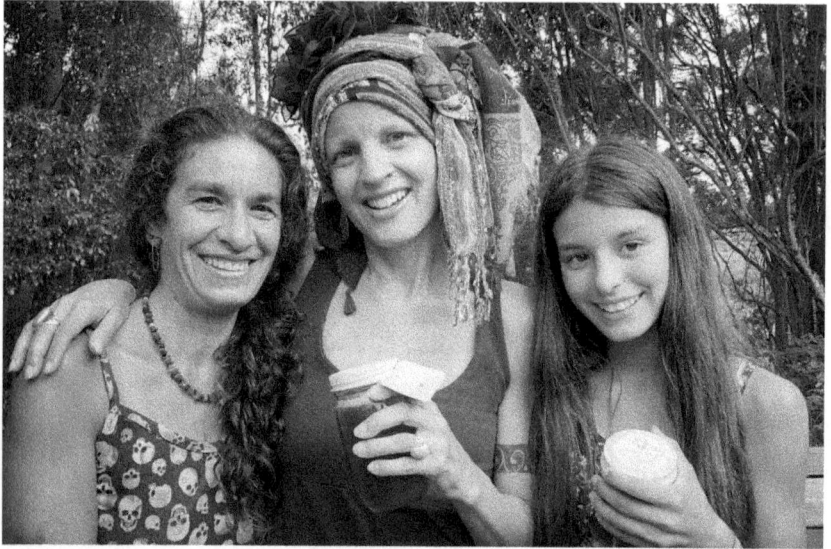

Michelle, me & Zenobia

10/4:

Praise beloved Michelle! This lovely bright being visited me in Kaua'i three times since I was plunged into the deep waters of my health crisis. Michelle has walked by my side through the hardest moments.

She's watched me puke.
She's made me food when I could eat only the blandest food.
She's been by my side when I was blubbering away, broken down by chemo and delirious with pain.

She's scrubbed my toilet.
She's danced with me when I felt good.
She's walked my dog for miles (as I can't now).
She's celebrated the highs and cried with me during the lows.
She's a true friend.

Treasure the dear ones who stick by your side through thick and thin. They're worth more than gold.

Michelle and I became fast friends twenty-five years ago when our boys were tiny toddlers. Now our boys are older than we were when we met in the heyday of our Grateful Dead dancing years. What stories we have to share!

My time with Michelle during her visit to Kaua'i was deeply transformational. Since Deb had died four years earlier, my heart was heavily guarded. During Michelle's visit, I allowed myself to open up to her in a vulnerable manner like I hadn't opened up to anyone since Deb's passing. This was a dynamic shift!

CONGRUENCY WITHIN RELATIONSHIP:

The dark and light dance together.
It's necessary to walk into the shadows to find one's light.

One of the blessings of chemo was the extreme mental clarity I found after each infusion. It gifted me with crystal clear vision to see the toxic behavior in those surrounding me. This allowed me to truly discern what healthy behavior was in all of my personal relationships.

I was looking at my relationship with my partner under a magnifying glass, trying to understand if it was truly a congruent situation for me.

10/5:

> Weeding toxic people and situations out of my life: This past month dealing with massive mold remediation in the yurt has necessitated I throw away an enormous amount of prized physical objects. Both my physical and mental reality are in alignment as I'm also clearing out toxic relationships that drain my energy.
>
> My relationship with my partner has been sweet yet loaded with stress at unpredictable moments. This last week was eye opening to these patterns! Last night, I tossed and turned, crying with sadness and hurt about angry words directed at me.
>
> I realized that this toxic behavior is very similar to the cancer in my body. If anger, rage, frustration, and repressed emotions are not tended to and released in a healthy manner, they can become like cancer (or ironically like mold) and take over a body with dis-ease. I must let go of any unhealthy energetics that pull me into the vortex of anger, fear, frustration, and hatred.
>
> I'm coming to understand that the key to handling the situation is to let go of my anger toward him. Then, it's important to create strong boundaries in the future for self-care. If I have firm boundaries, it will prevent future drama from consuming me in a negative manner.

My health and healing depend on it! I can have compassion for someone with toxic behavior but maintain a stronger line of compassion in the form of self-care for myself. I deserve it.

> *Hope abides; therefore, I abide.*
> *Countless frustrations have not cowed me.*
> *I'm still alive, vibrant with life.*
> *The black cloud will disappear,*
> *The morning sun will appear once again*
> *In all its supernal glory.*
>
> –SRI CHINMOY

CT SCAN RESULTS!

10/19:

I was scheduled to get CT scans every two and a half months. Every scan continued to bring stellar news with the tumors continuing to shrink! When the doctors would go over the scan results, it took an optimistic frame of mind to see cancer in so many organs and body parts and still stay positive.

This time, when I received the scan results, it clearly showed the lesions/tumors in six vertebrae in my spine. (I had known the tumors were present before, but this time the images were shocking to see! It was a reminder of the damage that had already been done to my spine.) It was as if Pac-Man came along to nibble on my bones.

Overall, the results were great! I was happy to see that the tumors in my liver, hip/pelvis, and everywhere in my body continued to shrink. The radiologist said that if my body kept responding well to treatment, I would have years left to live, which was euphoric news!

The reality of the cancer in my body was a constant reminder that my time could be very limited on Earth. It can be a heavy reality at times. One part of me felt great peace when I thought about death, but my mind was actively choosing to live daily. I wanted to be around for my son!

I truly wished to enjoy as many sunsets as possible before I met lady death. When it's my time to go, I will gracefully chant Akal. (Akal is the chant in the Sikh tradition when someone passes. See more info in the Explanatory Notes.)

TEMPERANCE:

I was grateful to be living on Kaua'i with all the healing magic she brought. My world was rocked with chemo, the dance with cancer, dealing with mold, and having to live elsewhere temporarily, but there were so many blessings to being present on my ancestral home island.

My curves were back! I was back to 125 pounds, which was my beginning weight before chemo. I was happy for the extra bit of chub around my midline, as it meant I was healthy. Getting down to a skinny 110 pounds was a scary wake up call. I decided to never criticize the chub again. Love your flesh, folks; it means you're alive!

I was back to using Frida, my lovely turquoise cane again. I was stubborn and fought mentally against using her. I went for two months without her, but then I ended up pushing myself too hard and had to embrace her support again. I used her occasionally when my hip/leg was sore. I had to accept that I wasn't the superwoman athlete anymore. I was striving to find temperance between my strong Amazon self and the reality at hand.

THE FINAL PHASE OF INANNA'S JOURNEY: IN THE DEPTHS OF THE DARKNESS

October 29 was a fateful day. I took Xaria to the vet for her regular heartworm test. During the entire time I was there, I was staying present to the fact that she's a strong, boisterous dog of 70 pounds. My cousin Stef said, "She's a bit of a bull in a china shop!" It was necessary to hold her firmly. As my body was regularly experiencing pain, I had to watch every move I made to make sure I didn't overdo it. Being in a state of pain was, unfortunately, a normal part of my everyday experience.

While I was inside the vet's office, I was extra diligent paying attention to her. Once we got to the parking lot, I briefly let my guard down. There was a small dog in the parking lot, which I noticed once it was too late. Xaria gave a small tug on the leash to say hello to the dog and I braced my body to hold her big fuzzy body back. The impact of bracing my body was the final straw for my fragile hip.

I heard a loud "Crack!" and felt a tremendous pain in my hip. My body immediately wanted to hit the ground with the shock of the pain. I couldn't hold myself up, so I fell into the hood of my car. Fortunately, two sweet older ladies were walking by in the parking lot.

When the ladies saw me, they were immediately concerned and kindly asked how they could help. I asked if they could please get my cane out of my car. They graciously got Frida and helped get Xaria in the car. Thank goodness for angels walking by in time of need!

I somehow managed to drive myself to the house I was staying in while the yurt was being treated for mold. Upon arrival, I hobbled inside while in tremendous pain, grabbed a morphine pill, and laid down on the sofa. I called Syris and my physical therapist, telling them what happened. My PT told me to go immediately to the hospital to get an X-ray. When Syris was free, he came to get me to take me to the hospital. The nurses gave me an X-ray and delivered the traumatic news, "I'm really sorry to tell you this, but your hip is broken."

What?

My hip was broken?! I was the impervious athletic superstar. How could this be? I was shocked! My PT had warned me how brittle my bones were with cancer metastasis and how I had to be careful while doing any sort of exercise. I never imagined that I might break my hip, though!

The nurses were surprised that I wasn't in tremendous pain. By this point, I was so used to living with massive amounts of pain that I was used to it, plus I had taken one of my emergency stashes of morphine.

As I had gone to a smaller hospital, I was whisked away by ambulance to Wilcox Health Hospital which was the main hospital on the island.

I had never ridden in an ambulance before! Everyone was very nice, and it actually was a pleasant experience. I had been through so much up till now that somehow my brain wasn't too freaked out; I was more stunned than anything else. The reality of my situation hadn't set in yet.

Once at the hospital, I had my own private room. I was told that, most likely, I would need emergency surgery in the morning. What?!

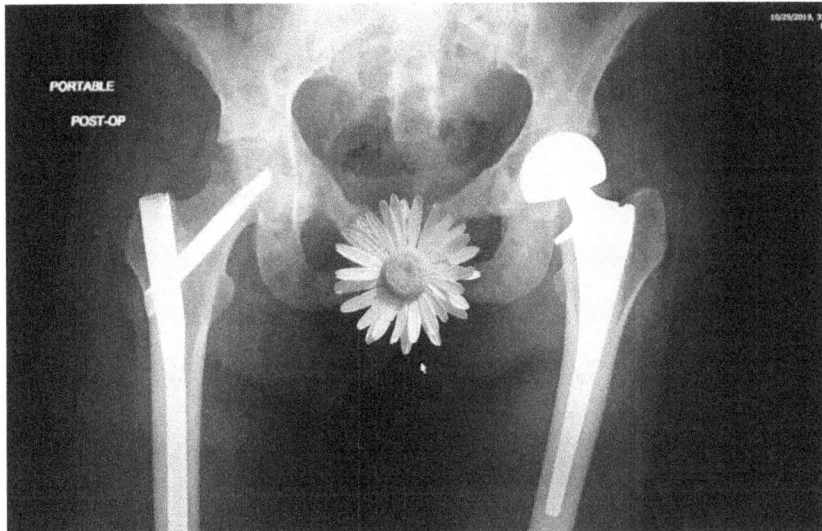

10/29:

These are my Jedi bracelets. At this point, I'm earning every badge of heroism that comes my way. I'm back in the hospital! These are the bracelets that were just strapped onto my wrist upon being admitted to Wilcox.

What happened? Let's just say I had a stupid dog accident and broke my hip!

Am I freaked out? Yes, a little. Am I scared? Yes, a bit. To be honest, life has been so wacky doodle crazy in the past year or so that this latest incident seems like just another thing to add to the list. I think I'm getting used to the universe dishing out absurd incidents to grow my soul from the inside out. For now, I'm calm in the center of the storm.

I'm hooked up to fluids and a beeping machine. They tell me I might have surgery tomorrow. I'm a complicated case, though, as I have bone metastasis.

My biggest fear is losing my mobility. I love being active. I'm focusing on the fact that I will overcome another hurdle! I will heal. I will overcome one more obstacle in my path! I won't let the demons of despair write my story.

I'm focusing on hope, faith, and healing. I see myself walking on the beach. My choice is to focus on my infinite healing potential. I'm not choosing to focus on my cataclysmic fears, which I won't even mention here, as to write them out is to give them power. I know my soul signed up for immense growth in this lifetime and this is one more growth opportunity.

The nurses are super kind. I've been impressed beyond belief with the care at Wilcox Health I've received. I place my faith in their care. I will heal with their help.

In no time, I'll be dancing on the beach again. Please help me visualize this. Mahalo!

***

In retrospect, when I read this post, I see how optimistic I was. It's hard to believe when looking back how I could have such a positive attitude. I really had no idea what my future looked like. If I had known the gravity of the recovery I was facing post-surgery, I might have been singing another tune!

When I was wheeled into the pre-surgery room, I talked to the kind surgeon. He explained that I would need a full hip replacement on my left hip due to the break. I was all by myself, as Syris was at work.

As I lay immobilized and frightened in bed waiting for surgery, the surgeon came back in to talk to me. He expressed that he also detected a faint hole in my right femur due to bone metastasis. He suggested, since I already would be going through the pain of surgery, that it would be wise to insert a titanium rod from the top of my right femur to my knee to stabilize my right side and prevent it from breaking in the future. He suggested that it was smart to do it now as, most likely, I would have to do it in the future. Why endure two surgeries when I could get it all done at once? He said it would be a hard recovery, but the benefit would be that I could endure all the pain at the same time.

WHAT THE FUCK?

I was completely freaked out.

An extremely compassionate nurse spoke to me and listened to my tears and fears. I called both Syris and Willow, crying and asking them what I should do. It was comforting to talk to both of them during this traumatic time.

I decided to go ahead and do it.

In retrospect, it was a good thing that I didn't know I would be enduring double hip surgery. When most people go through hip replacement surgery, they plan it months before. Usually, classes and educational presentations are attended to understand how to optimally heal post-surgery. I had none of that. One day I was dealing with a massive amount of pain daily. The next day, I was in the emergency room being wheeled into major surgery.

The surgeon told me that my left hip had actually been broken for a month, and I had no idea! No wonder I was dealing with so much pain daily.

The long road to recovery began.

As usual, I found my way to work with the challenge with a dose of humor. Humor was my coping mechanism during the most difficult moments.

*Due to the intensity of this time post hip surgery, I have decided to share the raw posts from this time as they capture the difficult reality of this time. While it pushed me to the edge of my mental and physical capacity, I also found a resilience within myself that I didn't know I possessed before.

11/3:

Oh, for the kindness of strangers! Having emergency hip surgery this week has turned my life totally upside down. I just had a conversation with a nurse about her experience going through breast cancer. By the end of our conversation, I had tears in my eyes at the incredible kindness of her soul. She radiated exactly the kind of positivity I needed to hear. It's been tough this week to be contained in a hospital bed day after day by myself alone with just my thoughts while dealing with extreme limitations in my body. This angel lifted me up and helped me feel less alone. She knows the demons I face every day with having a cancer diagnosis.

Thank you, dear angel nurse, for blessing me with your message of finding humor, going forward, and focusing on the positive outcome.

11/4:

The first days after receiving hip surgery were spent in a high level of pain. Morphine was my best buddy. Now I'm learning to walk again. Day by day, I pushed myself a bit farther, and today, I'm getting in and out of bed by myself, getting to the toilet by myself (BIG accomplishment!), and taking walks down the hospital hallway. I'm elated to be finding my mobility again!

I thought I would go to a rehab center in Oahu for a week, but I was recently told I wouldn't be admitted, as I've already surpassed expectations for how fast I would heal. The doctors are all blown away by how fast I'm healing, and, most likely, I'll go home tomorrow. Yay!

I'm very aware I have to take it super easy and curb my tendency to do too much. I plan to line up a crew of fabulous friends and family to help me during this time. I'm told I won't be able to drive for 6 weeks, but we shall see about that!

I'm so appreciative of the laughter and warm aloha I'm receiving from the staff here.

Next week: a marathon!

11/5:

Today, I left the hospital. Breathing fresh air has never been so exciting!

I'm super grateful for my dear cousin Laura, who has been an amazing support for me during this crazy week after breaking my hip! Lovely Laura scooped me up, helped me gather a walker and other tools needed for my recovery, shopped for food, settled me at home, and has been such a comfort during this stressful time.

A huge lesson of this cancer journey has been to learn to receive and ask for help. In the past three years I've learned this lesson repeatedly. Now, I'm recovering from a massive double-hip surgery and am stripped of all my independent, stubborn "I must do it all by myself" egoic self. What a gift it is to learn that I'm valuable enough to receive help and that others want to give it! It's ironic, as I was always the giver; now I'm stripped down to the raw state of having to learn to receive. This is really a blessing in disguise.

Other kind friends visited me at the hospital which was an immense help for my psychological healing. Gifts, flowers, deep conversations, healing sessions, food, medicine, and so much love were shared. I'm blessed with so many loving friends and family surrounding me. This week has been challenging but my heart is so full of all the kindness pouring down upon me. I'm certainly not alone. The healing power of LOVE and community is strong!

11/7:

I'm home! The escape from the hospital went smashingly well! Joking. I was told I was sufficiently healed enough post double-hip surgery to go home for my recovery there.

Day by day, I'll learn to walk again sans walker. I realize the universe is wanting to drastically slow me down to a snail's pace. I'm seeing that I'm meant to go deep into the healing process for another level of awakening within myself. I think I'm at the bottom gate of Inanna's journey to the underworld.

Did Inanna have to give up her bones and physical competence as part of her sacrifice for wisdom and awareness?

What better way to drop me into another level of healing than to stop my energizer bunny self? I have no choice but to lie still. This time of quiet and reflection is necessary for my hips to grow tendons and ligaments to support my new titanium superhero self. I will rise again, like the phoenix from the ashes!

I'm super grateful to just be alive! It's hard to deal with the pain post-surgery, limited to a bed, completely dependent on others, and shuffling with a walker, but I know this is just temporary. In fact, maybe the whole process of getting a new hip and titanium rod in the big picture is to help me feel less pain and have more agility overall?

Let the shuffling commence. This requires great perseverance and patience.

THE POWER OF THE MIND:

Being bed bound was extremely challenging for me, as I was a go getter and doer. I had to cultivate a huge amount of patience to be able to endure the healing I faced.

My long-time Kaua'i friend Richard Diamond stepped up to help me by visiting me a few times while I was stuck in bed. He thankfully reminded me of the powerful work of Joe Dispenza.

Joe Dispenza is the author of *You Are the Placebo* and other groundbreaking books. When he was twenty-three, he was run over by a SUV while competing in a triathlon event in Palm Springs, CA. The accident left him with six broken vertebrae. He decided against going through the high-risk surgeries and focused on philosophical inner healing. Miraculously, he had a full recovery from his healing!

I had known about Joe's work in the past through reading some of his books and listening to his meditations. Richard reminded me about the innate power of my mind to transcend a difficult situation. He helped me to see that even though I was bed bound, I would find my way through the hellish situation. It was up to me see beyond the limiting perspective of my mind that yearned to be running free rather than chained to a bed. He reminded me that I would be okay. As soon as I grasped onto this perspective, the reality of being jacked up on painkillers, having a hard time even making it to the bathroom, not able to run wild with my animals, and being dependent on everyone else for my food and transportation needs was a bit easier. I was incredibly grateful to be reminded of this peaceful pathway through the maelstrom of my mind!

While I was doped up on painkillers, the web that connected Syris and me was actively being pulled apart. We had survived my three-year journey with cancer, dealt with losing the ranch, moved 2,500 miles away from California to Hawaii, but the deep dive into chemotherapy and then breaking my hip felt like the last straw that broke our relationship.

Without going into personal details, as I truly do respect Syris and how he showed up through the roughest moments, I'll just say we reached a crossroads. It was apparent that it was time for us to go our own separate ways. It was horrible timing, seeing how I was chained to my bed and enduring the most challenging time in my life. But perhaps this was the perfect timing to make the dramatic shift that was necessary.

It was difficult, but, apparently, it was part of the medicine for my growth.

CRAWLING OUT OF THE CAVE:

I was slowly becoming more mobile! My brother Ted and his wife Renee generously came to Kaua'i to help me move things back into the yurt after the mold removal and renovation. During this time, I was elated to get out of the house, walker in hand to participate in my Hawaiian teacher's event. It was a special workshop to learn how to create our own ceremonial Kihei.

11/17:

I did something creative and fun today! It's been almost three weeks post double-hip surgery. After being cooped up in the hospital for a week, in bed covered with ice for two weeks, only getting out of bed for doctors' visits and hobbling around the house, I was in sheer bliss to attend my Hawaiian teacher's Kihei-making class today! I'm fortunate to attend a class about Hawaiian culture and spirituality at Studio HA'A from the wise and wonderful Kumu Kehaulani Kekua.

We all made Kihei, a traditional Hawaiian garment intended for sacred ceremony. We learned of the art form known as, Lau Kapala, and used native Hawaiian healing plants such as, Ti and Kukui Nut leaves to make prints on our cloth. I will attend a ceremony at the end of the month where I will use this sacred print.

Art is so healing, and it was wonderful to be out in the world again after being in my healing bubble.

It's such a balance to be present to the process of healing. I'm finding that too much time by myself makes me a bit stir crazy, as community is so important to me. Although, if I spend too much time in the world, I lose my own inner balance at times.

Grateful
Heart full
To feel part of something bigger than myself is extremely fulfilling.

Being able to attend this Hawaiian event felt like a gentle ascension from the depths of Inanna's cave.

11/19:

Healing takes time, presence, and patience! The physical therapist came today and said I can slowly transition to a cane, which is exciting! It's such a bizarre feeling to experience bones, tendons, and ligaments coming back together again. Sometimes, I feel a deep ache from the inside of my bones. The process of healing is getting easier. I'm patiently doing my PT exercises through the rain and all the variables of the tempestuous Kaua'i weather.

I'm almost ready to move back into the yurt, which I'm so happy about! It will be so good to be in my cozy mold-free nest.

I'm now staying by myself at nights. I've graduated to a higher level of self-care. I'm grateful for any level of independence I'm able to manage now. Ice bags are my new best friend.

So, it goes, cultivating seeds of patience as the bones knit, telling tales of future leaps and bounds and adventures yet to be had. I see myself dancing forever free on the beach.

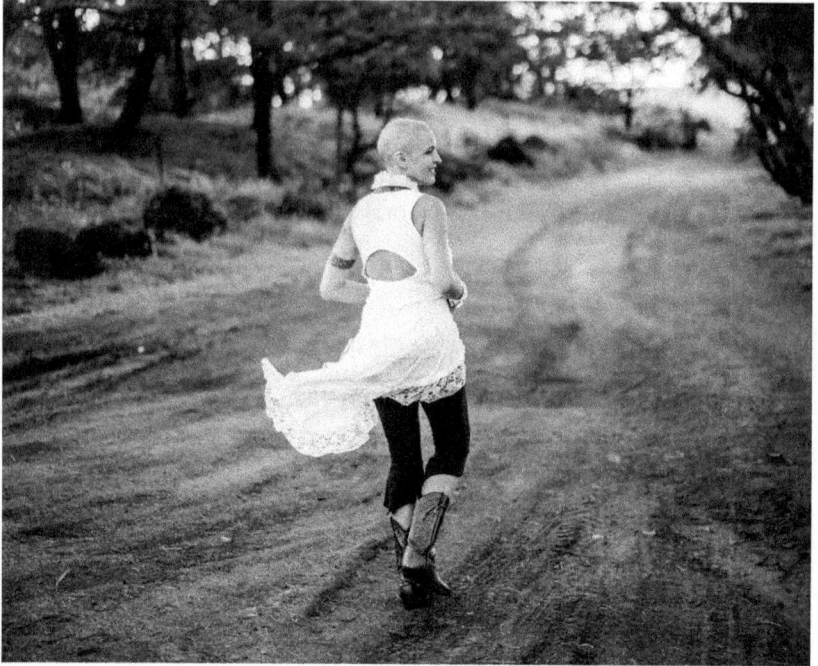

Photo by Bradyhouse Photographers

Breaking up with Syris merely weeks post hip surgery was dreadful. I constantly rode that fine line of allowing myself to feel the grief and not falling into a mental space of feeling sorry for myself.

Inanna continued on with her descent to the underworld. It was another symbol of letting go of Inanna's regalia by releasing the relationship with Syris.

I felt stripped of everything I held dear in order to be reborn again. My closest friend Deb died, Rowen passed soon after, my hair was gone, my ranch was sold, two horses were left behind, my partner was gone, my body has been altered, broken, bent, and now was healing. To find the source of light it was necessary for me to surrender completely to the dark.

My motto was: *"Inanna was born again and so will I, teal boots and all."*

***

It was a crazy time between the mold outbreak, break-up, and double hip surgery. I hadn't lived in my yurt due to the necessary renovation for two months. When it was time to move in, I was elated to be finally going back home to practically a brand-new yurt. Oh joy!

The 30-foot Pacific Yurt I lived in was put up in 1994 and was in a fairly rough state when I arrived in January 2019. As I was teetering on the edge of death then, the simple, dingy interior didn't really bother me. I was used to its worn-out state and it was home to me. The self-enforced remediation was exactly what it needed to make it a lovely living space. After twenty-five years, it was inevitable that a fancy tent in the tropics would become funkified!

11/22:

And just like that the clouds clear, the sun peeks out from the clouds, and life is flooded with its staggering, breathtaking beauty!

It seems like when the shit hits the fan it just means that brighter times, clarity, and resolution are on their way.

Time to celebrate! I'm moving back into my yurt today! It's been two months of being out of my cozy nest due to an unfortunate mold outbreak.

Best news of all! Many of you have been asking me about my writing project. "Tara, when are you going to write your book?" Well, I've found a fabulous online program called Self-Publishing School that will provide a structure to help me piece together all my years of blog posts and social media material to create an awesome life-affirming book. I hope it can help to bring hope, faith, and courage to others on the cancer journey and those facing difficult times. The most important element of what I want to share revolves around making peace and facing fear about death. (That book announcement was the seed of what you, dear reader, are holding in your hand!)

There are endless gems to be mined when fears are faced, and shadows are transformed to manifest the ultimate lessons of self-growth.

Keep shining through the rain, sleet and snow, and I promise the sun will come out again.

BRING IN THE COLOR!

When I finally started growing a bit of hair, I decided to have some fun with it and put some red color in. It was truly a joy to see the little peach ball patches of hair starting to come in again! My cousin called it "deer fuzz." Putting a dash of color in my hair was a way to reclaim what I had given up during the sacrifice of all my metaphorical Inanna regalia. I had given up my hair, but, at least, I could bring in some color with the little bit of fuzzy tufts I had!

BREAK UP CHRONICLES 1:

I was still processing the break-up between Syris and I. This poem says it all:

11/27:

Break-ups can be tough.
The tenderness of the human heart.
The instinctual push and pull that inevitably unfolds.

Taking one step forward in the effort to move on and forget,
staying positive, and seeing beyond the pain.

Then stepping back and remembering the love, laughter,
joy, and beauty.
It's a dance, this separation game.
Being grateful for the time shared.
Pissed off for the wounds inflicted.

What is truly real?
What is me?
What is a projection?
What is my own distorted version of the truth seen through
the wounded child's eyes?

There is the reality of going through a separation while on
social media.
The childish notion of "blocking" another in the effort to
wound, sever the ties, and lash out in blame.
As if blocking your beloved on Facebook is the end of the
world?
Might be to some.
Is this high school enacted all over again?

The sun still rises, yet with another view.

There are the friends that tell you to date.
What?
I'm all for living life and having fun, but this is a sacred time
of remembrance.
This is a time of grieving what was lost.
This is a time to be grateful I don't have to deal with the shit
that frustrated me for years!
There is much to explore in this Tara world.
I intend to mine the gems from this moment!

Bones knitting together,
Heart healing,
Cancer dissipating,
Just watch me fly!

This is all material to fuel the fire of growth,
Purify my heart,
Make me stronger,
And grow my capacity to love!

ATTITUDE OF GRATITUDE:

Staying positive and finding the good in every situation was a huge part of me getting through adversity. While recovering from major surgery, every little accomplishment was a huge victory.

Americans possess a great love of driving as it's such an expression of freedom. Being able to drive again post surgery was an exciting step to reclaiming my independence!

11/28:

I'm driving! There's so much to celebrate. After having a double hip surgery one month ago and being totally dependent on others, I'm jubilant to be gaining more mobility every day!

As it's Thanksgiving season, I'm thankful for this celebratory list:

- Walking: I've transitioned from shuffling with a walker to Frida, my beloved teal cane. Sometimes I even walk without the cane now! This is a big deal. Bye bye Johnny Walker!

- Driving: The ability to shop and make simple foods for myself.

- All the friends and family who stepped up for me this month to help me with things such as: dog walking, rides, food, house cleaning, juice, holding my hand through the tears and fears, moving, and so much more.

I wouldn't have chosen to break my hip and to undergo such a drastic transformation, but the gifts are limitless. I'm appreciative for the lessons of stillness, patience, and perseverance that I've learned. It makes the reemergence back to life all the sweeter!

12/2:

The reality of recovering from a double hip surgery is that it takes great stamina and patience to heal post-surgery. Tight muscles scream as they're stretched to their limit.

Bones, tendons, and ligaments knit together again, striving to make sense of the new titanium hardware in the body.

Walking is becoming easier each day. I'm still dependent on pain killers. This surgery was quite drastic with two hips done at once. I'm not the simple hip replacement candidate. I was warned that it was unknown how I would heal, but that hopefully it would bring long term relief and greater stability.

I keep going. My walker has been returned. I'm using Frida the cane less and less. I'm taking a plethora of bone building supplements to aid in the internal healing of my body.

I'm starting chemo again on Tuesday after a six-week break. I'm nervous to start up again with the combination of my hips still healing and then adding chemo on top of it. I know I'll be okay, but still it's a lot. Deep breath, Tara.

I take comfort in the belief that I'll get through this. Four or five more rounds of chemo to go. I'm close to the finish line and showing up for each moment the best I can.

It's important to stretch and move my body beyond its limitations but not go too far. If I do too much, I'm in pain the next day. There are so many lessons to be learned!

Tender is the body; tender is the heart. What a journey it is, being a spiritual being in a human body. Thank you, sacred body, for teaching me what it is to be vulnerable and alive. I'm showing up and listening.

BACK TO CHEMOLANDIA:

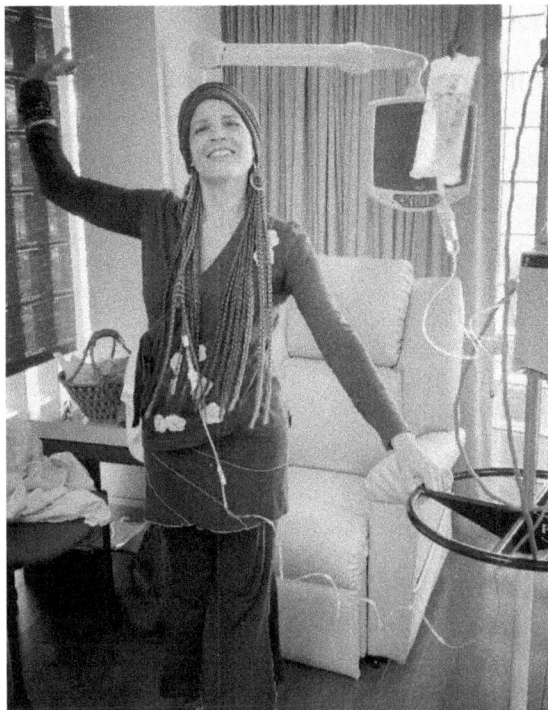

My pole dancing debut!

12/4:

My dancing partner is back! After a six-week break of no chemo, I'm blissful to be reunited with my dancing partner again. (Joking!) Let's just say I'm in acceptance of what's necessary.

This is what I wrote early yesterday am: "I can't sleep. It's 5:45 a.m. I'm restarting chemo again today and I'm nervous. It's like I'm willingly submitting myself to the boiling vats of hell in order to go through massive transformation. It's like Inanna who knew it was necessary to travel to the underworld in order to grasp the tiny tendril of life she held dear. Life is worth it. It's scarier than shit, though!

It takes time for the effects to hit. Surrender is necessary. There's no holding onto what's safe, as control is a total illusion. The best thing is to let go and enjoy the ride the best I can, even if it means I feel like crap. If this is what it takes to claim my life, I'm all in! No one said it would be a cake walk, but there are certainly brilliant rewards along the way. Here I go down the rabbit hole again."

12/7:

There's a kitty curling around my foot observing me as I recover from the effects of chemo. Taxol worked me pretty hard the last two days. The usual body pains I experience from the side effects of chemo were amplified due to the double-hip surgery I went through six weeks ago. My resilience was certainly tested last night as the pain killers didn't sufficiently chill the pain.

Ice,
Oxycodone,
Advil PM,
CBD/THC,
Brilliant, loving friend Kim, whom I called at 2:30 AM Hawaii time/8:30 AM Florida time,
A half-wilted apple banana, and
A leopard-colored cat
All got me through.

Riding the waves

The pain has passed, and I'm left with gratitude that the worst has passed. The talented, healing hands of Michelle connected my severed body through a nurturing massage.

Finding the breath,

Enjoying my space,
Defending and defining the lines of who I am after post break up spaciousness,
Let it be known that I'm happy now to be on my own.
It's easy to be in my own head with much less drama and no one to argue with.
I'm creating my own reality, moment to moment, without anyone else to worry about.
Total and complete self-love.
Aloha Mā.

Finding simple satisfaction with a feline friend contentedly purring while wrapped around my foot, mermaid toenail polish and all.

BREAK-UP CHRONICLES 2:

Processing the break-up continued. Writing has always been a cathartic way to process the deep emotions and I was grateful to have the outlet of social media to let it move on through.

12/8:

Words can hurt,
Daggers to the heart.
Seems that, with all the miles walked, moments shared, and obstacles overcome, parting with love is possible?
Why must it be downgraded to angry, spiteful words cascading out with the attempt to harm, to inflict the same pain that is felt?

I guess it just represents the space of mind, the reflection of the wounded self, unhealed trauma lashing out with a dragon forked tongue spitting fire in every direction.

I stand in my vulnerability, recognizing that I'm doing my best, as is he.
I retreat into my safe place, knowing that, ultimately, my healing is the most important thing, and harsh words are just an expression of the wounded boy.
It's not me.
It's a reflection of the pain felt in him.
Still, it hurts.
I acknowledge it and let it go,
Tears rolling off the back of dragon flesh,
Raw, scaly, green, and rough.

I will transcend this fire.

HORSE MAGIC:

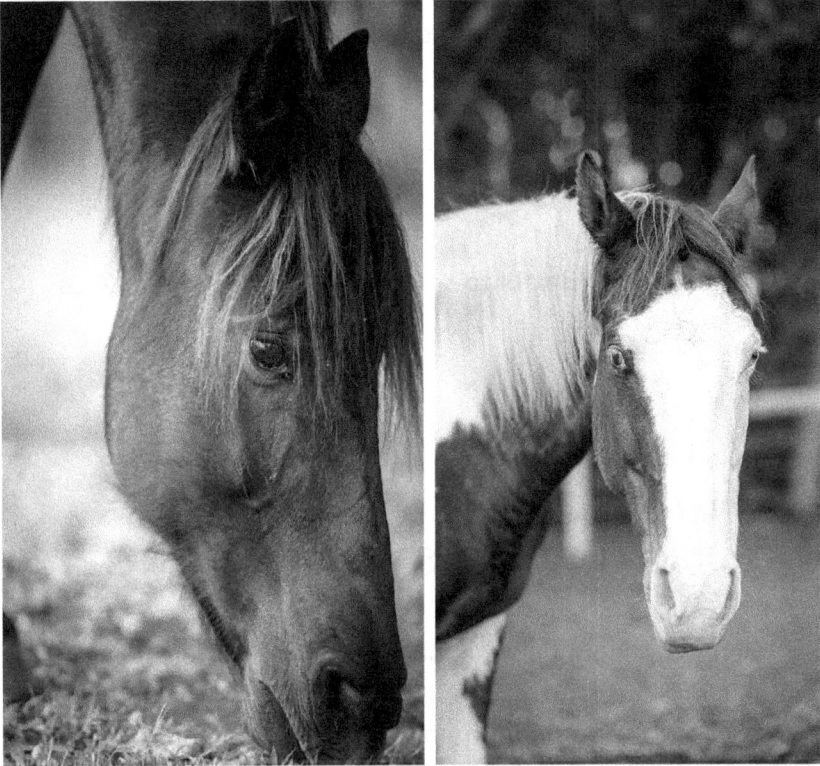

Comanche & Blue - Photo by Kalalea Photography

12/13:

Due to my double hip surgery, I haven't seen my horses for almost two months! That's an absurdly long time for a horsewoman to not see her beloved beasts!

My two horses roam free on over eighty acres, which is horse heaven for them. This means I either have to walk far to see them or wait patiently till they come to me. As I'm not walking so far these days, I was ecstatic that they voluntarily came to visit me at the yurt!

It was a complete JOY and surprise to see my fuzzy equine friends today. I miss them so much! I've been dreaming of resuming the Equine Facilitated Learning work I do, as it fills my heart with joy. It's truly profound and a remarkable honor to witness how horses help to transform human consciousness with their wise presence. My greatest hope is to continue this work.

For now, I'm thankful to share space with the herd. Such beauty to behold.

Love,
The horse-crazy girl

DATING WITH STAGE 4 CANCER

Here's a seldom talked about possibly HOT topic! Cancer, relationships, and dating. I've been out of my four-year relationship for a month now. To be transparent, I'm truly enjoying my solo time and giving myself space to grieve my relationship. It's fascinating to see how the mind works as I catch my subconscious self "looking" for another to fill the space that my beloved filled. I'm watching the impulses and staying as conscious to what my authentic self desires.

The truth is I love my own company, and it's much easier to be in my own head rather than wrestling with the frustrations that were abundant in my past relationship. No matter how hard I tried to find a solution, the same darn issues stuck like glue. Sometimes, I feel moments of loneliness, but that's natural. I'm blessed with a plethora of family and friends on Kaua'i.

I have some friends urging me to date. I wonder, what's the hurry? What's wrong with me taking time to decompress and heal from my past relationship? I'm not ready to navigate the depths of another relationship. It's a gift to have solo time, and I truly want to enjoy it! I'm aware that it's necessary to be present with the process of untangling the roots that Syris and I wove together. It's a heroine's journey to come back to oneself again.

I realize the friends encouraging me to jump back into the dating pool right away are coming from a place of caring and concern, but they have no idea what it's like healing from double-hip surgery and still completing chemo! Perhaps they're afraid to reside in their own company; therefore, they're urging me to find a replacement right away. Humans easily project their own personal issues upon others.

Then I wonder, who would date someone with a stage 4 cancer diagnosis anyways? I've been asking my friends this question as I'm curious to know what others think. It's brought up some fascinating points.

I would think a potential partner would be hesitant to get to know and date someone with a serious diagnosis. The reality is it takes courage to be vulnerable and open one's heart in general. If a partner is dating someone with a life-threatening diagnosis, there's a higher probability of loss than if they had no cancer diagnosis. Then again, no one is guaranteed everlasting life! As a friend pointed out, I could fall in love and lose my lover in a sudden car accident leaving me alone and still standing with stage 4 cancer.

If I personally were considering dating someone with stage 4 cancer, I would be open to it if I felt in alignment with the person. I would also be cautious, as I've already seen so many dear friends die from cancer. I would continue to remind myself that all we truly have is the present moment.

VICTORY
CONQUERING THE STAIRS!

I was slowly healing. It was a full-time job to adapt to my new post-surgery body. I had to keep stretching, do physical therapy, and constantly pay attention to my surroundings so I didn't re-injure myself. It required being extra vigilant. Around this time, I vanquished the stairs!

Undergoing a major surgery has gifted me with a fresh perspective about the things I always took for granted before.

12/17:

I never knew stairs could be so scary! This last week I've overcome my recent stair trepidation, as I had to walk up two long staircases. After double-hip surgery, stairs can be pretty terrifying with the necessary bending and strength required to propel you forward. Two weeks ago, I wasn't prepared for a long staircase. After walking up and down one, I endured days of pain. As of this week, I'm happy to say my body has healed sufficiently so stairs are doable!

It's important to celebrate the accomplishments however simple they may be. Onward and upward!

12/20:

In every moment, this path requires mighty perseverance and dedication. We cancer journeyers hit our edges at times.

The daily endless duties necessary to stay alive and heal the cancer bug is exhausting. I see it on other people's social media threads and empathize. There's no stepping back; it requires a razor's-edge vigilance to keep going.

Today, during my weekly vitamin and mineral infusion (IV) my doctor hit a nerve when injecting the needle. I'm usually a pretty tough cookie, but the pain was so intense I had big elephant tears rolling down my face. I didn't find relief till she took the needle out.

Keep going. Find the middle path, the way of least resistance. Keep rising above adversity. Some blessed days, everything works out perfectly and is easy. Other days, I feel like I'm as sensitive as a delicate glass sculpture and will shatter with the slightest touch.

In many ways, we're gifted to receive these lessons. Turn the challenges around to find the wisdom. If you can't find it, take the day off and curl up in bed. This too shall pass.

BREAK UP CHRONICLES 3:

12/21:

Last night was an invitation to travel into the depths of my shadows. Going through a breakup is a stellar chance to do inner work, though it's definitely not an easy one!

There's the wish to avoid the work. How can I distract myself? Often behavior such as shopping, food, being busy, drugs, alcohol, another possible partner, too much screen time and other addictive patterns are tempting to fall into. It's easy to avoid the opportunity for personal growth after a break-up. Many choose to not look at their personal patterns that contributed to the separation. Projecting blame on another is a common evasive approach.

Last night, I was looking at break up books online and discovered I had one in my Kindle from when my husband and I split six years ago. Lo and behold, everything I'm feeling is normal! It's nice to be validated for all the emotions I'm experiencing. Part of me feels like hiding and the other part of me doesn't give a fuck.

I'm aware of the massive amount of inner work I have to do during this sacred time, and I plan to do it! This is a great opportunity to reassess and look at similar themes that keep showing up in my relationships since I was a teenager. I refuse to slap on sticky layers of duct tape around my heart and pretend everything is okay. I intend to take this time to discover the wounded Tara I carry around from childhood. I will bravely puncture the veil of duality within myself. I will stop running away from the shadows that cloud my vision and boldly face them! It's time to date myself and give myself all the love and self-care that I've been desiring to receive from another. I will cherish this divine body, soul, and heart I've been given.

What else is there to do on the healing journey?

GRACE, GRIT AND GRATITUDE:

12/22:

The path of grit: I recently told a beloved friend who was exasperated about how difficult it is to have a stage 4 cancer diagnosis that we're like diamonds in the rough. It takes an extreme amount of pressure to create a diamond. This is what those of us dealing with a life-threatening diagnosis are dealing with daily.

Witnessing our bodies going through the side effects of cancer and cancer treatments is a daily roller coaster. In the last two months I had to learn to walk again after double-hip surgery; I'm ecstatic to say I've gone out dancing twice this week! This doesn't come easily, though. Each day, I battle with doubt in my mind that tries to remind me of my limitations.

I honestly don't even want to write down the doubtful thoughts, as that would give them power.

The truth is the cancer thriver friends I know walking this path are the bravest ones I know. To keep continuing forward with a positive attitude when a possible death sentence hangs over your head takes tremendous courage. Society is full of fear, stigma, and dread when it comes to the topic of cancer. It can be rough to be in one's mind with these daily thoughts, let alone handling the negative projections of others!

The reactions I receive when I'm asked why my hip broke are quite surprising and shocking! People generally have a stunned look on their face and don't know how to react when I tell them my hip broke from bone metastasis.

My thoughts are powerful. I have the ability to create my reality in every moment. Every day, I choose to see myself thriving with stage 4 cancer.

I'm not saying that just "thinking" alone will change one's health outcome, but it has been documented that the people who visualize themselves as healing are more likely to receive better medical results than those who believe they're doomed to die.

The medical community is starting to see having stage 4 cancer as living with a chronic illness rather than a death sentence.

We can rewrite the paradigm. It's possible to keep going, face our fears, and jump over each continual hurdle, even when life threatens to crumble the precious ship of our soul. It's possible to rewrite the story. Cancer doesn't have to be a death sentence!

Every breath you take,
Every thought you think is creating your future reality.
And if death is the final outcome, there's beauty in that too.
The final frontier.
Keep going.
Don't give up.

RETURN OF THE PRODIGAL SON:

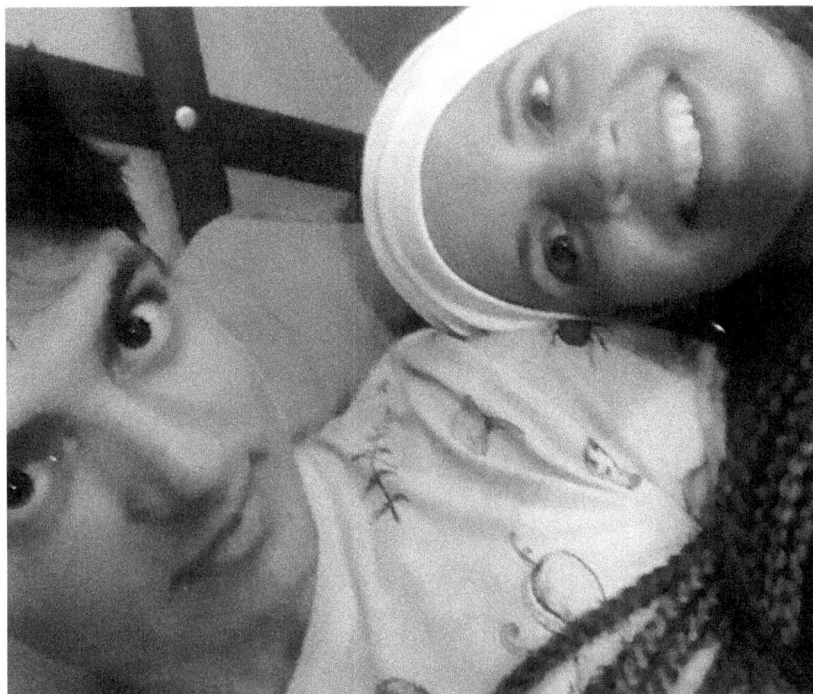

I was fortunate to have Willow come visit me for a short time during the holiday break.

12/23:

And my tall son arrives bringing light and levity on the heroine's path. For six golden days, I get to be with my brilliant boy. Yay!

Tomorrow morning (Xmas eve), I resume chemotherapy again. I have FOUR more rounds till I'm done! I'm thrilled to feel hope. It's been a major journey since I started chemo in May of this year. I'm ecstatic to be finished by the end of January or early February!

I'm feeling great overall, functioning normally, and walking without a cane. I'm very optimistic about my future. I've got exciting ideas brewing that give me hope about helping others through the grueling parts of this path. I'm just grateful to be alive!

The best gift of all is to see my son during the holiday season. Though I'm generally optimistic, it hasn't been easy. Having my Willow sprout here eases the intensity and helps root me back in my heart again.

12/30:

I'm crazy grateful for my cherished son and all he brings to my life. I had him at a young age, so we pretty much grew up together. I didn't know who I was when I had him. I knew I loved to dance, loved art, nature, the Grateful Dead, horses, writing, and Kaua'i.

I was a wild young hippy momma, moving her tow-headed baby around the world as we explored the cracks of our existence. I was reluctant to settle down, so we ended up moving every two years or so. By the time Willow reached high school, I realized that he desired firm roots in the ground and wasn't too fond of our bohemian lifestyle, so I decided that Willow would finish school in one location. That chosen location was Fairfax, California, where he had already spent four years in elementary school.

Now Willow is all grown up. He's a brilliant leader in the science community and getting his PhD in biochemistry. Can you say, "Smart"? He works his tush off and has accomplished feats beyond most kids his age. This momma is proud!

His life hasn't been easy. I raised him mostly as a single mom. His dad is one of those sperm-donor deadbeat dads with six kids who range in age from eight to thirty-two. I knew when I chose to birth Willow that I would most likely raise him on my own, but I had no idea how hard it would be. For the most part, he was an easy kid, and that was a divine blessing!

I feel compassion for him as both his mother and grandma are going through treatment for stage 4 cancer. I know it must be frightening. He's a deep, sensitive, and caring soul.

I have great respect for Willow's ability to keep going through adversity, finding opportunity within the challenges, and not giving up when times are tough.

Thanks for being my sidekick in this lifetime, Willow. Your momma loves you so!

2020

DANCE!

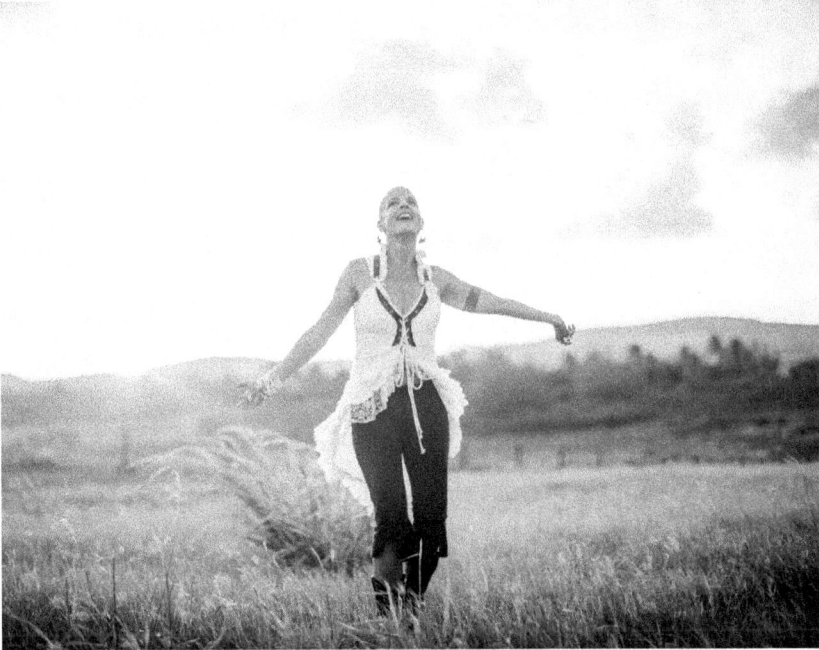

Photo by Bradyhouse Photographers

Dance is its own form of communication. Ever since I was a child, movement has been a healing tool of self-expression for me. Freedom of expression is my own version of bliss.

When Syris and I packed up to move to Kaua'i and my health was spiraling down, I let go of the magic of dance. I was just trying to survive and keep my head above water. Before I started chemotherapy, I went out dancing a few times on Kaua'i. Once I started treatment, my life was relegated to just making it to the next appointment.

January 2020 was my last month of chemotherapy. It had been eight months of wading through the heavy mud of the medicine, breaking my hip, dealing with mold, a break-up, and the trials of life. My goal to make it through the last month of treatment was to video myself doing one dancing video a day on Instagram stories. This practice would hold me accountable to my dancing practice and help me ride the waves of the rough moments. I called it #DancingForHope.

I even did a dance video with a chemotherapy infusion pole while I was getting a chemo treatment that went viral on all my social media pages! I called it "a pole dance."

The #DancingForHope practice was wonderfully healing and a joy to partake in. It was my way to proclaim that I WAS ALIVE and to celebrate all that I had come through. I was casting out the shadows and reclaiming my full expressive self again!

Another purpose for creating the #DancingForHope idea was to inspire others to work through their blocks, insecurities, and inhibitions through movement. I wanted to encourage others to fully embody themselves through dance in the way I found it liberating. I recognized that others might not be so brave to post a video of themselves dancing, but I encouraged them to step outside their comfort zone to at least try it. I encouraged people to just dance, move their body, and embody that creative part within themselves that often is caught up in fearful limitations.

It was exciting to see all the people who participated in #DancingForHope around the globe! I got a kick out of watching cancer thrivers and others film videos of themselves dancing in faraway countries such as Brazil and Australia!

As I got closer to finishing chemotherapy and saw encouraging signs that the treatment was working, it felt like my wings were expanding to find a new sense of freedom and joy.

***

I spent New Year's Eve going into 2020 calling in all that I wished to manifest the following year while dancing:

1/1:

Adios 2019! Aloha 2020! I danced harder and longer tonight then I have for months. For three hours I morphed my body into intuitive shapes moving and grooving to the beat as my mind freed itself from the limiting constructs of ego. I let go of a month's worth of frustrating limitations and self-imposed mental paradigms. I had so much fun!

I released the struggle of moving, dealing with mold remediation, breaking my hip, double-hip surgery, the immense strength and patience it took to learn to walk again, chemotherapy treatments, the tumultuous painful breakup, and the pain and shock of my dear momma being diagnosed with stage 4 cancer. I let go of all the unreleased shit through maniacal wild dancing, bare feet pounding the ground, and didn't stop until my body screamed for rest.

AWARENESS:

The truth about living with a stage 4 cancer diagnosis is:

- You never know how much time you have left to live. You plant your feet firmly into the ground and affirm life while, at the same time, making peace with death.

- This reality of accepting your death is a profound gift to understand how precious life is.

- You come to accept pain as part of the daily process of being alive. Discomfort in the body is normal and the everyday reality. "Quality of Life" means to focus on how to manage the pain and enjoy your life.

- The reality of loving and appreciating your friends and family takes precedence over drama and petty disagreements, as you realize your days with them may be numbered. Appreciation is more important than discordance.

- Acts of kindness and generosity take on a significant importance, as you have a profound understanding of the sacredness of each breath.

- Important life accomplishments (like finishing this book!) become crucial to complete when the clock is ticking loudly above your head. At the same time, you have a deep acceptance, surrender, and understanding that, in the big picture, pushing yourself to achieve doesn't really matter.

- Understanding sacred, spiritual information and what it truly means to be alive suddenly makes sense. This is hard-won wisdom.

- You would sacrifice your soul to prevent the pain of what you most dread, leaving behind your loved ones with your possible death. The thought of causing your beloved friends, family, and, especially, your golden children pain with your death is heartbreaking.

- Tears flow easily when touched by the hand of death. How can you not cry at the simple beauty of life?

I share in the hopes that others can understand some of what us stage 4 cancer journeyers go through. Sadly, there are many of us walking with a serious cancer diagnosis and there will be many more. Cancer is a reflection of our toxic environment.

Life is short, live large!

Please don't waste a moment.

NEARING THE FINISH LINE:

1/6:

Tomorrow I do another Taxol chemotherapy treatment.

I'm ready to be done with these treatments, but I will hang in there till I know I'm done. The last time I received treatment, my hip was too painful post hip surgery, and my compassionate oncologist told me I could take a break. My hips are healing considerably well, so I'm hoping the pain will be easier this time.

It's like being in the Boston Marathon, knowing the race is almost over, but there's still Heartbreak Hill to climb. I'm on that hill and determined to finish, yet I'm listening to the limitations of my body. I can only handle so much. I think my bone marrow and body are tired of being poked, prodded, and given a gazillion different medicines in the name of healing.

I'm inspired to live! I don't know how much time I have left on Earth. I hope my life far exceeds my fiftieth birthday, but I have no idea. (Does anyone ever?) I've been surrounded by so much death that part of me expects to die at a young age, but the other part of me believes in the possibility that I can defy conventional medicine's predictions of how long I will live. I believe in miracles and have been steeped in the work of Dr. Joe Dispenza. I know radical remission is possible! It takes GREAT FAITH to believe that, even with the diagnosis of cancer in my breast, liver, lungs, bones, and adrenal glands, I can live. I'm going to give it all I got!

I have a mission I want to accomplish while I'm here, and I'm putting the pieces together to bring it into fruition. Maybe this is why I barely escaped death this summer? Maybe I've been given a precious gift that hopefully will help others find faith and courage while journeying with cancer? I truly hope that my message can help others, as there's potent material for growth here.

Great wisdom and beauty are born from pain.
Don't push away the lessons that strive to melt away the inhibitions.
All that you struggle with is meant to make you whole.

Embrace the pain.
Be brave enough to look at the fear that threatens to capsize your reality.
Question your beliefs.
The world is waiting for you.

1/8:

I Faced major FEAR this week:

F - False
E - Evidence
A - Appearing
R – Real

There was a new oncologist at Wilcox Hospital. I felt incredible trepidation about meeting him. When I lived in Grass Valley, CA, I experienced terrible manipulation, threatening and unprofessional behavior from the oncology department. My general experience at Wilcox has been vastly different and I have felt the aloha spirit in every doctor and nurse I've met here.

When I met the new oncologist, I was pleasantly surprised! He is highly intelligent, offering me explanations and new ideas I hadn't heard before. He was caring, loving and took his time with me. He told me he's a straight shooter and he said that with my current situation, test results, and his approach I have many years left to live. Those were musical words to hear! I think he's the perfect new oncologist for me considering I'm soon to finish treatment.

I have three more rounds of Taxol, as I did one yesterday. I'm in the home stretch!

My hair is starting to flip out in all sorts of curly directions! Let me be clear, this isn't a complaint, I'm thrilled to have hair! My wacky, noncompliant hair makes me laugh.

I'm loving the practice of #DancingForHope. It's helping me get through the last treatments. It's an incredible practice to get me out of the mud puddles of my mind!

1/11:

I lie in my bathtub letting the intense Taxol waves move through me. This pain is indescribably excruciating. It feels like my body is being crushed, my bones are being mauled, my joints ache and my muscles are twisted in indescribable shapes. Thank goodness for the warm water and Epsom salts that bring soothing relief.

Last night a friend who is visiting and I went out to an event. As I hadn't done treatment for a while, I forgot that Taxol usually hits me hard on Friday evenings. The debilitating pain began when I was actually at the dance event. I retreated to my car with delirious elephant tears pouring down my face as my hips, legs, and feet were bombed by sharp needle-like pain. Fortunately, my friends Martin and Eugene talked and texted me through the spasms as I rode the waves of pain.

When I was stuck in my car during this traumatic pain episode, I couldn't even walk to tell my friend that I wanted to go. I couldn't drive. I could barely talk as the sobs and delirium took up all the space. This morning, I woke up to full-body excruciating pain. More tears. More delirium.

The chemo journey is a fucking hard road. If it's the price for life, I'll endure it. With my high tolerance of pain through giving birth, getting large tattoos on my body, and surviving double hip surgery, experiencing chemotherapy takes the cake. Even I am crushed by the immensity of it.

I'll continue to keep walking forward on this heroine's journey in the face of daunting adversity.

I think I'll stay in my bathtub all day.

1/15:

Weekly vitamin and mineral infusions dripped slowly into my veins to keep me healthy while on this chemotherapy healing regimen. I fully believe now that an integrated approach (standard and natural medicine) to healing cancer is the best method. In my case, I tried everything natural and nontoxic for two and a half years. I had endless fundraisers and spent an obscene amount of money. I was stubborn in my belief to not do any conventional medicine until I was staring death in the face. I had to decide if I was willing to die for my beliefs or choose life. My love for life, my son, and all whom I hold precious keeps me tethered to this earthly plane. I'm joyful to still be here and am doing everything in my power to thrive!

In the last year, I've gone through massive transformation through selling my beloved ranch and horse retreat center, moved back home to Kaua'i, was close to death, came to peace with allopathic medicine, let go of my four-year relationship, had to throw away many of my physical objects due to a mold outbreak, my mother received a stage 4 cancer diagnosis, I broke my hip and underwent an emergency double-hip surgery! Need I go on?

I'm honestly elated, as I feel that the worst of the storm is over and I'm finally settling into a place of ease and true happiness. Being able to dance and move again is the greatest gift. I'm dating and falling in love with myself instead of focusing on others, and I'm loving the process! I'm surrounded by so much abundance and loving friends and family who are helping me receive in an entirely new manner. I can honestly say that this is the happiest I've ever been, and I have this cancer dance to thank for it! Knowing your time is limited is an immense gift to truly wake up to what matters.

Treasure your time, friends. Life is a gift. Don't wait till you have a life-threatening diagnosis to teach you that. Celebrate and embrace each moment while you can, as you never know when your time might end.

***

The following section illustrates the deep loss of control I experienced every time I accepted the chemotherapy into my body. Like Inanna releasing what was important to her, the surrender to chemotherapy was a surrender to whatever mind worms or painful body sensations came my way.

1/17:

The slow descent into chemo land. The brain starts becoming foggy, it's like wading through cotton candy clouds that block clarity of vision. It's the ultimate lesson in letting go.

Are you trying to function normally? Not a chance. The best thing is to surrender to the exhaustion, body pain, and inability to think and function normally. To resist it just creates more pain and discomfort.

Jump on the chemo train. Pour toxic chemicals willingly into your body to kill the cancer that threatens your life. Knock out some brain cells and create early signs of aging within your body. This is what we do to live, to cling to the life we hold dear.

The Earth continues to spin. The ants go about their busy body lives accomplishing, building, and creating, but you're exempt while you're on the chemo train. Everyone understands and fears the words "cancer" and "chemotherapy," which gives you an automatic ticket to take a break from life.

Then there's the waiting for the pain and discomfort to arrive, knowing it's an inevitable part of the journey to feel the pangs of contraction as your knees, shoulders, hips, and joints are being bitten by a thousand internal fleas. You breathe through the pain until it becomes so bad you ask your friends for a magic potion to put you out of your suffering. Exhaustion comes from sitting for hours with pain. Trust in your beloved friends and family to hold your hand through the worst of the nightmare.

This is my greatest challenge. Oh, cancer, I bow down and receive these lessons with grace. Give me the strength to finish. Remind me I will dance again on the other side. This is all just temporary, a necessary initiation to stay tethered to this precious body I hold so dear.

**

Despite the hard experience of chemo, I learned brilliant lessons of wisdom when I was in the pit of the experience. To find my way out again, I had to reach into my deepest strength to find my light. These next three entries perfectly illustrate this experience:

1/18:

Chemo slams either my body or my mind hard. Last week, I was physically ground to the bone with pain. This week, it's my mind freaking out, finding the parameters of its limits.

Here comes superwoman Tara, the one who gives and shows up for others. She's the strong one, the one you can count on. She holds the weight of the world on her shoulders.

Here comes the breast cancer guru who cuts down any shred of attached ego identity. It reminds me I need to learn to ask for help and we're all dependent on one another.

I fight.
I cling to my identity.
I can do it all.
Slow down, child; you have limitations.
We're going to break your hip and throw you to the ground so you learn how to receive!

Even in the depths of chemo when my body is in pain and my brain can't function, I still stubbornly go forward determined to take responsibility for tasks that others won't follow through with. My pattern is to do it all, even at the price of my health.

Thank you, cancer guru, for your lesson of codependency. I'm stuck in the habit of trying to fill a wounded part of myself that desperately needs to learn self-care. I remain that little girl who is still searching for attention from her father. Being the eldest child, I learned about impenetrable strength. If someone told me I couldn't do something, I had to prove them wrong. I can be stubborn and oppositional to no end.

Time to let it all go.
This illusion isn't serving me anymore.
Time for vulnerability, heart healing, and self-love.
I set down my sword and retreat to my cave, humbled by these lessons.

1/19:

Dancing through a tunnel of darkness. This is taking all of my internal and external strength to keep the faith, while the demons of chemo hell poke and prod the essence of my soul with fiery hot tongs. Waking up with the physical pain of hammers slamming my knees, shoulders, and hip joints is one thing. Combine the physical pain with the mental worms that come from chemo medicine, and it's a full-on attack of your body, mind, and soul!

This is truly a hero/heroine's journey.

According to folklorists and other narrative scholars, the hero's journey forms the basic template for all great stories. Described at length in Joseph Campbell's, The Hero with a Thousand Faces, *the hero's journey serves as the tale every culture tells. The journey's path is described variously, but in general it includes the call to adventure, a supernatural aide or mentor, initiation by trials and adventures, victory, and return. Many fiction- and screen-writing courses focus on the hero's journey, and its universality can easily be seen in fairy tales and other traditional tales, as well as in such popular culture offerings as J.R.R. Tolkien's* Lord of the Rings *trilogy and George Lucas' Star Wars.*[13]

Joseph Campbell created the archetype of the hero who goes on a journey to face the daunting monsters, hairy spiders, and trolls that threaten to boil you alive. I think of all these monsters as being an example of the demons of the mind. All the myths and stories we've been raised with from Star Wars to King Arthur follow this story line. Right now, I'm in the phase where I'm beaten down and the figurative dragons continue to threaten to extinguish my precious light. Like Inanna, I am rising up from the darkness and the last of the shadows are creeping out of the cracks.

I now understand why chemo can bring the most solid person down to their knees and evoke incredible negativity. It's what petrified and prevented me from doing chemo when I was first diagnosed, as I saw the physical and emotional suffering my bestie Deb went through when she danced with leukemia.

I find myself dancing on that same razor's edge. Eugene reminded me last night in a late-night phone call that this mental struggle is normal. The physical battering of the body is much easier to endure than the darkness of the mind.

This is exactly why, in my everyday life, I'm so positive and upbeat when I'm feeling good, as I'm not struggling with these side effects. When I feel normal, I'm just grateful to be alive and feel like my regular self. I would love to step away from this medical roller coaster and constant time spent in the hall of mirrors. I yearn for a sense of regularity.

I'll keep going. The hardest part is to feel the grief from the death of my dear friends, Deb and Rowen who died young. I've cried a river of tears for their loss; yet there are more!

To show up in each moment in an authentic manner requires a profound adaptivity of the soul. To not hide, be courageous, and face whatever challenge presents itself is what it means to be alive. This isn't always easy.

1/19:

Chemo dance: As I find my way through the quagmire of this healing nectar, I wrote a piece as the pain was slamming my body. I write to transcend the pain. I write to live.

Journeying through the hall of mirrors
Deep in the chambers of my mind,
I face self-doubt, fear, insecurity, terror.
All the demons that lurk beneath the shadows rise to challenge the essence of my soul.
The criticisms of the peanut gallery ring loudly when the evils of illusion are pulled forth.

I'm just trying to make it through.
With every breath, I wade through the poison threatening to darken my soul,
Holding onto the light with all that I hold dear,
Believing in what feeds my soul,
Knowing the demons of the mind are just fear parading as authority.

The pain can wrack my body.
My bones can crumble.
My light will not be dimmed.
In every breath, there is hope.

The heart, the reality, the love of this dance is what is real. Nothing else matters.
It is all an illusion trying to dim the divine light which is LOVE.

ALOHA MĀ:

Self-care/self-love/Aloha Mā was ultimately the biggest lesson of my healing journey. There was no lack of lessons that came my way in this regard!

1/20:

The lessons of self-care and over giving. Where do I stop and you begin? I've been diving in deep to the lessons of codependency. A friend pointed out years ago that I might have work to do around it. I laughed at that notion, but, oh Nelly, I was wrong!

I'm Tara, codependent girl, big sister, single mom. My Chinese sign of the dog makes me strong and not willing to give up till I know it's necessary. My pattern is to give to others, as I get a sense of purpose for being the strong, solid one. Need something? I'm here and will move mountains to help you!

No more please! This is the time to learn the sacred art of self-love! How can I give to anyone if my cup isn't full? How does giving serve me if I'm too depleted to tend to other's needs?

This is one huge reason why this cancer dance is a huge gift. My life is on the line, so I must unapologetically give to myself lest I end up early in my grave. It took having a life-threatening diagnosis to realize this!

I share this in hopes that you realize how important it is to tend to your needs and not over-give of yourself. Be self-full! There's nothing wrong with loving yourself and giving yourself what you deserve; in fact, it's necessary for true evolution. Don't wait until a nasty diagnosis to learn this, please. You can learn it now and avoid the whole shebang!

Aloha Mā as my Ke'oni says: self-reflective love.

ALMOST DONE!

I was elated to be almost done with chemotherapy! This was a huge milestone that seemed endless to get through. The last months were the hardest moments to endure, as I was so close to being finished with treatment.

1/20:

One more chemo session left after tomorrow! I was waiting for my blood test results today to find out if my white blood count was going to be high enough to receive treatment tomorrow. This is a huge deal for me because, for months, my bone marrow wasn't producing the sufficient blood cell count to be strong enough to receive chemo treatment.

The A/C chemo I did from May to July hit my bone marrow hard, so my treatments from then to December have been inconsistent. The double hip surgery, my mom being diagnosed with stage 4 cancer this summer and deciding to travel to California all threw the infusion schedule off.

The pattern has been to do one or two treatments and then discover I need to wait a few weeks for my body to recover. The fact that my body is bouncing back is great, as it means my body is staying strong despite this strong medicine!

Even though I would rather not receive more Taxol tomorrow and endure the body pain and mental struggle that comes with this medicine, I want to be done! I will endure. I will make it through. I will finish. I'm so close. I GOT THIS!

The last time I did chemo was an experience I documented in great detail. It was the end of a very long journey. Like Bilbo Baggins about to return home after a long time away, the end of an epic tale is usually imprinted in the most vivid detail.

1/25:

Self-portrait of Pisces girl with three weeks of accumulated Taxol chemo in my system on a Saturday:

I'm hanging out in a dilapidated tent whose demise was the Xmas eve tropical storm. The cat is hilariously climbing the wobbly tent legs in pursuit of a cute, little wiggly lizard, while the dog is loyally by my side, offering her comforting endless white fur to ride these waves.

My body feels like Gumby when I walk, sore and loopy. My brain is like a sieve, so I sit here giggling with friends on the phone, making the best of my chemotized state.

My shirt says, "Love Your Now." Part of me resists this slug reality, but then I also know there's nothing I can do but embrace it, so I'm doing the best I can. The accomplisher in me and the doer has to take a back seat, as there's nothing to do but BE today, and that's the gift. I've been surfing this wave for so long that I've finally learned to let go.

At least there isn't the excruciating body pain I felt two weeks ago when a friend came over to rub my feet and assure me it would pass.

All I have are the birds, roosters, leaves blowing in the wind, horses far away upon the hill, and this wacky reality. Today is a day of comfy sweatpants, non-air-brushed photos, and goofy laughter. There's no one to take care of right now, except for me, and that's a gift. Self-care. Self-love. Scratched ancient sunglasses and kitty paws attacking my feet.

When going through difficult moments writing has been my saving grace. Here's a poem I wrote to help transcend the shadows:

1/26:

Unsuspecting pain waking me up at 2:30 am
Like woodpeckers in my joints, hammering away at bones, tendons, and ligaments
A jab in my hip, pounding in my neck vertebrae
Feeling the layers of discomfort circling my soul.

Apparently, my spirit chose this path for rapid evolution,
Letting go of defiance,
Drinking in the soreness.
Why resist what persists?
Surrender to the sensation.
This unholy sting is what leads you to your wisdom.

I did not choose this road:
Early menopause,

Bones breaking due to metastasis,
Cancer mutinied.
Some say, "Fuck cancer."
I say, "Cancer is my Guru."
Though I did not consciously choose this,
My spirit called in this expeditious growth.
All I can do is accept it and ride the waves,
Fast and furious earthquakes of torment,
Which leads me to transformation,
The path of the Jedi.
Wounded warrioress
Chiron enraptured with the dance of darkness.

Take this pain and make me whole.
To accept is the golden doorway of awakening.
I will continue on,
Jumping the hurdles,
Till my bones fall loose from my skin,
Phoenix rising from the flames,
Rising white into the light.

There is no such thing as death,
Only life being born in every moment.
The dragonfly's wings sparkle on.

As I got close to the end of my treatments, I felt a need to visit my relatives at the graveyard. As it had always been one of my favorite places to visit since I was a child, I derived great comfort from visiting.

1/26:

Today my world was rocked by the third week of chemo in a row, so I went to the graveyard to pray and ask for strength, as I felt whittled to the bone. I was shaken and needing the comfort of being with my ohana.

I'm grateful to live in a place where I have such deep roots. I'm held in the ancestral realm. They guide me when I need assistance. In the darkest moments, I know I'm never alone.

I felt slightly bonkers by this point. I was burnt and questioning doing more chemo, even though I just had one more infusion left. How much more could I endure?

DANCING AWAY THROUGH THE CHEMO CLOUD

I was almost done with chemo and my #DancingForHope challenge.

1/27:

As chemo has a cumulative effect, the last chemo treatment was particularly challenging. Between the body pain and the quagmire of my mind engaged in what I call an Advanced Shadow Dance, I was pushed to the absolute edge of my sanity. When I was dodging immense mind worms, I saw another breast cancer sister in Brazil made a dance video and tagged me in it! Tears poured down my face when I realized that this novel idea of mine was reaching others across the globe. I didn't feel so alone due to her share.

I'm almost to the end of my month practice and I have one more treatment. I'm taking this week off of doing chemo, as, honestly, I would go totally insane if I did one more in a row.

Movement is Medicine!

1/28:

Oh, the ups and downs of this crazy cancer path. I saw my new oncologist for the second time. All looks good so far!

The oncologist said my bone marrow is recovering extremely fast, considering all I've endured. I attribute this to keeping my natural protocol strong with weekly vitamin infusions, CBD/THC tinctures, healthy lifestyle, tons of other supplements, love, support, and lots of inner work. I believe moving back home to Kaua'i played a huge part in my healing too. I'm much happier here and have a stress-free life compared to my previous life in Northern California.

After treatment is over, I'm getting a full body and brain CT scan to witness my brilliant progress! (See how I'm framing that I'm going to have positive results? That's part of my tactic. Wink wink.)

He said the median time for the cancer learning how to find its way around the drugs he plans for me to take is eighteen months. The trend is that the cancer eventually comes back. He knew someone for whom it took four years to come back.

I will be the anomaly and be on the longer time scale! I also believe that radical remission is entirely possible. I firmly believe with that, with all the awesome life choices I've made and the powerful healing work I'm doing, I can defy these odds!

It's a daily mind trip to sit with the thought, *Will the cancer come back and when?*

I'm so grateful to be alive, as I would have been dead without these conventional treatments. I'm showing up each moment the best I can!

The lessons kept coming in fast and furious! There was definitely more to let go of on Inanna's heroine's journey of surrender. In the last week of chemo treatment, there was a robbery where I lived. I was heartbroken to realize that my precious, antique one-hundred-year-old German violin was stolen! Ten years earlier, I had saved up for many months to purchase this deliberate and sacred purchase. The iconic Zahrah red wig was also stolen. I shook my fist at the universe with the acknowledgment that the lesson of surrender was again at play.

ODE TO COMANCHE:

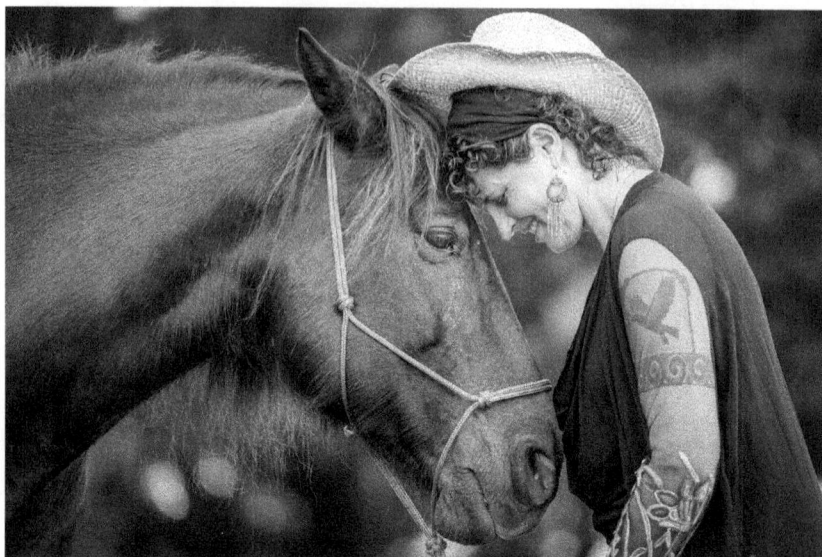

Photo by Kalalea Photography

Beloved Comanche. Your eyes pierce right into my soul. You were there from the beginning when the castles in the sand I had so carefully constructed began to crumble.

You were the first horse, my soul mate, and the impetus to sell my Pilates and Gyrotonic business. You helped me create the impossible dream, my business Wind Horse Sanctuary.

You were with me when Tom and I separated, through Deb's diagnosis and death, Rowen's death, and my own diagnosis.

You've stood by my side through the hardest of times. You served as a gentle sentinel for hundreds of people at the ranch.

You breathed life back into my lungs when I realized I couldn't have more children. I was adrift and broken down by the loss of a dream. You helped me claim my joy again!

When life brought another harsh curveball, I was forced to sell your one and only home, the one you first came to when you were a yearling. Your first owner, Lynlee, got you from a mustang herd around the Reno, Nevada area. She trained you with great love, recognizing the depth and priceless beauty of your soul.

I brought you and your buddy Blue across the ocean back to my ancestral home on Kaua'i. I worried that the journey across the ocean in a cargo container, not seeing sun for five days and no soil under your hooves would be too much for you and Blue. Your journey from California to Hawaii was three weeks in total. When you and Blue arrived at our home in Kaua'i, you immediately did a celebratory roll on the grass as you both were so happy to feel the earth again! That was the last moment I saw Blue's white coat be its authentic white color. Ever since then your blue-eyed friend has been stained red with the iron rich, red soil of the Garden Island.

After three weeks of chemo and dealing with a break in, I was raw to the bone. You visited me yesterday and brought immediate comfort to my tattered heart.

The wisdom and love in your eyes have no ending. You and Blue bring me home again and again.

You're like an old Indian soul contained in a gruella colored coat with a stocky, strong Mustang body.

Thank you for the gift that is you. Tears pour down my cheek as I write this. Such salvation in the eyes of a horse. I'm never alone with you by my side. Of this, I'm sure.

THE BEAUTY TRAP: VULNERABILITY

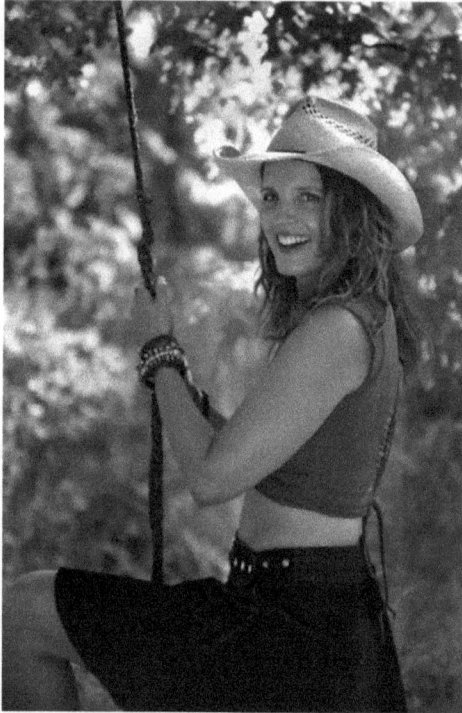

Wind Horse Sanctuary days - Photo by Meridian Brady

One of the greatest gifts of cancer has been to truly own that I'm a complete, worthy human being, separate from the viewpoint of anyone else. At a young age, I learned to gain validation from others from my physical appearance.

I was an insecure little girl. When I was about twelve, I started receiving overwhelming attention from the boys at my school. Due to growing up in an academic family where I was the artistic black sheep, I thought there was something wrong with me as I didn't fit in. I sincerely thought I was "stupid." Basking in the attention of the boys, I latched onto the concept that I had a value in my physical appearance. In my tween mind I reasoned that I was daft but, at least, I was "cute." I learned to gain self-worth from my outside appearance as many young girls do.

When I was twenty-nine, I lived on Kaua'i and did a shitload of therapy to realize that I wasn't actually stupid! I saw that it was a false assumption I learned from society and my family. I shifted my thinking to believe that I was worth far more than how others perceived me.

Fast forward to the cancer diagnosis and deciding to do chemotherapy to save my life. I lost my hair and twenty pounds, and there was a plethora of other unpleasant side effects. The changes in my body were scary to witness. I asked myself, *Who was I without my hair or my strong, athletic body? Was I still the same person after all these changes?*

The gift of this experience is I don't need anyone to validate me but myself. I'm a sovereign being. I dance only for me, not to attract a man, but to shine my light solely for the purpose of my own joy. I'm alive! I won't base my own identity on society's projections. I don't need a man to be okay. I'm brilliant and perfect just as I am.

Losing my hair and this limited perception of beauty is a powerful gift. I was dependent on my beauty for my self-worth. Now that my hair is short and crazy curly with chemo curls. I'm much happier now than I was then!

I give thanks for the lessons that challenge the growth, I'm worth far more than a self-identified image of perfection!

Sometimes, the most difficult experiences can bring the greatest gifts.

EMERGENCE:

2/3:

Today, I feel small, scared, vulnerable, and sensitive. I'm feeling the immense weight of the world. The reality of walking with constant uncertainty in my life, the fragility of my dear mother at the age of eighty-one with a stage 4 diagnosis, my own health journey, and this wounded world is heavy at times. I see pain, love, and beauty everywhere I look. It's an unpredictable time to be alive. These are days of accelerated growth when the darkness mingles so closely with the light.

Tomorrow marks my last chemo treatment! It's been a long journey since I started in May.

My darling stubborn mother is flying to Africa now. She and my father have led wildlife safaris around the world for forty years. The willpower to visit their favorite countries, Kenya and Tanzania, keeps them going. Even with stage 4 cancer and her body blasted with chemo, she's unstoppable. She's fragile. She's brave. How I wish I could wrap my winged arms around my parents and let them know everything will be okay. Yet, I'm only a mere mortal and don't possess that power. I feel shaken about the uncertainty of it all.

Yesterday, I heard of a mother here on Kaua'i with three kids recently diagnosed with an aggressive brain tumor. My heart hurts. I wish to save everyone from pain and suffering.

Being brave enough to engage in a shadow dance is what transforms the soul.

Dive into the dark and you'll find the light.

Tears of salvation.
Tears of hope
Reborn in the breath of the Gods

2/6:

I greatly identified with the last Star Wars movie. The main character is Rey, the female Jedi knight. Like previously mentioned in the framework of the hero/heroine's journey, she faced her internal darkness and chose the power of the light over darkness and fear.

Through this chemo journey, I feel like a Jedi warrior facing the daunting shadows. These shadows are chemically induced and solely within my own mind. I know I'll make it through.

Last dance with chemo,
I'll be celebrating soon!
I will do the most glorious dance ever.
One more journey into the darkness,
I'm almost out of the underworld, the vast darkness of Inanna's cave.
I will face these shadows that plague my vision.
Light saber in hand, I continue on.

For my last treatment, my devoted friend Michelle flew out to help me through the final initiation. She had already visited four times in the past year to help me through treatment and knew the tenuous territory well.

When I moved back home to Kaua'i and my health was declining, Michelle made it clear she was brave enough to face my fear of chemo, death, and the effects cancer was having on my body.

Cancer is a brilliant opportunity to weave hearts together. Instead of reacting from a place of fear, it's an invitation to expand into limitless love.

***

On my last experience with chemotherapy, I did one more dive into Inanna's silver cave to claim my last treasure in the darkness. I wrote this poem to capture the expression of the experience:

> The art of being human,
> Waking up at 3 am, feeling like my femur bones are crushed.
> This is the result of chemotherapy.
> I'm walking a shaman's path.
>
> I trust that this feeling of being all alone is exactly where I need to be.
> I'm surviving this gauntlet of pressure and pain.
> It is rebirthing me in every breath.
> It is not easy but certainly an adventure worthy of merit.
> Waking in the wee hours of the morning, these poems are my salvation to carry me across the river of unbearable pain.
> This aching in my sternum bone, like my ribs are crushed from the inside out; it is the remnant of the cancer that once resided there.
> It's been so long without a partner by my side.
> This joyful expression of fully embracing me is a gift.

No distractions.
Just me recreating my story in the realm of hard-won wisdom through the tunnel of discomfort and mental anguish that forges the toughest of warriors.
I embrace this opportunity to rise above adversity, to stop the endless chatter of the wanting mind.
I will transmute this agony, like the Phoenix rising from the flames.
The memory of my death has disappeared.
Immortality is real.

Keep beating the drum that is my heart.
It will pound till it is clear it's time to go.
Until then, I'll embrace each shadow that calls my name,
The beacon of hope that is reborn in every breath.

RISE WARRIORESS

The troubles that you complain about serve to carry you to your next plateau of growth.
Each challenge an opportunity of growth.
Rise beyond each breath.
Seize your sword.
Your light won't be extinguished.

2/9:

I'm so blessed to have a friend like Michelle, who is near and dear to my heart. This devoted friend has seen me when I was facing my possible impending death, deciding whether to do chemo or not, moving due to mold infestation, breaking my hip, and the dark shadows of chemo. We have laughed, cried, and danced on the razor's edge of our love for twenty-five years now.

The last two days have been rough with bone breaking Taxol induced pain and the dark shadows of chemo influencing my usually optimistic brain. After a 4-week run of this I have hit places of mental darkness that's rare for me to touch. I faced the emotions of doubt, fear, frustration, anger, and intense negative thought spirals.

Yesterday, this tender spirit ran a bath for me to help get the shadow of dread out of my body. Strong Italian hands gently caressing the pain off my tenacious soul. Today, Michelle held me as I cried, pain wracking my body due to Taxol hell. How I love this lady so!

The truth is that it's been hard to walk the last road of the chemo journey without my partner by my side. It's been three months since the break-up, and, overall, I'm much happier to be without the drama of that dance. But when I'm plunged into the toxic effects of chemo, it's very difficult to navigate it on my own. When I realized that would be the case, I asked Michelle to visit me for the last treatment. I needed a strong hand to pull me through the gloom.

I'm fucking done! I'm tired, but I'm still shining!

2/10:

What makes you vulnerable?
What stops you from opening your heart?
Why not take a chance to expose the tender core that makes you human?
The gift of feeling,

taking a chance
sharing your truth
falling on your face
and then
getting up again.

This is the delicate reality of being truly alive.

People tell me that I'm inspiring.
I'm told that I glow.
I say, why not seize life in all its tragic beauty?

I have danced with death.
I'm grateful to be alive.
I'm blessed to have seen the shadows
I'm fortunate to have a body
I'm battered,
But I'm still dancing!
I'm still alive!

"Open up and live
Let that sweet love come in
I go forth into the heart
Aloha spirit through the dark
You learn more the more you give
Open up and let that sweet love come in"

–TREVOR HALL MUSIC

BIG ISLAND TRIP

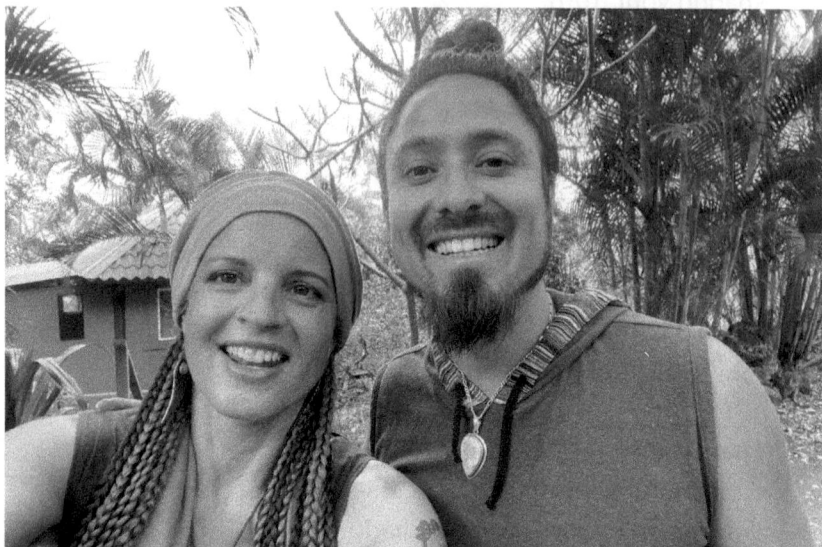

Me and Ananda Yogiji

I believe it's important to set a goal to have something to look forward to when going through a difficult time. Having a metaphorical carrot to reach for has always been a part of my coping mechanism for getting through challenging moments.

When I was in the gauntlet of chemo treatment the previous August, I decided to make it my goal to visit the Big Island (Island of Hawaii) in February, the following year to spend time with my cherished musician friends Jaya Lakshmi and Ananda. When I heard they were offering an event combining their ephemeral music with kundalini yoga, swimming with dolphins, whale watching, and nutritious food in a community setting, I was determined to manifest this magical reality!

I had known Jaya Lakshmi for twenty-five years. We were both young, single-parent hippy moms finding bliss on the beaches of Maui. I had been listening to her uplifting music ever since that time.

Ananda was her musician partner. I had been listening to the combined music of Jaya Lakshmi and Ananda for nine years. Their music was the background of my life and brought me through all the turbulent ups and downs.

I had even gotten my cherished friend Deb into their music when she was on her twenty-two-month jaunt with leukemia. It definitely helped to inspire her through her difficult moments. At Deb's memorial, we even had Jaya Lakshmi and Ananda's sacred music playing in the background.

I had attended this same event in Oregon three and a half years previously which was one month before I was diagnosed. Who would have thought all these years later, I would have the amazing opportunity to swim with dolphins with them as a celebration for thriving post cancer treatment!?

Life goes in cycles. It felt like a perfect circle of closure to have experienced the magic of their event right before I was diagnosed and then within two weeks of finishing such a grueling chemotherapy adventure.

When I decided to sign up for the event, I honestly didn't know if I would be alive to make it!

It was an epic gift to give to myself as something to look forward to while in the midst of heavy cancer treatment. Through challenging chemo treatments, healing from double-hip surgery, and a relationship break-up, this lovely adventure was my reward for all the hard work I endured. It was a positive affirmation of my healing to be able to attend.

2/11:

Lately, I've been thinking how the mind likes to separate what's safe and comfortable from what's unknown and scary. For example, if I'm in a new group of people, I can choose to isolate myself from others due to whatever thought form is rippling through my head. Thoughts like, I'm too fat, too skinny, too black, too white, too weird, my butt is too big, my butt is too small, I've got (insert some diagnosis here), they're too smart, or they're too stupid can serve to separate myself from the experience of connecting with others.

Tonight, in a new group of people I watched how my mind was clinging to thoughts so I could feel safe. I noticed how I mentally separated myself from the group with my current health situation. Fortunately, I caught this thought pattern and made myself be present. I chose to actively not separate myself from others out of insecurity. I'm sure the others in the group had their own version of stories running through their head too. It can be anxiety producing to meet new people in a group.

We're all connected despite what individual path we choose to walk. It's the labels that make us different.

It seems it would serve society to focus on what unifies, rather than what divides.

BE YOUR OWN BELOVED:

The musical event happened to fall on Valentine's Day! As I attended the event as my single fabulous self, my focus was on self-love. After all, so much of my inner healing had been focused on learning to love myself in a vibrant, new manner.

2/13:

It's so easy to want to look outside oneself for fulfillment in our Disney-coated culture of searching for perfection in a mate. If you're single on Valentine's Day, why not give yourself the love that you're wanting from another? Please don't buy into society's viewpoint that there's something wrong with you if you're single and unattached. Challenge yourself to see beyond the limited cultural paradigm.

Self-love brings awareness. Ultimately, it teaches you to fill your own cup of self-sufficiency, which, in turn, makes you much more attractive to others.

Find the answers in yourself rather than looking for it in someone else.

2/14:

I swam with dolphins today! Today was a day of facing major fears and blissfully dissolving them.

I walked into waves on slippery rocks, which is potentially terrifying for someone still recovering from hip surgery. (While undergoing healing, unstable surfaces could have potentially knocked my new titanium ball and socket joint out of alignment. This would mean I would have to do another dreaded potential surgery and have more time in the hospital.) Ananda generously held my hand over the rocks and helped me face this fear.

After I got in the water, I swam in deep water farther than I've swam in years to get to the dolphins. My heart was pounding fast. I wasn't sure how the muscles that were cut through during surgery and my titanium hip would handle a long swim. I think, in general, the reality of being in deep water takes great courage.

As I swam farther out into Kealakekua Bay, my new friend Marine swam next to me. Her gentle giggles helped me relax. I felt held by mama ocean's unending glory.

Then the dolphins came! I watched a pod of around fifty dolphins split up into two different groups beneath my snorkeling flippers. They were playfully making figure-eight designs with their bodies in the sparkling bay. I found out later on they were swimming in their sleep. I could have cried witnessing their sheer beauty and bliss as they swam around me. Crying tears of joy with a mask and snorkel on isn't possible I realized!

My thighs, glutes, and hips loved being in the water! It felt so natural, effortless, and healthy.

Jaya Lakshmi stayed by my side as I watched the dolphins frolic. She knew I was pushing my comfort zone, and I so appreciated her presence.

When I knew my hip had enough time being in the water, I swam to the shore by myself, as I've learned to not overdo it.

The feeling of swimming with these magnificent beings was one of total peace. Words cannot express the joyful reverie I felt here.

Do you know that dolphin sonar can dissolve tumors?

Here's to facing fear and truly living!

**

Magical Heiau Moment: I don't usually pick up hitchhikers, but I was in a place of trust while on the Big Island. I saw a local man in his 30s walking on the road. He had tattoos all over his brown arms and neck. I didn't think twice about my safety and immediately pulled over to pick him up. Instinctively, it just felt right. I trusted my gut! We started talking and I had time to spare so I ended up driving him twenty minutes away to his destination, an avocado farm. During the ride, he told me he'd never been off the Big Island his entire life.

Somehow, the topic of the heiau in Kealakekua Bay came up. A heiau is an ancient Hawaiian sacred site and temple. This particular heiau, named Hikiau, is the largest contained heiau I've seen on all the Hawaiian Islands. Its stunning presence holds an overpowering amount of mana.

The man told me his Tutu (grandma) was the woman who took care of this sacred site. As Kealakekua Bay is a tourist destination, she would protect the heiau to make sure it was given the respect it deserved. My deduction was that his grandma was a kahu or spiritual caretaker, descendant and holder of sacred Hawaiian knowledge associated with

Hikiau. It was a profound revelation to meet him, as he was the grandson of someone very special.

I told my Hula teacher, Kehaulani Kekua about this auspicious event. She made the connection that the day I was there was the anniversary of Captain Cook's death. He died in a location very close to this heiau on February 14, 1779. I was there exactly 241 years to the day of where Captain Cook was killed! What an auspicious connection.

I feel extremely fortunate to be living on the Hawaiian Islands. I hold great respect for the indigenous Native Hawaiian culture of the Islands. The mana in the 'aina is powerful. I give thanks every day to be given the opportunity to heal here. The magic keeps unfolding! I feel truly alive here on this sacred ground.

I'm so grateful to Jaya Lakshmi and Ananda for this sacred week. It has deeply nourished my roots.

I hadn't traveled for pleasure for years! The responsibilities of owning a ten-acre ranch and retreat center for five years prevented pleasure travel due to the immense cost and work the ranch and the four horses required.

This trip to the Big Island to spend time with my beloved friends Jaya Lakshmi and Ananda was a precious gift. Having my heart set on attending this event got me through the grueling months of chemo treatment, breaking my hip, and double-hip surgery.

The fact that I could swim in deep water, walk, dance, travel by myself, and ride on a rocky boat is a total miracle!

My advice: If you want to do something, just do it! If you love someone, tell them! Life is far too short to waste a moment. If you're unhappy in your life, shift your reality!

You deserve to be happy and love your life.

All that you love and hold dear can be taken away in a moment. Don't wait to live your life! Seize the moment.

Life has many surprises. Every moment there's an opportunity for transformation!

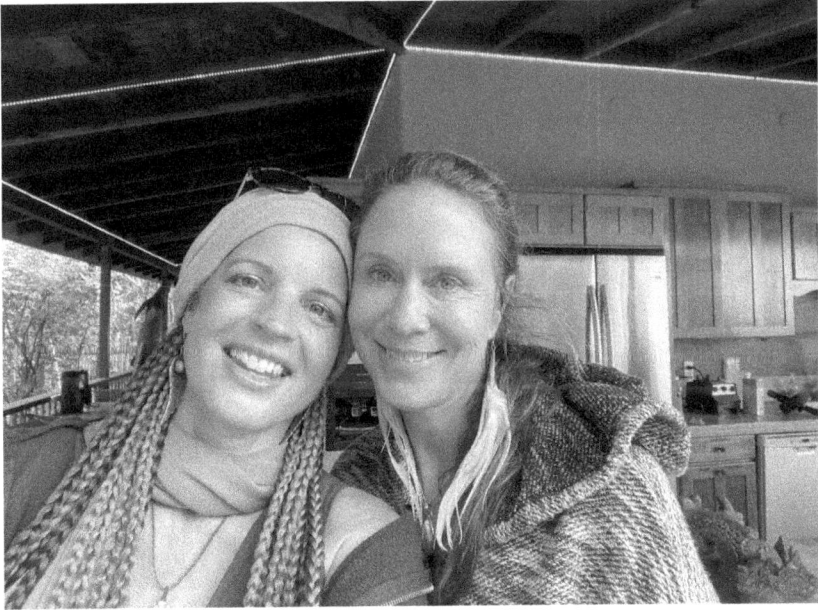

Me and Jaya Lakshmi

ASCENT

Immediately after getting back from the Big Island trip, I was due for my full body CT scan and MRI brain scan. I had never had a brain scan before, which my new oncologist at Wilcox was surprised about. He said with the extent of how many places the cancer spread, it was shocking that no one had checked my brain. He said that when the cancer spreads to the lungs, the next place it goes is to the brain. This was news to me, and, in retrospect, I'm glad I didn't know, as it would have been anxiety producing!

Scanxiety is real! It was a nerve-wracking experience to get a scan that would demonstrate whether nine months of intense treatment had worked. Was it successful? Did I go through hell and back for nothing? My blood tests progressively looked better month after month, and I was feeling remarkably better than I had the year before. Still, it's so easy for the mind to fall into doubt. The brain is designed to spin circles around itself.

The acknowledgement of death is always present when you're walking with a serious cancer diagnosis.

2/18:

REQUESTING PRAYERS & VISUALIZATION PLEASE: There have been literally 10,000 or more of you through my combined social media pages walking by my side through the last three and a half years of this cancer journey! You have stood solidly by my side, sending love, support, and prayers, donated to my many fundraisers and been extremely loyal friends. I wouldn't be doing so well without all of you. You have made a huge difference during my darkest hours. I'm profoundly touched, honored, and deeply grateful for all the love!

My full body CT and brain scan are tomorrow. At 6:30 AM Hawaii time, I go in to drink the noxious banana flavored radioactive sludge that will show the prognosis after nine months of intense chemo. At around 9 am, I will receive both scans.

Please join me in imagining the cancer gone from my body, my brain cancer free and overall immaculate results. Please visualize my bones, liver, lungs, adrenal glands, and brain clear, and all cancer gone from my body.

It's taken all my strength to get through this extreme treatment. I have never felt so much physical pain and discomfort in my life. My mind has been pushed to the edge. It's all worth it, though, as I'm alive!

It's my hope, dream, and desire to dance on this beautiful Earth for many more years. To see my beloved son grow to his 30s and beyond would bring me extreme joy! I have so much more I want to do on this sacred planet. Please visualize me healing and thriving!

So far, all my scans and blood tests have been stellar. Please see this trend continuing with me.

Without a doubt:
I will HEAL.
I will LIVE.
I will LOVE!

My cousin Laura went with me at a godawful early time. I forced myself to drink the horrible radioactive barium banana shake for the CT scan results to be accurate. Why do they even try to flavor it when it's so putrid tasting?

I survived the experience.
Then there was the long wait.
Day after day, I wondered what the results would be.

The scan results would give me a clear picture of how much time I had left on Earth.

Life with stage 4 cancer is like balancing on the razor's edge. On one hand, I'm very realistic, as I've had a plethora of friends die from cancer and know how fragile my situation is. On the other hand, I hold tremendous hope, faith, and courage. My test results have been stellar so far. I'm feeling great, yet it's all very raw, real, and scary when I allow myself to fear. At the deepest level, I have to trust that all is perfect. The only thing that's real is the present moment. I remind myself that now is truly all there is.

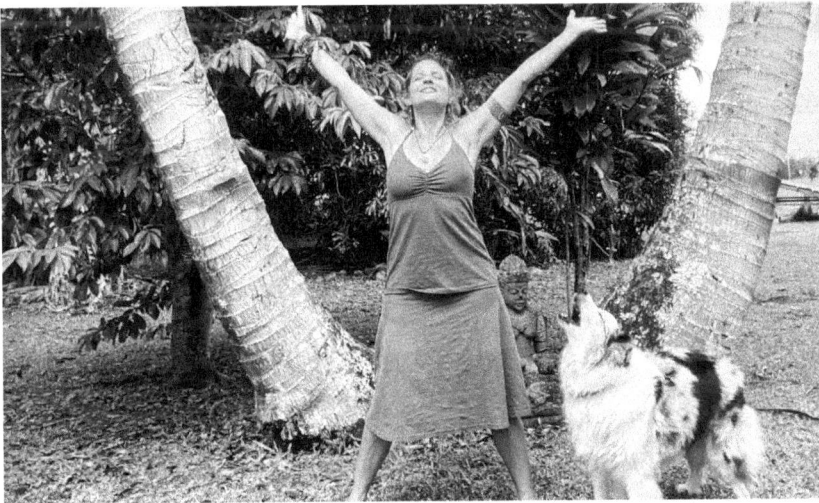
Celebration!

2/24:

Today, I get the final results of my latest CT and brain scan. Last night, the fear and apprehension crept in, and I ended up having a fabulous conversation with a dear friend for three hours last night, laughing tons, crying a bit, and feeling the depth of my emotions. This is the astrological season of Pisces which can be a deeply sensitive time for me as I'm a tried-and-true fish girl. The waters run very deep. I sometimes feel it all, which is why I become possessed, must write, and/or make spontaneous babbly videos!

I'm a bit scared. Vulnerable. Cracked open. Praying deep. Laughing loud. Doing silly John Travolta moves on the beach, not caring a fuck what others think. Why not?

Whatever the results may be, this is my life, and I'll live it large till it's clear I can't anymore. I've walked with death by my side for years now. I'm so close to her that I know the texture of her hand when I'm holding it. I don't fear her. Yet, I love my battered earthly form and will hold onto my delicious brown shell of a body until I can't anymore.

I'm fierce momma, doing what I can to be present for my son who knows only me as a parent. I'm the daughter who adores her parents. I'm friend. I'm lover emerging. I'm Artemis galloping on her wild mustang on the hard-beaten red dirt of my mother island Kaua'i. I'm confident. I'm love. I'm light.

I hope to chant Wahe Guru at the top of my lungs and celebrate my great news by spinning ecstatically in the waves. I will choose to be at peace with whatever the results are.

Release expectation.
Surrender.
Keep dancing through the thunder and rain.
Continue on.
Live fearlessly!

BEST POSSIBLE TEST RESULTS!

2/24:

I'm elated to say that my latest CT and MRI results are stellar! My wonderful oncologist said that I got an A+ and defied all odds! He shared that most people don't respond as well as I did to treatment. He was surprised at how resilient I was through the entire experience.

The results of the tumor cell count test (CA 27.29) are normal; this means there are no cancer cells in my blood! When I first started chemo nine months ago, the numbers of this test were over 950. Cancer free is under 40. My number is at 35.6!

The tumors in my lungs, liver, bones, and breast have all shrunk. There's still some cancer in my body, but blood tests show results faster than scans do, as the physical tumors take longer to dissolve. The blood stream clears faster than tumor masses.

I didn't expect to be cancer free, as I'm very realistic about how much the cancer had spread. The results are exactly what I was wishing for!

He also said it was a miracle it wasn't in my brain, considering it had already spread to my lungs.

Now, I'm going on a series of monthly shots. I will be getting Faslodex (hormone blocking medicine) and Xgeva (for metastatic bone strengthening). I will keep taking my natural supplements, IVs, CBD, and everything else I'm doing as I know it's keeping my immune system strong.

I'm very aware of the reality of how cancer comes back. I know I'm incredibly fortunate to have defied the odds. I'm going to actively wield the tremendous power of my mind combined with the healing mana of mama Kaua'i to keep my earthly body alive and kicking! I'm so incredibly grateful to have more time on Earth!

SURVIVOR'S GUILT

At the time of this writing, it's been four wonderful and turbulent years since my cancer diagnosis. During this time, there have been many deaths of beloved friends also on a cancer journey. Each time I hear of another death, it temporarily shakes my world.

Recently, there was the death of a dear friend, Debbie, who was diagnosed within the same month as me four years ago. We had the same diagnosis, stage 3 hormone driven breast cancer. We both dove in to treat it naturally and refused the standard route of treatment.

I created a secret cancer group on Facebook, and she was one of the founding members. We communicated fairly regularly talking a few times on the phone, texting, and being in touch via social media. She was bright, resilient, and a powerhouse.

Debbie's death was a harsh blow, as she and I were on such parallel journeys. Few of us who started out on this health journey are still alive today. This is why I choose to see each day as an incredible gift, as I know how swiftly the path can change.

Survivor's guilt is a real thing if you're the one to defy the odds with a life-threatening diagnosis. When a beloved friend dies, I ask myself, "Why am I still alive and they have passed?" I have to trust that each of us has our own fate and destiny, despite what treatment we choose.

I've been on this healing journey for so long now. It has been heartbreaking getting close to others on this path and then finding out they have died. Due to this repetitive circumstance, I've learned not to get too close to others with cancer.

As I've been in the public eye for the entirety of my journey through blogging, videos, and social media, other cancer patients reach out to me. Somehow, they think I have all the answers, which I frankly do not. If I opened my heart to every person who reached out to me as I did for the first few years of my journey, my heart would be constantly tattered into smithereens. I would be most likely among the countless friends who have died, as I wouldn't be able to bear the weight of the sorrow.

For this reason, I learned to erect a mini barricade around my heart to people who reach out to me. I care for everyone. I have a generous nature and would save everyone if I could. I'm well aware of the perilous ledge that I stand upon. I also have dear family members who are relying on me for support. I only have so much of myself to go around. Self-care has been one of the biggest lessons of my journey. Therefore, strong boundaries are necessary.

This is why I don't participate in other online cancer groups, except for the secret cancer group on Facebook that I created and lead. Occasionally, I'm tagged by others in online groups, and I will answer questions, but I don't spend time in those groups. I find that many people in those groups are caught up more in the "cancer is my story" mindset.

I also choose to relate to other cancer thrivers who see their journey as a path for transformation, rather than being in the "victim" mindset. If I spent time talking constantly to the cancer patient with a "victim" state of mind, then that mode of thinking would bleed over into me. Many on the path use their cancer diagnosis to feel sorry for themselves and are jealous and skeptical of your good results. I know this is a touchy subject and I don't want to offend anyone, as I know this path is extremely hard. We all choose what paradigm we want to be in, even if we're struck with the worst life-threatening diagnosis.

I don't want cancer to be my story. My story is that I'm living as large as I can within the parameters of what my body goes through on any given day. My story is that I love living with horses and my animals in Hawaii. My story isn't about cancer. My dear friend Martin (DJ Dragonfly) taught me this at the very beginning of my journey. It was the best advice I ever received.

I choose to be a victor, not a victim. Yes, I've gone through some tough shit. Nine months of heavy chemotherapy and going through a break-up after double-hip surgery was hell, but I choose to rise above the challenges that come my way rather than be crushed by them. When I was stuck in bed with two titanium pieces put in both of my hips I was pushed to the edge of my mental and physical comfort zone, but the attitude I chose to have was, "Okay, here's another fucking growth opportunity!"

We choose our story in every moment. Whether you're facing a life-threatening diagnosis or not, you're creating your thoughts which frame your reality.

Which story are you choosing today?

2/25:

I got the news yesterday that my precious light flame that was almost snuffed out last year will continue to burn brightly for years if I keep my mental and physical agility on point. I will keep continuing to defy predictions!

The immediate response upon the good news was tears in the oncologist's office. I was so relieved!

When I drove back home, there was a flood of tears as I thought of my dear friends who died young from cancer. They call it survivor's guilt.

Why do some of us make it and some don't? Rowen and Deb live on in my heart. As I was crying, I knew they were celebrating my happy news. They want me to live! There's only a thin veil between the dead and the living. I know our souls will dance again.

So many beloved friends haven't made it. Many were much younger than me. There have been countless words of encouragement and information shared between us. We're warriors of the heart. We bond deeply. This connection comes to a harsh end when one of us bright souls leaves the Earth far too soon.

I will continue to live fully for those who can't. When you dance with death so intimately, your love of life is strong!

Feel the grief.
Express it.
Dance with life.
It's a choice.
You decide.

For all of you on a health journey, I suggest you dig your feet deeply into the ground and find your courage. You have a tremendous well of strength and can jump over any hurdle. You're so much stronger than you think you are.

It's not easy, though. This path can push you to the edge of your sanity. Your body could experience the most discomfort you've ever felt.

It will either grow you or destroy you.

Every obstacle is an opportunity for growth. You can get through any adversity that comes your way.

Reach out for help. You're not alone. Others on this journey want to help you if you're open to receiving it.

LIFE AFTER TREATMENT: PTSD

Going through standard cancer treatment is tough. It's normal for layers of trauma to be triggered post treatment.

Fabian Bolin is the creator of the ingenious "War on Cancer" app, which is based in Stockholm, Sweden for cancer patients and their family.

After being diagnosed in 2015, at twenty-eight years of age, Fabian began documenting his cancer battle on a blog, which made him realize the true power of storytelling and how sharing his story helped him cope with his "cancer trauma." It helped him to process what he was going through emotionally and psychologically but also gave him a sense of purpose he had never felt before. This, together with a strong urge to help others affected by cancer, became the foundation for the War on Cancer app, a social network aiming to radically improve the mental health of everyone affected by cancer.

Fabian shared with me regarding PTSD:

> *Studies have varied in the assessment of patients for the full syndrome of PTSD (i.e., all DSM criteria met) or only some of the PTSD-related symptoms. Thus, incidence rates have varied accordingly. The incidence of the full syndrome of PTSD ranges from 3% to 4% in patients recently diagnosed with early-stage disease to 35% in patients evaluated after treatment. When the incidence of PTSD-like symptoms (not meeting all diagnostic criteria) is measured, rates are higher, ranging from 20% in patients with early-stage cancer to 80% in those with recurrent cancer.*

Clinical depression affects approximately 15% to 25% of cancer patients and is believed to affect men and women with cancer equally. Individuals and families who face a diagnosis of cancer will experience varying levels of stress and emotional upset. Depression in patients with cancer not only affects the patients themselves but also has a major negative impact on their families.

Immediately after I finished treatment, a huge wave of stored trauma from all that I had endured washed over me. While I was in active treatment, I was just trying to get through the day. Now that I was finished and had successful results, I could drop into a parasympathetic peaceful state of being. Dropping into this state of mind required me to also be present with the unexpressed emotions that were left to process.

I posted a photo of myself with the synthetic braids that I wore while I was crying:

2/26:

Vulnerability: You can't tell from this photo, but tears are pouring out of my eyes. I never have shown a photo of myself crying on social media. Society encourages us to present the strong, positive, capable, inspiring self at all times so others won't see the soft, scared, and tender self.

Today, I allowed myself to collapse and be held with the total exhaustion that hit me post treatment. As the tears fell, I realized how impenetrable I've had to be, especially in the last year of treatment. Last year, when I was told I would probably die, I had to find my deepest strength and embody my warrioress self.

Then I broke my hip and had double-hip surgery. Two weeks after hip surgery, my partner and I split up. During this time, I was learning to walk again while dealing with the physical pain and mental distortion that comes with chemotherapy.

I prayed deeply for the results I got two days ago. It was beyond my wildest dreams to hear how much the cancer had receded.

I know I'm strong. What I truly want, deep down, is to feel safe in the world. I want to be held and told everything will be okay. (Don't we all?)

I deserve to rest. I want to let my guard down in the face of accomplishing such a huge feat. I want to be vulnerable.

NOW WHAT?

Immediately after treatment, I had a sense of *What do I do now?* After putting so much emphasis on survival, it was a transition to go back to regular life.

3/1:

It's been almost one year since I was recommended to go into hospice. This past year has been spent literally fighting for my life. I don't use the word "fighting" lightly, as I know it embodies war, strife, and conflict, but, in this case, it's true. I've been clawing through the mental and physical hell of cancer treatment to hold onto this spark of life I value so dearly. All those weeks of gearing up for the battle of chemo and now I've got the most stellar test results possible! What happens next?

I'm definitely celebrating my life! While I'm in joyful reverie, I'm allowing my feet to slowly settle on the ground. This is a strange transition.

All the emotions that I've had to push away to get through each grueling week are now tapping me on the shoulder, saying, "Hello, we're still here! You still need to deal with us." There are layers to deal with around my mother's stage 4 cancer diagnosis and my recent break-up.

Part of me is totally exhausted by the extreme strength it took to get through each day. I want to crawl under a rock in the ocean and hide like a clown fish in the warm embrace of a sea anemone. Part of me is excited to reclaim my life, continue my horse work, and make a difference helping others going through cancer.

I know I must find balance. I must recognize how much work it took to get here, release the mental and physical toxins accumulated to survive chemo, and move forward with grace.

I'm tender,
Sensitive,
Blown open,
Raw,
Reborn,
Soon to have a major birthday & still dancing!

GIVERS & TAKERS:

One of the most profound lessons of my healing journey was to learn how necessary self-care is. When my brain and body was being pulled apart by the side effects of chemo, it made me stand up for myself like I never had before. I realized that I was important and worthy of impeccable self-care!

These hard-won lessons of chemotherapy and hip surgery led me to end my relationship, which I didn't have the willpower to do for several years. Even though some elements about the relationship were lovely, ultimately, other aspects were toxic for my spirit.

In the winter of 2020, two guests visited me who took advantage of my generosity in letting them stay for free on the islands. Challenging behavior played out that led me to sever the friendships. This was extremely perplexing and upsetting for me, as I pride myself on being able to work through the most difficult communication issues in most of my relationships.

It was particularly disturbing to have these two incidents happen close to one month apart during my last month of treatment. I was extremely depleted and worn out. I had to trust that everything happens for a reason.

1/24:

There are givers and takers. Both sides can operate from a dysfunctional sense of deprivation.

I tend to be a giver. I recognized years ago that sometimes, the impetus to give to another originated from a place of needing to feel valued. If I'm needed, then I'm worthy. This is coming from a place of deprivation, as I'm needing some sort of acknowledgment for my own self-worth. I'm proud to say that I'm able to recognize when this pattern arises a little more easily now.

Takers also act from a pattern of deprivation. They feel a lack of self-worth; therefore, they can have a sense of entitlement and needing something from others.

Both these ways of being derive from the pattern of codependency. When you're reliant on others for your self-worth, you're setting yourself up for trouble!

My giver self experienced a blow this week when I offered a friend who was having a rough time a place to stay here in Kaua'i. I hosted him for two and a half weeks and ended up getting the short end of the stick. He left without a goodbye, leaving the place a mess, and not even saying thank you for staying for free at my place.

The lessons keep rolling in! I was shocked by this behavior and quickly looked to find what I could have done better to prevent the situation. I try hard to keep my relationships clean and value clear communication.

Discernment: I surround myself with high-caliber people who have strong moral values. I assume that everyone is like this, but when I experience a situation like this, I realize this is merely an idealistic assumption. Many walking wounded aren't taking responsibility for their actions and end up blaming others for what's their responsibility. I assumed my friend would be like the other appreciative friends and family I've hosted. This was my mistake. He was a new friend, and I extended the same trust to him that I naturally gave to my long-term friends. I gave too much to him without setting firm boundaries and expectations.

I'm grateful for these lessons of self-discovery. Though his actions hurt, I now see it had nothing to do with me!

Then another disturbing incident happened with a girlfriend who had been a dear friend for years:

2/27:

The ties that bind and the fissures that separate. I was on cloud nine two days ago from the impeccable results of my latest scan. A friend had recently arrived to help me sort through my personal belongings that were still not organized after moving one year ago.

Certain behavior went over the line of what felt healthy for me. Words were shared that felt inappropriate and extremely insensitive, especially given the reality of all I had just gone through. I was pretty cracked open with my brain and body still processing the toxins of chemo. I was still finding balance after the incredible maelstrom I was recovering from.

This incident felt like being tripped and thrown to the ground. It reopened other wounds that ultimately go back to having a father who was occasionally intimidating when I was a child. I love my dad dearly; he's a remarkable father. But we all have wounds from childhood, and his large Portuguese personality was daunting to my little girl self.

I learned how to retreat within the safe cave of my quiet, frozen façade to defend myself in the face of such intensity.

The incident with my friend was an opportunity to reach into that cave and let the little girl within me know she wasn't alone. Through the tears and bewilderment, it was an access point to the part of me that wanted to be healed.

All these years later, I can still reach in and soothe the tiny child within me who is yearning to be seen and loved.

We all are walking wounded. None of us are exempt from the misperceptions of childhood. What we choose to do with our wounds makes us who we are.

I'm letting go of this friendship. The boundary crossing was too severe, and I decide whom to allow in my safe bubble. While on a deep-healing path, it's imperative that I surround myself with healthy, supportive, and loving people. It doesn't mean that I'll run away from conflict. Quite the opposite, it means that I have the right to choose who I'm around. This, ultimately, is very empowering and healing!

I wish her well. I let her go. May we all grow and heal our fractured hearts. It's possible to operate with an open heart and clear boundaries.

THE NEW NORMAL

3/4:

I ride the waves of indescribable joy and sorrow that bend and break the soul only to birth me to a brighter and stronger self. I'm left without parameters of meaning again. I take this medicine to "save" my life, but it ultimately throws me to the ground and leaves me feeling like shit. It's a constant reminder that I'm not invincible. I'm limited in this human form. I must listen. Rest. Heed the body that's processing heavy chemicals.

Yesterday I had two huge shots of Faslodex (hormone blocking medicine) in my hip area. Ouch! I had a shot of Xgeva (given for bone metastasis) on my arm. I feel it all, being the sensitive fish I am. I'm knocked down once again, dreaming of running with wild horses. Crawling precedes walking. Running follows walking.

I want it to be done. I wish I could return to a normal life. I envy those who can go to a predictable job. It's true! You have no idea how blessed you are to have predictable normalcy. With my stellar test results, part of me wished to be done with the pills, shots, tests, and the endless medical quagmire. I'm starting to see that this is my new normal. If it's allowing me to live longer (which it is) then I'll keep going, as the gift of life is so precious. It's not easy, though.

We're all being pushed to our limits. Life on Earth is a testing ground so our souls can evolve.

Can you keep the faith?

Can you keep your heart open and not fall into fear, hate, anger, resentment, doubt, and despair?

I have deep compassion for all of humanity and the struggles we're facing.

Stay open.
Don't give up.
Remember to love.
Find the points of connection rather than the walls that separate.

Choose love over fear.

***

And the point is to live everything.
LIVE the questions now.
Perhaps then, someday far in the future,
you will gradually,
without even noticing it,
live your way into the answer.

–RAINER MARIA RILKE,
LETTERS TO A YOUNG POET

METAMORPHOSES:

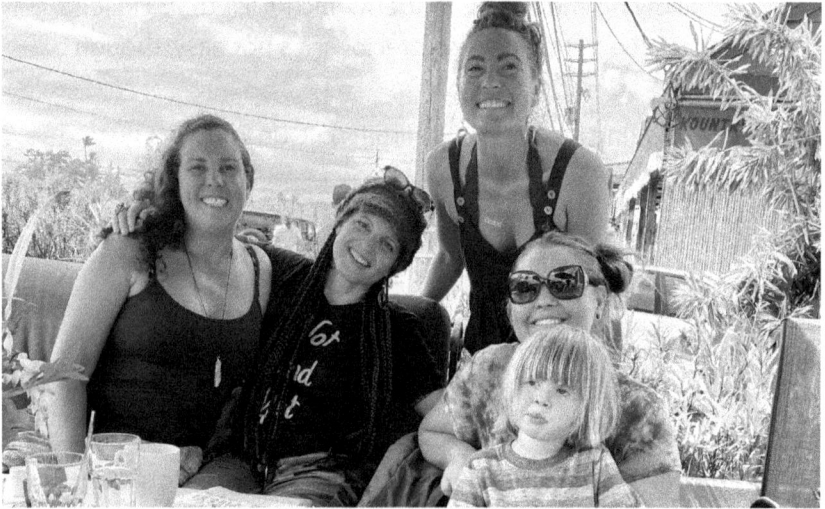

Kaua'i ohana: Laura, me, Stef, Emma & Atreyu

3/4:

A big birthday is coming up on Saturday. It feels like I'm standing on the edge of a cliff with massive winds careening through my pixie hair. Every moment is a decision and challenge to stay present.

The world is pulling at me. I used to be actively in the public eye before moving back home to Kaua'i one year ago. I was sharing my journey of "healing cancer naturally" on multiple social media platforms, blogging, making videos, and doing interviews until my health went downhill. I stepped out of the limelight, as I was just struggling to survive. Now I'm hearing the call to make videos and share my story, as I have an important message to express. I believe this is part of my kuleana, my mission, and why I've been given a second chance to live.

The question is how to maintain balance. It's easy to be sucked dry when you're in the public eye. It's vital to maintain my sacred sovereign self while I also share my light with the world.

3/6:

My dear momma is having a bone marrow biopsy to see if there's progression with the cancer in her bones.

Tomorrow is my birthday and my beloved parents (who have been together for fifty-seven years!) are shining all sorts of love on me. It made me feel special when I got a message from my dad right after my mother's procedure that said, "We think you are very brave. We love you and stand strong with you. Lots of love, Dad."

I'm blessed to be so adored. I give thanks for the infinite abundance of life. Even in the midst of a so-called tragedy, there's so much beauty and love.

I have been blown away by the tenacity and courage my parents have displayed since her diagnosis in August 2019.

My dad is a loving, tender, and patient caretaker. My mother has an impeccable positive attitude. They could have crumbled in fear, doubt, and misery, which is what happens to many others. They both are such bright, inspirational forces for me. I'm so fortunate to be their daughter.

Thank you, Mom and Dad, for birthing me, for always being present, for enduring my rebellious hellion teenager days, for loving my son when he didn't have a dad, and for being such solid rocks in my life. I love you so.

3/7:

I had a stellar fiftieth birthday doing exactly what I wanted to, which is the ultimate gift of self-love. My beloved ohana took me out for breakfast and then I went out to hike on a dazzling beach.

My goal is to rest more! I'm so wired to achieve, accomplish, focus, and manifest, which often comes at the expense of my health. I'm still recovering from the massive doses of chemo and new medicine I'm taking. After the hike, I had a delicious nap for three hours. It was so good.

Life is grand. I'm so happy to have another whirl around the sun. Each day is a gift, and I intend to live it fully! I'm fifty and fabulous!

Don't take a moment for granted, dear friends. It can all end in the blink of an eye. Each breath is sacred.

3/9:

Full Moon intensity,
Riding the waves,
The indomitable human spirit
I refuse to give up.

Realizations,
Growth,
Awakening,
Walking with the Gods and Goddesses is not easy but must
be done when your life is at stake.
I continue on
One foot in front of the other,
Finding the precious light,
The joy in the shadows.

TRUE BEAUTY:

Today I saw three surfer/hippie girls in their twenties with long
curly blond/brown ocean-kissed hair. I immediately felt a pang
of envy seeing their long locks cascading upon their perfectly fit
and tan bodies. I thought, *That was how I used to look.*

Women in western society are programmed to automatically
compare themselves to other women. At the age of thirteen, I was
obsessed with *Seventeen* magazine. Being glued to the airbrushed
pages of young women who looked faultless taught me that I had
to look perfect all the time. I had to have a slim body without an
ounce of fat on me. My hair, clothes, and face had to look spot on
in style at every moment.

When I look back at my life, I see how critical I've been of my
appearance. This is heartbreaking to me. When I see old photos

of myself, even from a year and a half ago, I see how gorgeous my body and face looked. There will always be someone to compare yourself too, even if it's a younger version of yourself.

Now I'm fifty years old. I've barely escaped death a few times in the last year. Every day, I remind myself how fortunate I am to be functional and able to care for two horses and a small piece of land all by myself. My hair is coming in crazy curly after nine months of chemo that gave me a second chance at life. My body was slammed into menopause due to the heavy medicine. It was always easy to get into shape, lose weight, and look good in a bikini. Now I find myself coming to acceptance of my new post treatment body. Recovering from double-hip surgery was deeply humbling, as I was reliant on others for a short time. As a proud, independent woman, this was a new record for me in asking and receiving help.

All of these experiences have shaped me to realize that every second is a gift! The fact that I can hike with my dog, pick up endless piles of horse manure, care for land, and dance is a minor miracle. Without modern surgery and medicine, I would be dead and/or in a wheelchair. I'm deeply grateful for my life. Cancer has gifted me with this profound realization.

Still, with this newfound wisdom, I sometimes fall prey to the comparing mind when I see young people with their flawless bodies and long hair. When the bite of envy creeps under my skin, I remind myself that I'm still beautiful, and I had my time of immaculate youth. It's important for me to acknowledge these emotions and then let them go. If I don't acknowledge the pang of jealousy, then it will continue to bleed through every encounter with a gorgeous young woman.

I share this so you know you aren't alone. If you're experiencing the reality of aging and grieving the body you once had, I see you.

If you've gone through or are going through cancer treatment and have had to sacrifice your tresses, I understand. This is the same theme as the goddess, Inanna. In order to save her life, it was necessary to let go of all her precious gems, garments, and all the symbolic objects she held dear.

I often feel like Inanna. In the last five years, two of my closest friends died. My marriage faded away to dust. I let go of my beloved ranch, two of my horses, and a business I worked so hard to manifest. I've been surrounded with the deaths of dear friends I came to love on the cancer healing journey. Last year, I had to throw away some of my most sacred objects due to a terrible mold outbreak. My bones have been broken and I've risen from the ashes once again. All of these sacrifices have helped me realize the precious opportunity of my life. My hair and body are the least of these sacrifices. Even in the depth of tragedy, I'm surrounded by miracles. My life is the greatest gift.

My hope is for future generations of women to let go of the comparing mind. It seems like a terrible waste of time to not appreciate your golden youth when you have it. If our society taught us to celebrate our beauty rather than constantly criticize ourselves, the beauty industry would quickly go out of business. Who would pay for plastic surgery and endless piles of makeup if all women exuded a sense of self-confidence and inner beauty? We would know we were gorgeous no matter how we looked, whatever our size was, and how old we were.

Today, I claim my beauty: wrinkles, imperfections, extra weight, an occasional limp in my step, gray short hair, and all. I know that if I'm privileged enough to make it to age sixty, I'll look at how I look now and see the beauty that I didn't appreciate in this moment. What a waste of time that would be!

I think that true sexiness comes from a sense of self-confidence rather than how you look. If you know you're drop-dead gorgeous, you'll radiate that sense of exuberance. The most striking super model could feel deeply insecure, not owning her inherent beauty, and others would instinctively sense her low self-worth.

Why not embrace the gift of how you look? Regardless of the extra weight you're carrying or the fact that your butt or breasts may be too big or small, you're complete. You're brilliant as you are now! Your body, your face, your hair, all of you is divine, so why not celebrate it!? What are you waiting for?

In March of 2020, the United States and the world dramatically changed due to the virus that took over the world. Our predictable reality was shattered within a moment's notice.

We thought it would just be a two-week lockdown.

Two weeks turned into months which turned into complete upheaval with the brutal murder of George Floyd, the Black Lives Matter Movement, the turbulent fracturing of the Kundalini Yoga community with shocking news about Yogi Bhajan and the sexual predatory allegations toward him, and the insanity that got increasingly more bizarre with the United States Presidential Election approaching in November, 2020.

What seemed completely impossible suddenly became a reality in 2020.

As toilet paper rolls sold out in stores across the country with the terror that we wouldn't have enough of this soft commodity to wipe our derrieres, we became accustomed as a society to a growing sense of isolation with the new rules of "social distancing."

Dissent was increasingly more common between people who believed that face masks were necessary to stop the spread of the virus and those who felt that mandating mask mandates were limiting our civil liberties. All these beliefs were fed by the upheaval stirred up by the media and the various political parties aiming to make their point to sway possible voters to cast their ballot either for Trump or Biden. Communities and neighborhoods that normally were close were torn apart by these various belief systems.

Nothing was normal anymore.

As the death toll rose with the virus spreading around the world, some didn't believe it was real and that it was a conspiracy for those in power to make money on a new vaccine.

During this time, I had a pretty sweet personal off-the-grid yurt bubble on Kaua'i on the land with the horses. I was fairly shielded from the discombobulation stirred up by the virus as all the Hawaiian Islands had a mandatory two-week quarantine time for any incoming visitors and residents who had traveled off island. The quarantine greatly limited the number of tourists on all the islands. Due to this, Hawaii was safe and, throughout the pandemic, had the lowest number of cases and deaths; Kaua'i, in particular, was the strictest island travel-wise, so it was relatively untouched by the virus.

As the Hawaiian Islands have been reliant on tourism since the sugar cane and pineapple industry moved their operations to third world countries where agricultural labor and production is cheap, Hawaii's economy was hit much harder than the mainland USA. Unemployment was at an all-time high in the continental United States, but it was worse in Hawaii.

I was grateful that I was living simply in my humble yurt home on Kaua'i. I understood why the universe used a meddling neighbor to boot me off the ranch in Nevada City back to my roots on the island. In retrospect, if I had been trying to run my business like I was with workshops, private sessions, and renting out the cottage on Airbnb, once the virus hit, I would have been in a terrible economic situation. It was already incredibly challenging to make ends meet financially when my workshops were wildly successful, and we were solidly booked with guests. Due to the high cost of running a ten-acre ranch with things constantly breaking, needing maintenance, feeding and caring for four horses and the high cost of my natural cancer healing regimen, I never had enough money!

The neighbor who turned us into the planning department was actually an angel in disguise to get me home to the 'aina. Due to my simple off-grid lifestyle, it was easier to afford my island lifestyle than the high cost of living in Nevada City. I was grateful to be living on Kaua'i once the virus shook the world!

I loved living on the red earth with my animals. After so many trials and tribulations, I was finding a place of true happiness. Perspective is everything. You never know when tragedy will turn out to be your greatest blessing!

RETURN OF THE HORSES 2

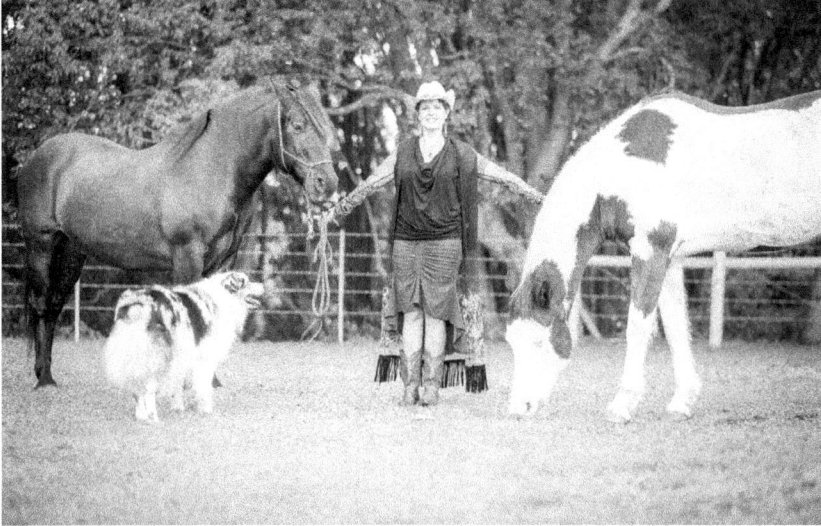

Comanche, Xaria, me & Blue - Photo by Kalalea Photography

The horses had been roaming freely on more than eighty acres for a year after they arrived on Kaua'i. As they lived on the property next to the yurt, I was fortunate to see them occasionally. They would show up during the most auspicious tender moments when I was needing some extra love. They were magically tuned into me!

Due to how consuming and tiring chemotherapy treatment was and not being able to walk far due to my hip breaking, I hadn't seen them often since they arrived. I missed the daily rhythm of caring for them. For the previous seven years, everything in my life had revolved around the horses.

I had suspected there was something wrong with Blue's eye for a while. On the rare occasions I saw him, he had a pus-filled inflammation around the edges of his gorgeous blue eye.

I first met Blue when I was searching for a more "spirited horse" for the EFL work I taught. I wanted a horse that was a bit of a boundary pusher. The other two horses I had then were Comanche (the famous mustang) and Spirit (a seventeen-year-old Arabian gelding). Both boys were extremely gentle and easy to work with. In Linda Kohanov's work, she has active leadership exercises where participants learn about the nature of boundaries. It was important to have a horse that could challenge clients to step out of their comfort zone and face their fears.

When I was looking for a new horse, I searched on various online sites that listed horses for sale. One day, I stumbled upon a unique looking paint horse named "Slugger" that piqued my fancy!

I went to see him and immediately was drawn to his unique character. He had a wacky, off-beat personality, and I could tell he was the type of boundary-pushing horse I was looking for. He cost more than I was looking to spend, but I was smitten with him and was determined to manifest him however I could. As other horse owners know, it's easy to acquire more horses. It's hard to pay for them once you have them! I ended up taking out a small bank loan to purchase him.

When I brought Slugger home, I immediately wanted to change his name. The name Slugger wouldn't work for a horse designed to practice EFL with clients. Many people are drawn to the Eponaquest work to heal their trauma with horses. Having a name like Slugger brought up violent images. Slugger needed a kinder, gentler name. I decided to name him "Blue." The name seemed to fit him; it was fun and spunky like him! He also had the unique blue eyes that gave him natural character.

Blue was the boundary pusher, the curious one, and the wild card of the herd. If the handyman drove into the field with a truck full of boards where the horses grazed, Blue would walk up to the truck, lift the boards up with his mouth, and drop them onto the ground! He was the firecracker, the unpredictable one. One time, when I was teaching a workshop, he suddenly bolted out of the gate when I was getting another horse out. He ran straight into the rope that the other horse was attached to, which then became wrapped around my finger. With the full weight of Blue's large body up against the rope, it yanked hard on my finger! The painful incident ended up breaking my finger. Ouch!

Despite his unpredictable nature, he was the one that many clients in my workshops would fall in love with. He was the friendliest horse, as he was so naturally curious. When there was an exercise during a workshop that required the participants to gather around the four horses outside the large, fenced riding arena, Blue would be the one to amble up to each participant and nibble on their shoulders. He would try to be as close as he could to my clients, he would have climbed on their lap if he could! Some people loved this characteristic about him, and some feared him. All these traits made Blue an extremely endearing horse.

When I brought the two horses back home to Kaua'i, they lived on a slice of over eighty acres of horse heaven. They shared this property with two other horses, cows, donkeys, wild pigs, and the flora, fauna, and vast insect empire of East Kaua'i. I was happy to see that the horses adapted easily to their new tropical life. As I didn't see them often, I was dearly missing them.

The rare times I saw Blue, one of his eyes had goop and a light bit of blood around it. This obviously concerned me. I was eager to try to help him out, but there wasn't sufficient space around the yurt for the two horses to comfortably live.

The yurt where I lived in Kaua'i had two and a half acres around it with a small area sectioned off for the horses. I wanted a larger pasture area for the horses to freely roam around in. I hired a local guy to fence a larger area that would be available for the horses to be in.

2/28:

I love the synchronous interconnectedness of all things. I'm putting up a horse fence so I can be closer to my two boys. This is a huge celebration for me! I've been waiting for my treatment to be finished and to be healthy enough for this next manifestation.

A local Portuguese guy comes to give me a quote. Of course, he's big, dark skinned, tattooed, and resembles my father (minus the tattoos)! We start "talking story," and, of course, he's a cousin of mine! The common phenomenon of having family from the small island of Kaua'i and being Portuguese is that everyone is your relative. I love that everywhere I go there's ohana and a vast web of interconnectedness through family genealogy.

It's fairly typical when I mention that my family's last name is "Bettencourt," that locals recognize me as kin. I'm immediately accepted and no longer an outsider. When you have family roots going as far back as the 1870s, that's a good reason for instant acceptance.

The fence builder became immediately open to me, as he knows I'm part of the historical pod on Kaua'i. He knew my great Uncle Eddie and other family members.

As we're talking, this big, robust guy gets tears in his eyes as he shares about having to put his beloved mare down years ago.

We horse people speak the same language. We understand how these magical beasts touch our hearts and move our souls. Even the most hard-boiled man melts within the gaze of a horse.

When the fencing was finally done, I was excited to bring the horses back again!

3/30:

This might not seem like a big deal, but the fact that I have hay bales in the back of my messy truck brings me incredible happiness!

While the world melts away with panic about the virus, I'm still focusing on my goals and what brings me joy because that's what keeps me sane.

Getting anything done on island takes massive patience and persistence as the pace is so slow here. You know the term, "Hawaii time"? There's truth to this! To get the area ready for the horses, I fenced off a large pasture area. Then, it took weeks to get piles of hazardous junk removed from the area. How many times can someone tell you they'll do something tomorrow and not follow through? Tomorrow can be a very vague word!

Blue is needing medical attention. This is my motivation to get this project done. I have dearly missed my horsewoman lifestyle.

I'm so close to finishing this project! Stay tuned for happy horse photos. Someone is figuratively itching at the bit!

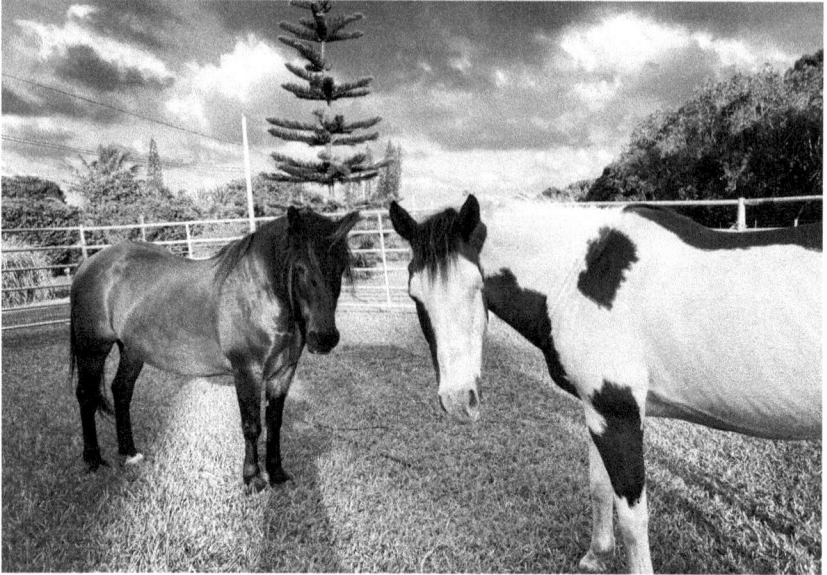

4/13:

Something magical happened today!!

Since the summer, I've been trying to manifest a round pen. (A round pen is a metal circular pen usually used for horse exercises.) Trying to find a used round pen on a dinky island in the middle of the Pacific Ocean was impossible. I literally tried bargaining and bribing with owners who owned one of these precious commodities, putting "wanted" ads on Craigslist, asking every horse person on island, and the answer was always the same: "No." When you live on the mainland, you can drive to the next town, city, or state to purchase something, but this was impossible when you're surrounded by 2,500 miles of ocean. I tried, and it didn't work.

In September, I was told by the feed store that the business only placed one large order per year for round pens. This was during the month of March. Back then, March seemed like an eternity away, but as there was nothing else I could do, I waited patiently. I was so patient that once fateful March rolled around, I almost forgot to inquire! I called the feed store at the last possible minute. Lo and behold, one of the kind owners found a display model in Oregon for me. It took a month to ship to Kaua'i, but in the grand scheme of things, time is irrelevant. It was a huge accomplishment to be able to get one!

It was assembled today. Horse friends, you understand how exciting this is. Having a round pen means I can play, run, and dance with them. This is one of the freest most exhilarating sensations in the world! Hopefully, one day, when the virus passes, I can return to my horse work. I gave up a huge part of my soul when I sold my ranch. Words cannot express how happy having the horses close and having a round pen makes me!

It's equivalent to Inanna regaining some of the precious regalia she had to sacrifice in order to claim her life.

I had finished with the new pasture area for the horses and was ready to bring them to their new spot!

4/16:

I faced some major fears yesterday! Engaging with large animals such as horses and cows can be unpredictable. It requires an adept awareness to not be stepped on or unintentionally run into. In the last six years, I had more broken bones due to horse accidents than the sum total of incidents in my whole life. I had broken my finger, my arm, and almost been stepped on and knocked over multiple times.

I went to go get the horses yesterday off the large piece of land adjacent to the yurt property. I usually have help and I haven't fetched the horses by myself in over a year and a half! I knew it was risky to do it by myself, because if I got hurt, no one would know. It took extra courage for me to fetch them, especially because I'm still recovering from double hip surgery six months ago.

My heart was beating mighty fast when I went to go get them as I also had to fend off a large herd of cows. I hiked down to the pasture with a bucket of feed to lure the horses back and was immediately surrounded not only by Comanche and Blue but thirty cows trying to get the food! Imagine a large herd of bovine beasts that weigh in at 1,000 pounds or more each lunging at you trying to get a small bucket of feed. I had to keep shooing the boisterous cows away.

I led the horses up the hill toward the yurt property with a trail of hungry cows mooing at me and yearning for the food. I was the mad cow piper cowgirl chick!

Once we got up to the main gate of the pasture, I swiftly let the horses in, while simultaneously trying to keep the cows out, and gave the horses the grain. I was ecstatic to have performed this feat by my little old self. It was tremendously empowering.

I'm officially a cow wrangler!

BLUE

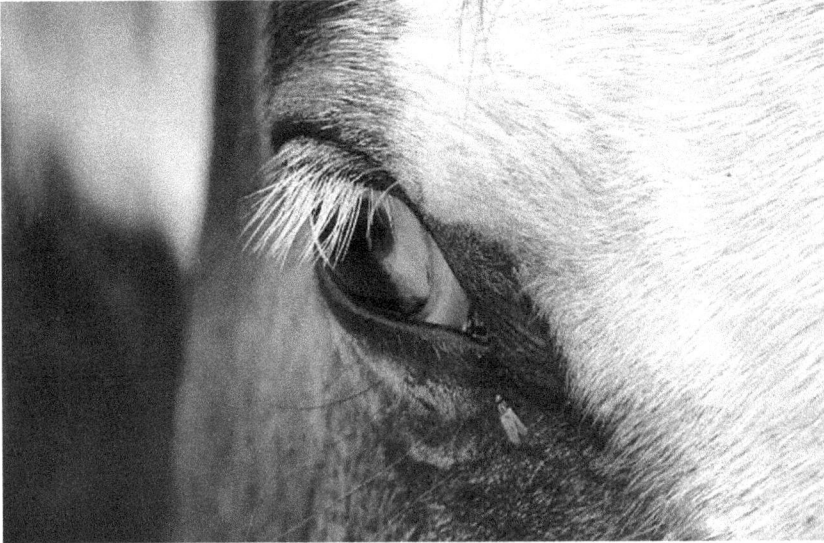

Photo by Melinda Vienna Saari

Once Blue and Comanche were safely contained in their new pasture, I could focus on finding out what was going on with Blue's eye.

After the vet visited, I found out crazy news.

Blue had cancer.

What?!

More cancer?

I was shocked!

How could another being in my immediate close circle be diagnosed with cancer?

I didn't understand.

4/16:

I just found out that Blue has cancer. Due to his light pigment and the hot Hawaiian sun, two squamous cell carcinoma tumors began to grow around the edge of his precious light blue eye. I've been absolutely stunned today. The amount of cancer in my life has been staggering.

My animals are like my family. The shock, anger, raw and real grief of another family member affected by cancer has pierced my heart.

Cancer, go the fuck away. I know you're here to teach me huge lessons of impermanence, but enough already! Seems like every time I get over one huge hurdle, there's another to jump. I know my soul signed up for accelerated growth in this lifetime. I'm grateful for the lessons, but it truly hurts my heart at times!

I'm digging in deep for another heroine's journey, this time with my beloved horse Blue.

RESEARCH:

After I got over my disbelief, I sprang into action researching different modes of treatment. I was pointed in the direction of a woman in Australia (Catherine of McDowell's Herbal) who creates herbal remedies especially for horses with squamous cell carcinoma. After exchanging a plethora of emails, she generously gave me a complicated nutritional and herbal protocol for how to treat Blue.

The difficulty was that as the Hawaiian Islands were in such a remote location, it was challenging to find the necessary nutritional remedies. It was possible to find the items on the mainland, but then paying the shipping to the islands was incredibly expensive. I spent two weeks doing major research for the necessary items while experiencing a fair amount of frustration due to this. I finally figured out a plan of treatment that I was optimistic would help him.

The vet offered a treatment plan for Blue that was prohibitively expensive and dangerous to give him. I instinctively felt it wasn't the right plan of action, as it would put his life in danger. Fortunately, a month or so later, the vet found another treatment option that was more affordable and easier to implement.

It was necessary for Blue to wear a UV mask every day that would protect his afflicted eye from the strong rays of Hawaii's sunshine. This would shield his eye from future damage and reduce the growth of the current tumors. The mask would be put on in the morning and removed in the evening.

While I was overwhelmed with the reality of another beloved with cancer, raising money for his care, the time and energy it took to feed the horses three meals a day and all the various complicated concoctions I gave Blue, it was also a blessing. There's always the silver lining if you choose to look for it.

Due to Blue needing constant care, I had to really step up and be present with my horses again. This helped me touch into the same rhythm of my life at WHS that was abruptly ripped away from me. The daily care of Blue and Comanche helped to root my feet back onto the earth again and come back to center. As the horses are my heart and soul, this was an opportunity to care and love them in the way that also nurtured my spirit. This was incredibly healing for me after surviving such a horrendous year.

The vet was wonderfully surprised with how well Blue was healing with the integrative approach! It's my belief that if you give the body the nutrition, space, and energy it needs to heal, it will repair itself. I found this true with my own body and I was witnessing it with Blue as well. This was a joy and a great affirmation of my belief system.

LIVING WITH HORSES:

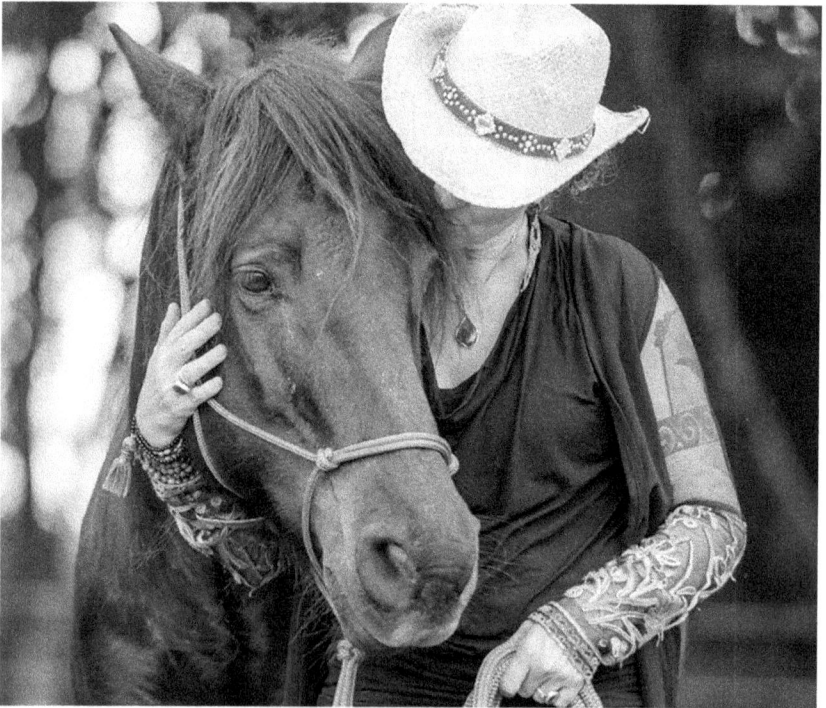

Photo by Kalalea Photography

My life took on an incredibly rich cadence after Blue and Comanche were back on the land again. I found a deep satisfaction in the everyday care of the land and animals. Taking care of horses with the necessary feeding three times a day, daily poop scooping and tending to a sick horse is hard work, but it gave my life meaning and purpose. I loved it. It was a true labor of love.

Being close to the land that my prudent great grandpa purchased in the 1920s was a potent act of returning to my roots. The ʻaina nurtured my soul. I felt like my body could relax into a deeper level of trust. This was the most profound healing I could possibly experience. There was no way I could have dropped into the same sense of belonging while living in California. My island home possessed the magic I needed to defy all medical expectations.

I would often close the gate to the main road adjacent to the property and let the horses roam freely on the land. This meant that I would wake up with Blue or Comanche standing right outside my door, waiting to be fed! It is my slice of heaven to observe horse behavior free of the confines of a barn, stall, or other self-contained human creation. Sometimes, I felt like the Jane Goodall of the horse world, except my two boys had been domesticated!

I'm sure if Blue could, he would wander right up the stairs into the yurt, plop down on the sofa, and start talking story. Hawaii has a languid lull to the language where people spend time chatting without a rushed sense of time. This is one reason why island life is deeply relaxing and healing!

The horses and I had many enchanted moments together. One time, when I was recovering from my monthly shots for cancer treatment, I came outside to find Blue and Comanche in deep sleep together.

I wrote:

Something powerful happened the other day. When I get my monthly shots for cancer treatment, it knocks me out for a few days. During these treatment days, I don't plan anything and just rest. My brain and body need time to absorb the side effects of the medicine. I'm used to this schedule and surrender to whatever the medicine has in store for me. After the Herculean strength it took to get through chemo treatment, the injections are fairly easy. I'm grateful for this medicine that's keeping me healthy.

I had the front gate closed so the horses could freely wander wherever they wanted to on the property. It's rare to see horses sleeping. Horses are prey animals and must be constantly vigilant to possible predators. They've adapted as a species to live with the awareness of danger, while still living harmoniously within their herd. Horses have much to teach humans if we're open to listen.

My head was spinning with the side effects of the drugs. I stumbled outside my door to find Blue languidly sleeping on the ground and Comanche sleeping standing up, acting as a sentinel for Blue. In the wild, one horse will be a sentinel to watch over the others for possible danger when they sleep. Usually, horses will sleep standing up, but occasionally, if they feel extremely safe, they'll lie down. To see a horse lying down to sleep is to witness an incredible act of trust.

When I saw Blue passed out on the ground, I felt a profound sense of awe about the trust he exhibited toward me. Both of them were intentionally close to me while the waves of drugs coursed through my veins. I covertly took a video of them and hobbled back to my bed.

About an hour later, I went out to the same exact spot and was shocked to find both Blue and Comanche sprawled out on the ground! Comanche rarely lies down. In the eight years I've been with him, I can count on my hand the times I've seen him like this. This was a phenomenal sight!

Horses are perceptive, energetic beings. My understanding about what was happening was they felt the dramatic effect the drugs had upon me. They voluntarily put themselves in a deep state of slumber and energetically aided me through the gauntlet of my experience. They knew what I was going through and generously entered the void to be present with me.

It was a powerful act of trust to have both of them lying down on the ground at the same time. This meant they trusted me as their sentinel. We were all present with one another in a benevolent spiral of support and love.

There's the energetic realm of the horse tribe that exists beyond past, present, and future time. I do believe that horses are actively aiding humans for the evolution of our consciousness. I use horses to work with humans in a therapeutic manner because horses are magnetic, sensitive healers.

I quietly spent time with the both of them while they were sleeping and appreciated the opportunity to witness such a wondrous, rare sight.

I'm grateful every single day for the presence of these boys. They gently hold my heart and help me thrive through every challenge that comes my way.

HOME IS WHERE THE HEART IS:

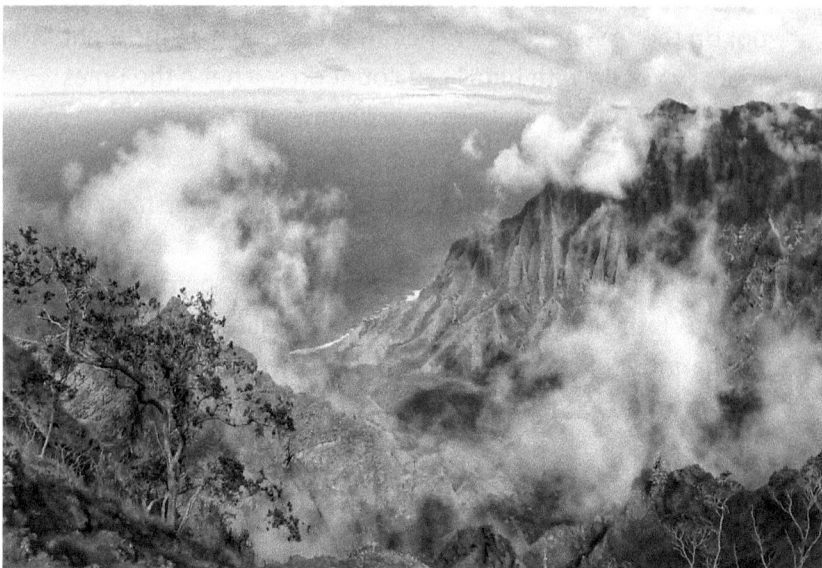

Kalalau Lookout, Koke'e State Park, Kaua'i - Photo by Danny Hashimoto

I realized that my life on the land with the horses, Xaria, and the cat Kismet was my dream environment. It was a very similar lifestyle to what I had experienced at WHS without the expensive overhead and stress of holding frequent workshops and taking care of guests. I had a similar life in Kaua'i with the added benefits of being in a nurturing, tropical environment that was also the home of my ancestors.

I was home!

I had worked so hard, fighting with nails clinging deep in the red, iron-rich dirt of Kaua'i to reclaim my health after being so close to death. As I slowly opened my eyes post treatment, I saw that I was exactly where I had started from many years earlier when I had moved to Kaua'i with my blond-haired baby boy Willow. Life had brought me around full circle!

A slow realization dawned on me that I was incredibly happy!

Everything was perfect the way it was. The terrible neighbor who had turned me into the planning department was actually an angel in disguise who brought me back to my incredible island roots again. In fact, the neighbor most likely saved my life! With the high cost and stress of maintaining the ranch, the lack of attention I received from the medical world in Grass Valley/Nevada City, and the dysfunction with my partner, I would have never been able to get up my courage to do chemotherapy in my old life. Being home on Kaua'i allowed me to drop into a sense of relaxation and experience the healing mana of the Hawaiian Islands. I was able to reinvent myself and gather the courage to do what I feared the most: chemotherapy. I would have most likely died if I had stayed in California.

Note: One can move to Hawaii and be in a negative mind space and consequently not heal as I did. Your thoughts and state of mind are vitally important for the body to drop into a parasympathetic healing space. Being in a mental state of fear can cause dis-ease and prevent healing from occurring.

Never underestimate the gifts that are birthed from tragedy. You never know when the most horrific situation could turn out to be your biggest blessing!

DEAR MOTHER:

In March 2020, an extreme wave of fear and the virus swept across the world. I was caught in a turbulent tide of emotions due to my dear mother having stage 4 cancer. For a while, she was doing fairly well, but then her health started going downhill around early summer.

The world was in lockdown. I lived 2,500 miles away on Kaua'i with my beloved family in Northern California. Never had the distance felt so far between the mainland and the islands. The Hawaiian Islands had a mandatory fourteen-day quarantine in effect. This meant if I travelled off island, I would have to stay on the yurt property, not going anywhere for two weeks straight. I couldn't comprehend how I could travel to California during a deadly pandemic, put my parent's life at risk and also my own with my already compromised immune system. Despite these obstacles, I was pulled like a magnet to visit my parents, especially when it looked like my mother's health was declining.

Due to the massive fear circulating around the virus and the rules around traveling, many people advised me not to travel to California. I was told that I could be put in a "camp" if I contracted the virus and never be allowed back home again. I was warned not to take the test as it would infect me with the actual virus. I was told I was risking my life if I chose to travel. The fear was so thick you could tangibly cut it with a knife.

I struggled with this reality for months. My heart was torn to pieces hearing what was going on with my parents and feeling powerless to do anything. Of course, technology (Zoom, online conference calls, phone calls, and texting) made it easier to be in touch. I was grateful for these modern modes of communication during this fractured time, but that didn't replace the one-on-one connection of being in the presence of a loved one.

Being that I was a natural caretaker, I felt split at the seams, knowing that for me to risk going to California might not only expose my parents to the virus but also might make me sick. My main root to the Earth is my beloved son Willow. I didn't want to risk him losing both his grandparents and his mother in one fell swoop from a visit to the mainland.

I sat with the decision. I did "The Work" of Byron Katie about it. I heavily questioned my greatest fears about the trip. In July 2020, my mother had a bad fall, became heavily bruised and then landed in the hospital where the virus was rampant in the Bay Area. I knew I had to travel to California or risk not seeing my dear momma alive again.

I decided to visit.

Once I made up my mind to go, I didn't feel tortured by the reality of being so far away. I went into action mode. How could I best prepare for my trip? How could I keep myself and my family safe during such a perilous time traveling? I created a logical plan and I stuck to it.

I ended up going to California twice in the period of three months. I realized it was important to see my family as much as I could, and I wanted to avoid traveling during the cold winter weather. I also had a storage container that I was spending far too much money on monthly that needed to be emptied.

The trips to California were wonderful. I learned from the experience of these trips that the fear of traveling was far worse than the actual experience. Isn't fear like that?

F – False
E – Evidence
A – Appearing
R - Real

It was actually easy to travel! I was careful by seeing minimal people, getting tested for the virus before seeing my parents, and was extra cautious when it came to pumping gas or shopping for groceries.

The leap of faith it took to get on an airplane and travel was worth the experience of spending time with my family. This experience can be summed up with my favorite cliché:

Choose love over fear;
Love always wins!

In August, my mother's health balanced out after a roller-coaster ride of possible scary situations. She started taking the steroid Prednisone, which gave her a general higher level of energy. I got to witness a new side of my mother during these visits. I saw how stubborn, resilient, and positive she was in the face of difficulties. She was as "tough as nails," which was the same term my oncologist had used for me.

It's a bizarre situation having two family members journeying with stage 4 cancer. I think both my mother and I inspire each other to keep going. Perhaps we both made a pact on a soul level before we embodied to share this experience together. Like a mother/daughter defying-all-odds soul journey. I'm deeply inspired by my mother's optimistic attitude, and I know she's equally touched by mine.

Life goes on.

HONOR THE EARTH:

Right before the 2020 presidential election, I created a ten-minute short film entitled *Honor the Earth* about climate change and equated it to my own health crisis. I also made an environmental resource page, listing solutions to address the climate crisis. My impetus to create a film was witnessing a profound sense of apathy around the important issue of climate change and the nerve-wracking buildup before the election. The dyed-in-the-wool environmentalist upbringing I had emerged when it seemed like it was most needed.

I wanted to give people a sense of empowerment around the overwhelming and daunting issue of climate change. I believe when people feel empowered, they're more likely to take a stand in what they believe in.

I wanted to give people a sense of hope about the future.

I fervently wished to educate others that the issue of global warming must be addressed for the children of the future.

I was delightfully surprised to see *Honor the Earth* had far more viewings on YouTube than I anticipated. It even won a few awards at environmental film festivals. I put countless hours into its creation, so it was a lovely surprise to see it gain recognition far beyond what I had originally imagined!

REBIRTH

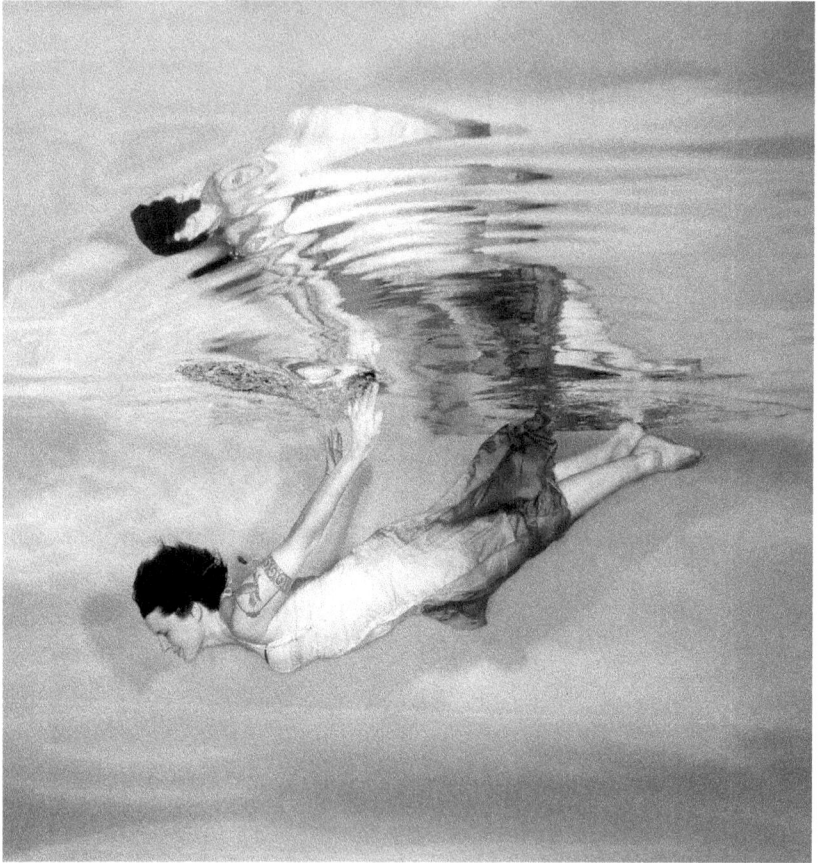

Photo by Erena Shimoda

Living with a serious cancer diagnosis is a daily reminder of how blessed each day is. I take nothing for granted. I know I've defeated the odds, and with all my heart, I hope I continue to do so.

Throughout this experience, I've learned how strong, vulnerable, and worthy of love I am. At times, I felt like I would be crushed by the experience, but I just kept going.

My attitude is that every challenge is a gift for my growth. I continually dare myself to face my fears and transmute them for transformation.

I would have never wished for a cancer diagnosis, but I can honestly say cancer has made me appreciate life like never before.

For those of you who are on the cancer path, I know it's not easy. Some days are simply horrible. I encourage you to take it one moment at a time. The more you surrender to whatever hardship you're experiencing, the quicker it will pass.

I encourage you to find the beauty.

Find the joy.

Surround yourself with what makes you happy. You deserve it now more than ever.

Most importantly, I want to remind you that you're so much stronger than you think you are.

"You are braver than your deepest fear
You are wise beyond your years."

–NAHKO BEAR/PUA CASE

***

I completed writing this book at the end of 2020. This is an astonishingly turbulent time on Earth for all beings. Whatever time you're in while reading the passages of this book, I'm praying for more peace, stability, balance, and unity in the world for future generations and ultimately, for the health of the planet.

I do believe that even during these crazy times, there's still so much to be thankful for. I'm full of gratitude for my life, animals, family and friends, and all that I hold dear.

Blue is thriving on his alternative healing cancer therapy. The two tumors around his eye have completely cleared up and the vet is happily surprised with how well he's doing! I continue to give him a nutritionally rich diet with various herbs and supplements to support his continued recovery.

More than anything, I'm grateful for the benevolent presence of the horses I've been fortunate to live with. I'm constantly in awe of the comfort, wisdom, magic, and beauty they bring. These beloved equine friends have been my rock of support through such a painful and challenging time. I wouldn't be thriving without the assistance of Comanche, Blue, Spirit, Daisy, and the energetic force of the horse tribe.

From the moment of the fracturing of the relationship between Tom and I, to Deb's and Rowen's illnesses, to my own journey with cancer, the horses have been my beacon of light throughout the darkest shadows.

BEDOUIN HORSE LEGEND

And Allah took a handful of southerly wind, blew His breath over it, and created the horse.... Thou shall fly without wings, and conquer without any sword. Oh, horse.

May my words give you hope, inspiration and resources for your own healing journey.

EPILOGUE

July, 2021: Tara continues to get impeccably clear blood test results, the tumors continue to shrink all throughout her body and her bones are growing back. She is incredibly grateful to be alive!

Thank you for reading

Māhalo for reading my book! I hope you enjoyed it.

Now that you are finished, I would love your feedback. Please consider leaving the book an honest review on Amazon.

The link below will send you directly to where you need to go. Thank you!

https://www.amazon.com/dp/1737247402

About the Author:

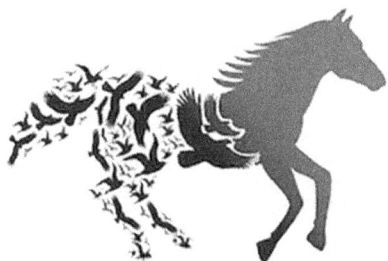

Wind Horse Sanctuary

EQUINE ASSISTED PERSONAL DEVELOPMENT

Tara Coyote was like a lot of horse-crazy little girls, constantly begging her parents for a horse. Despite her desperate pleas, it wasn't until much later in life, after a traumatic event, that she was able to fulfill her dream and experience the redeeming love of horses.

Tara created and ran a horse retreat center named Wind Horse Sanctuary in Nevada City, Northern California for five years with her four healing horses. She was fortunate to be trained through Linda Kohanov's organization, Eponaquest, as an Equine Facilitated Learning teacher. Tara also trained as a life coach through Lisa Murrell and Schelli Whitehouse at Equine Alchemy. After the death of her best friend, Tara created and led "Grief Rituals with Horses" to aid others in a healthy expression of grief. Hundreds of adults and children attended workshops or private sessions at the ranch and at conferences around the world.

When Tara was diagnosed with cancer in 2016, she immediately started sharing her health journey on social media and her web page Cancer Warrioress. Her mission is to spread the message that cancer can be a powerful force of transformation and a growth opportunity. She has written several published pieces, been featured in numerous interviews and podcasts, and coached many cancer thrivers.

Tara now lives on the island of Kaua'i where she continues to offer Equine Facilitated Learning sessions, as well as online coaching to clients. When not writing, teaching, or tending to the land and animals, you can find Tara enjoying the tropical beauty of her father's homeland in Hawaii.

To find Tara please go to:

www.WindHorseSanctuary.com
www.CancerWarrioress.com
www.youtube.com/c/TaraCoyote
www.instagram.com/taracoyote
www.instagram.com/windhorsesanctuary
www.instagram.com/gracegritgratitudebook
www.facebook.com/windhorsesanctuary1/
www.facebook.com/cancerwarrioress

Acknowledgments:

I have been held by an incredible community of humans, animals, and the divine guidance of spirit throughout my journey. If I thanked each being who assisted me on some level, then this book would be encyclopedia sized! From the moment I announced my diagnosis on social media, I was surrounded by angelic humans stepping up to help me in ways that I would never have dreamt of. I have been humbled by all the love, caring, fundraiser support, and friends going beyond the call of duty to help me.

Learning that I am worthy of being loved and accepting help has played a huge part in my healing. It is truly humbling to learn how to receive. Cancer has cracked my heart open to learn I am worthy of love and shattered my amazon woman's shield to see that true strength lies in vulnerability.

If you've been walking by my side through following me on social media, sending me encouraging messages, donating to one of my many fundraisers, helping me in person, or praying for me, please know that you have made a PROFOUND impact upon my life. Words cannot express how grateful I am for you. Mahalo for stepping up to help and caring for me in my darkest hour. I would not be doing so well without you!

Thank you to my scientific, adventurous, loving family for standing by my side. Even though I know you might not always agree with my choices, I love all of you beyond belief. I was blessed to be born with creative parents who took a chance to do what others only dream of doing: starting a wildlife safari business that travelled to every continent of the world. Because of their courageous leap of faith, I was fortunate to see untrekked territories at a very young age. Mom and Dad, you are such supportive, loving parents; I'm so grateful to be your daughter. *Please see the poem I wrote to my mother after the acknowledgements.*

Thank you to my brother Ted for your warm heart. I'm sorry for any lingering trauma when I pretended you were a horse and put a bridle on you when we were kids. Thank you, Renee, for your constant, loving presence. You are the embodiment of courage.

To my magnanimous son: I am so proud of you. You took the most putrid lemons and made the most enchanted lemonade. Thank you for your giving, grounded nature. You are my reason for continuing on this wild & windy road.

Thank you, Jasmine, for being my precious niece.

Tara's Healing Calls: Thank you to my generous friends who held twice monthly group Zoom and phone calls for me when I was most needing support. Your prayers and visualizations of healing truly made a difference! Amity Hotchkiss, Wendi Kallins, Mary Lou Perry, Andy Peri, Devi Peri, Julie Simonsen, Christopher Campbell, Dalila Cunha, Martin Webb, Michelle Russi, Kim Mears, Anny Owen, Eugene Turner, Wendy Botwin, Peter Belt, Sandy Shea, and Lindsay Wood. You all are incredibly special to me, thank you for showing up for me through thick and thin!

A special mahalo goes out to my special "Dream Team" - four individuals who carried me when the mind worms of chemotherapy threatened to mentally and physically break me. These altruistic souls patiently accepted my phone calls at 2 AM when I questioned my sanity and my body was wracked with pain.

Eugene Turner: My angelic big brother spiritual ally who continually reminds me of my light. Your life, story, and being are a constant inspiration for me.

Kim Mears: Queen of selfFULLness who shaved her head with me to show solidarity around the shock of losing my locks. Your zesty spirit always makes me smile!

Martin Webb: Thank you for being such a solid friend, the laughter, insight, and all you generously give me, my dear metal piggy.

Michelle Russi: You physically held my body through the worst of the pain, scrubbed my toilet, made me rich pasta when I could hardly eat and visited me four times in the course of a year! You are limitless embodied love. Thank you for making me feel less alone during the hardest journey of my life.

Mahalo to my Kaua'i ohana, my wild group of sister cousins who carried me through hell and high water. Portuguese blood runs deep, and I'm grateful to be a part of your clan! Stef: for your endless containers of nurturing chicken soup when I struggled to eat and for your selfless care of fluff ball Xaria. Laura (Lu) for taking care of me post-surgery when the simplest tasks were Herculean chores, for holding me at night through the depths of bone-breaking, drug-induced pain and your immense help with my book production. I dub you social media queen! Emma & Atreyu for your presence: I love our shared rainbow unicorn aumakua power! Lisa, for your kindness. Cameron for helping me to put my yurt back together again after the mold destroyed it. Lurline for your evanescent, jubilant, and constant loving self. You all have hearts of gold!

Although not in animate form, I want to give a big mahalo to my Kaua'i ancestors who came before me, especially: Uncle Eddie, Great-Grandpa Joe, Great-Grandma Rosie and Grandma Myra. In many ways, their lives became my legacy. They planted their Portuguese roots so deep in the red dirt of the 'aina which made it possible for me to easily put my own roots here. I believe they continue to guide me towards my ultimate healing potential. Note: The next book I write will be about my Portuguese ancestors' history here on Kaua'i! It's an endlessly fascinating topic to me.

Ke'oni Hanalei, mahalo my dearest brother for your endless wisdom, fern medicine, humor, and sharp reflections. You inspired me and showed me I could rewrite my transformation from death back to life again. All the blue jade in the world could not express my joyous gratitude to you!

Kumu Kehaulani Kekua for your knowledge, wisdom, and warm aloha and pule (prayers) for my mother and me. You honor me with your presence. Being a part of your world was a huge inspiration and assistance when I was in the depths of the shadows.

Thank you Syris for helping me with the immense responsibility on the ranch, your loving support when it felt like the world would cave in on me, wisdom, playful monkey ways, photo editing, poops scooping, techno wizard help and for the endless gallons of rainbow juice you altruistically made for me. When all is said and done, I am grateful to be your lifelong friend. Your soul shines like gold.

I wouldn't be alive right now if it hadn't been for the wonderful Bethany Webb (Please read her book *My Guru Cancer* and check out her class and private session offerings!) and "The Work " of Byron Katie. Bethany helped me face my paralyzing fear of doing chemotherapy. Your humor, wisdom, and love are a lighthouse for me. On that same note, a big thank you goes out to Helena Montelius for "The Work" and getting me through the shock of my diagnosis when the shit hit the fan.

Thank you to my fellow cancer thrivers and admirable members of the "Conscious Cancer Collective" for your support, love and wisdom on this wild and winding path. United together, we are reminded that this path is here to grow us, and we're ultimately never alone. I'm incredibly grateful to walk this path with you.

Thank you to my wise and loving teacher Linda Kohanov (who kindly wrote the foreword to this book!). Amongst tremendous opposition, you were incredibly brave to write the book *The Tao of Equus* and introduce the world to the healing power of horses. Your books quite literally saved my life and helped me rekindle my love of horses. You're a remarkable guide for me in this lifetime!

Thank you to all the students and clients who visited Wind Horse Sanctuary to attend workshops and private sessions in Nevada City, CA. It was a profound honor to share the magic of the horse herd with you.

Thank you to the kind-hearted and brilliant Véronique Desaulniers (Doctor V) who also benevolently wrote the foreword to this book. Your book, *Heal Breast Cancer Naturally* was a beacon of hope during a time of great fear after my diagnosis. Your guidance along with the lovely De'Ann Richter taught me that walking with breast cancer wasn't such a scary path. The love you both gave me was a constant affirmation that everything would be okay. Thank you for all you are and all that you give.

A big mahalo goes out to my dear long-time big sister friend Siena McCarthy. Your laughter, wisdom, and mutual Leo children kvetching are a blessing to me. I'm so grateful I get to spiral with you in this lifetime!

Thank you to Terry Tenzing, my other big sister, horse lover, family friend whom I've known since I was a wee baby. Your knowledge and presence reinforce the simple, yet challenging truth of choosing love over fear.

This book would not be complete without a huge thank you to Jai Dev Singh, Simrit, and The Lifeforce Academy. Your Kundalini Yoga classes, prayers, wisdom, music, and support over the years of Deb's decline and death, and my eventual diagnosis, when I was close to death pulled me through the toughest moments. Your magic ripples out and transforms more people than you can ever imagine. Thank you for shining your benevolent light upon the world!

A huge thank you goes out to all the doctors and health professionals who have given endlessly of their wisdom, healing energy, and expertise over the years. These exceptional people provided knowledge, care, and hope when I struggled with the dire statistics of the diagnosis: Virginia Osbourne, Lisa Hosbein, and Lisa Mandelbaum in Grass Valley/Nevada City. Carrie "Karu" Hodder, my lovely Leo friend whose acupuncture needles and presence bring immense comfort. Carrie Brennon, who is a delightful doctor while providing life giving medicine, wisdom, and insight to keep my body vibrant and flourishing.

Mahalo to Michelle Soto at Aloha Moon Massage in Kapa'a, Kaua'i who has helped keep my body relatively pain free for years now. Your heart is as glorious as the jade plants that bloom outside your door!

Thank you to all the healers not directly mentioned here who have aided me through the toughest times.

Mahalo to the wonderful oncologists (there have been a few!), doctors, surgeons, and nurses at Wilcox Medical Center. When my body was breaking down and I was most afraid, you provided hope and comfort, which gave me the strength to continue on. Thank you all for your generous hearts that give endlessly to your patients. The aloha spirit is alive and well at Wilcox!

I would not have written this book without the help of Self-Publishing School and their proficient support for new authors like me. Your Zoom classes, seminars, online material, exceptional coaching by Ramy Vance, Brett Hilker, Michelle Gano and the handy dandy journal (I filled four of them when writing this book!) helped to birth this book. (See more info about SPS at the end of this book!) Thank you to Wayne Purdin, fellow inspirational cancer thriver with the astute editorial skills and extraordinary patience to whittle down my excessive verbiage and my endless emails! Thank you to Carlene Vitale for your incredible cover design. Thank you to Trisha Fuentes for your formatting help and incredible patience with my complicated book! A big mahalo goes out to Jay Golden, storyteller extraordinaire who planted the seed for the Inanna part of the story and for your helpful guidance over the years.

Thank you to my helpful launch team members who read my book before it was published and assisted me in the birth of my book baby.

Thank you, readers, for taking precious time out of your day to read my vulnerable story. I truly hope my story can help inspire you in some fashion!

Last but certainly not least, the biggest thank you goes out to my animal clan: Leilani, Spirit, Daisy, Comanche, Blue, Xaria, and Kismet. The benevolence of your animal spirit love carries me like nothing else in this lifetime. Thank you for showing up for your wacky, intense human being with your constant loving, wise, patient, and compassionate spirit. I wouldn't be here without you.

POEM TO MY MOTHER:

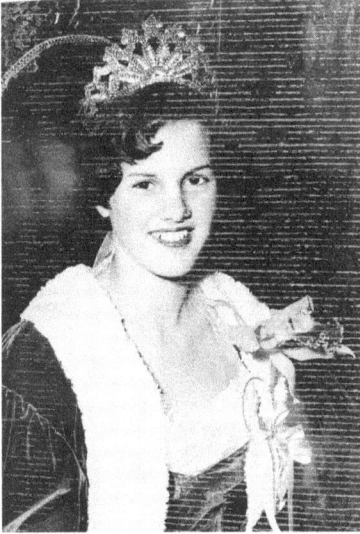

To my twin soul and mother in this lifetime, Gail the queen of Conway, New Hampshire, who
has consistently shown up for me in a truly selfless and kind manner.
For all you withstood to hold your beloved family together.
For the emotional trials you endured seeing your beloved daughter's flame of life almost snuffed out.
For the myriad levels of discomfort you have weathered in the last two years since journeying with your own stage 4 cancer diagnosis.
For your bright, courageous, inspiring spirit that refuses to give up even in the most trying moments.
For your intrepid creative soul that knows the song of every bird in East Africa.
As a teenager, I once thought you were weird, but now, I know you are the most magnanimous of them all!

I honor you and all that you have taught me.

Please know that your life matters.
You have made a profound impact on all who surround you with your luminous heart.
I love you to infinity and beyond.

Explanatory Notes:

General Word Reference Section

Akal: Part of a beautiful ritual in the 3HO (Yogi Bhagan) and Sikh Dharma communities that's done when someone dies. Whether it's a beloved friend, relative, or someone we never knew, this ritual assists the departing soul in her journey home and gives comfort to those left behind.

At the time of death, we chant *Akaal* three times. *Akaal* means 'Undying' and refers to the soul that is being released. This sound current helps to guide the soul to pass out of this worldly realm and into the *Akaal Purakh,* the Undying Being.[14]

"The chanting of *Akaal* creates a vibratory frequency that assists the departing soul on its journey through the ethers to final liberation." –Shakti Parwha Kaur

EFL: Equine Facilitated Learning

EMC: Emotional Message Chart

Eponaquest: Linda Kohanov's (best-selling author of *The Tao of Equus*) organization that trains students in Equine Facilitated Learning. This is where I studied.

Gelding: Male horse that has been castrated (not a stallion).

Mare: Female horse

Port definition: A chemotherapy port (also known as a "port-a-cath") is a small device that is implanted under your skin to allow easy access to your bloodstream. A port can be used to draw blood and infuse chemotherapy drugs. It can also be used if you need transfusions of red blood cells or platelets.

Wahe Guru: A Kundalini Yoga phrase that's derived from the Sikh tradition and 3HO (Yogi Bhagan), which is exclaiming joy over an accomplishment or something that ends up happily in your favor. Wahe (Wha-hay) means "Wow" or "Ecstasy." It's sort of an exclamation of the joy of existence. Guru (goo-roo) means that force which brings one from darkness into light.

Hawaiian Reference Page:

'Aina: Sacred Earth/land

Aloha Mā: A term I learned from my Hawaiian friend Ke'oni Hanalei which means self-reflective love. This term took on a profound meaning for me in my health journey. To me, it meant tapping into a deep sense of self-love for myself, which felt like the essence of true healing.

Aumakua: A personal or family god that originated as a deified ancestor, and which takes on physical forms such as spirit vehicles. An 'aumakua may manifest as a shark, owl, bird, octopus, and other creatures. It also can show up as inanimate objects such as plants, clouds, or rocks. (From Wikipedia)

Cuz: In Hawaii, the slang word for cousin is cuz. In Hawaii, everyone is your metaphoric cousin!

Heiau: A Heiau is a Native Hawaiian sacred site. "Pre-Christian place of worship, shrine; some heiau were elaborately constructed stone platforms, others simple earth terraces." (From 'Hawaiian Dictionary' by Mary Kawena Pukui & Samuel H Elbert)

Kihei: Kihei is a sacred Hawaiian cloth used in ceremony. "Shawl, cape, afghan: rectangular tapa garment worn over one shoulder and tied in a knot." (From 'Hawaiian Dictionary' by Mary Kawena Pukui & Samuel H Elbert)

Kuleana: "Kuleana is one's personal sense of responsibility. The person possessing Kuleana, believes in the strength of this value and will be quick to say, "I accept my responsibilities, and I will be held accountable." Kuleana speaks the workplace language of self-motivation, ownership, empowerment, and the personal transformation which can result. Effective delegation becomes about the sharing of Kuleana with others, recognizing where it rightfully belongs, or where it can facilitate hands-on learning."

http://www.managingwithaloha.com/19-values-of-aloha/kuleana/

Kumu: teacher, coach, guide

Lauhala: A tree that grows in Hawaii that's used to make hats, mats, and more. Pandanus leaf

Mana: "The spiritual life force energy or healing power that permeates the universe. Anyone or anything can have *mana*. It is a cultivation or possession of energy and power, rather than being a source of power. It is an intentional force." (Wikipedia)

Menehune: Mythological dwarf people in Hawaiian tradition who are said to live in the deep forests and hidden valleys of the Hawaiian Islands, hidden and far away from human settlements. https://en.wikipedia.org/wiki/Menehune

Ohana: Family

Pau: Finished, done, over

Talking Story: Slang for hanging out, telling stories, talking, and shooting the shit

Tutu: An endearing term that means grandma or elder in Hawaiian

Wahine: Woman

Resource List:

Websites:

1. Doctor V – Breast Cancer Conqueror:
   https://breastcancerconqueror.com/

2. RGCC/Greek Test – RGCC (Research Genetics Cancer Center): https://www.rgcc-group.com/tests/

3. Dr. Joe Dispenza - https://drjoedispenza.com/

4. Pacific Yurts- https://www.yurts.com/

5. War on Cancer app: https://waroncancer.com/

6. Linda Kohanov/Eponaquest:
   https://www.Eponaquest.com

7. McDowellsHerbal – https://www.mcdowellsherbal.com/

8. The Gerson Institute – https://gerson.org/gerpress/

9. Life Force Academy - https://teachings.jaidevsingh.com/

10. Simrit Kaur Music - https://simritkaurmusic.com/

11. Cheyanna Bone -
    https://www.facebook.com/cheyannabeecraft

12. Tamara Wolfson -
    https://ladybeebotanicals.com/about-us/

13. Heather Luna - https://www.acornherbschool.com/

14. Bethany Webb - - https://bethanywebb.com/

15. Helena Montelius - : http://www.lookwithininstitute.com

16. The Work of Byron Katie - https://thework.com/

17. Schelli Whitehouse - https://www.schelliwhitehouse.com/

18. Zahrah Sita – http://www.ZahrahSitacom

19. Pohala Botanicals (Ke'oni Hanalei) - https://www.pohala.net/

20. Studio Ha'a (Kehaulani Kekua) - https://studiohaakauai.wixsite.com/mysite-1

21. Stormy May - https://stormymay.com/

22. Gene Wei - https://anticancer360.com/

23. Jaya Lakshmi & Ananda music - https://jayalakshmiandananda.com/

Books:

1. *Heal Breast Cancer Naturally* by Dr. Véronique Desaulniers

2. *You are the Placebo* by Dr. Joe Dispenza

3. *Becoming Supernatural* by Dr. Joe Dispenza

4. *The Wild Edge of Sorrow* by Francis Weller

5. *Close to the Bone* by Jean Shinoda Bolen

6. All the books by Linda Kohanov

7. *My Horses, My Healers* by Shelley Rosenberg

8. *The Language of Emotions: What Your Feelings Are Trying to Tell You* by Karla McLaren

9. *A Cancer Therapy: Results of 50 Cases* by Max Gerson

10. *Hands of Light: A Guide to Understanding Human Energy Fields* by Barbara Brennan

11. *Song of Increase* by Jacqueline Freeman

12. *My Cancer Guru* by Bethany Webb

13. *The Business of Coaching with Horses* by Schelli Whitehouse

14. *The Path of the Horse* by Stormy May

Films:

1. *The Path of the Horse* by Stormy May

2. *Honor the Earth* by Tara Coyote - https://www.youtube.com/watch?v=ZbRnsjrK6R8

Linda Kohanov

Eponaquest
Connections 101

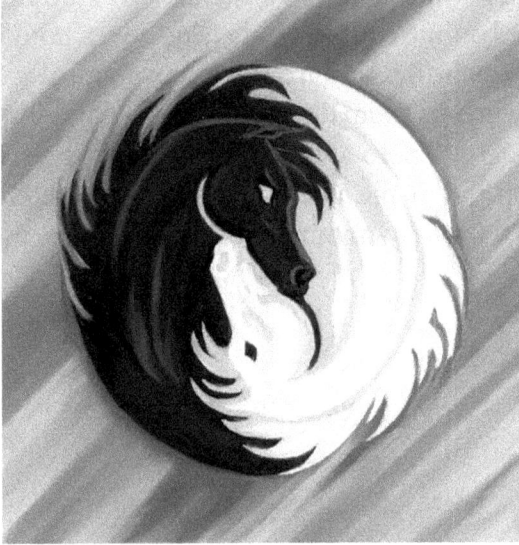

Linda Kohanov, best-selling author of Tao of Equus, founder of Eponaquest has created an exciting new online course called Connections 101! If you love Linda's books and want to explore the depth of the human/horse relationship, I highly recommend you take this fascinating online course!

Course Content:
Through her work with horses, Linda Kohanov has spent her career helping people better understand themselves and others' verbal and nonverbal cues. In this course, she shares research on emotional and social intelligence, leadership, and some of the more adventurous aspects of consciousness through the lens of horse behavior. She teaches skills that you can immediately use at home, at work, and in larger community contexts, skills that enhance all your relationships, help you manage stress, and

allow you to help others manage their emotional and behavioral responses.

Course Structure:

Connections 101 is a new adaptation of workshops that Linda has been teaching to thousands of individuals over the past decade. In this self-paced online course, Linda takes seven hours of lectures, storytelling, scientific background, and practical exercises and conveniently breaks them down into three major lessons over 33 bite-sized videos. There are also handouts, suggested readings, and a relaxing and inspiring music video composed by Linda and her husband, Grammy-nominated ambient music pioneer Steve Roach.

For more info go to:
https://university.nelda.com/courses/connections?ref=7a1fd4

Self Publishing School

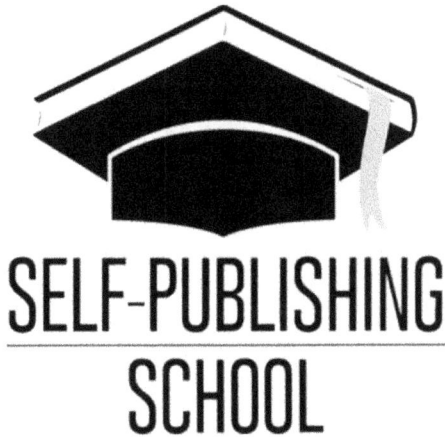

This book would not have been possible without the Self-Publishing School. Their online course, coaching, weekly Zoom classes and journal all helped me with the massive task of birthing this book.

You can get a FREE copy of the book 'Published' via this link: https://self-publishingschool.com/friend/

If you choose to join a Self-Publishing School program (listed below) you'll get $250 off and I will also receive $250 as a thank you from SPS.

Become a Bestseller
Fundamentals of Fiction
Sell More Books
Course Building for Authors
Children's Book School
Full Time Fiction
Publicity & Speaking

Be sure to include my name for who referred you!

End Notes:

3. https://www.annahalprin.org/biography

4. http://www.2012-spiritual-growth-prophecies.com/mount-shasta.html

5. https://principia-scientific.com/dr-max-gerson-a-cancer-cure-that-cost-his-life/

6. https://www.learnreligions.com/energetic-perspective-on-breast-cancer-1724413

7. https://radhinaturalhealth.wordpress.com/2011/10/27/breast-cancer-the-louise-hay-perspective/

8. https://beebuilt.com/pages/top-bar-hives

9. http://www.kamboclear.com/what-is-kambo/

10. https://www.anoasisofhealing.com/uvbi/

11. https://www.ancient-origins.net/myths-legends/descent-inanna-underworld-5500-year-old-literary-masterpiece-007296

12. Ibid.

13. https://www.cancerresearchuk.org/about-cancer/coping/physically/breathing-problems/causes-of-breathlessness/fluid-on-lungs

14. https://www.merriam-webster.com/dictionary/homeopathy

15. https://www.chegg.com/homework-help/definitions/heros-journey-41

16. https://www.3ho.org/3ho-lifestyle/lifecycles/first-and-last-breath/chanting-akaal-time-death

Appendix

My Healing Protocol:

Physical:

1. Monthly shots of Faslodex (hormone blocker) & Xgeva (for my bones)
2. Weekly general vitamin & mineral infusion (IV)
3. Medical protocol of CBD/THC
4. Amethyst biomat - Daily use - http://taracoyote.biomatnetwork.com/
5. Various vitamins & supplements:

From Cymbiotika:

A high-quality brand of liquid vitamins that I highly recommend
For more info about Cymbiotika: https://cymbiotika.com/
Use the coupon code TaraC to get 15% off

A. Vitamin C
B. Vitamin D3 + K2 + CoQ10
C. Vitamin B12
D. Nexus
E. Golden Mind

From LifePlus:

Another high-quality brand of vitamins I recommend
For more info about LifePlus:
https://www.lifeplus.com/vibranthealth

    A. Daily BioBasics
    B. DNA Immune
    C. Proanthenols 50
    D. Ome Gold

General Vitamins:

    A. Calcium
    B. General multi-vitamin
    C. Digestive enzymes
    D. Magnesium

    6. Weekly acupuncture & Chinese herbs

    7. Daily coffee enemas (Yes daily!)

    8. Strict ketogenic diet

    9. Shot glass full of Noni (Noni is a therapeutic plant grown
       in Hawaii that tastes like dirty socks)
       https://www.wailuarivernoni.com/
       (Tell them Tara sent you)

When you buy through links in my book, I may earn a small affiliate commission, at no cost to you.

Mental:

I believe it is vitally important to address the mental aspect of healing along with the physical. You can receive the best medicine

BUT if you're a wreck emotionally, you won't heal as effectively. I try my best to do my emotional work. When issues come up, I try to feel them, process them, and let them go. I reach out for help from others if I need it.

The work of Dr. Joe Dispenza and Byron Katie (check out Bethany Webb) has been vitally important for me in SEEING the tumors shrinking (they are!) and continuing to heal (I am!).

I don't feed fear! I don't waste my time worrying that C will take my life. I strive to enjoy each moment.

I honestly believe a huge part of my healing is being with my beloved animals: Comanche, Blue, Xaria, and Kismet. They generously balance my energy.

I try my best to rest and allow the parasympathetic nervous state to be activated, rather than the flight/fight/freeze state of the sympathetic nervous system. I choose to be around people who nourish me, not drain me.

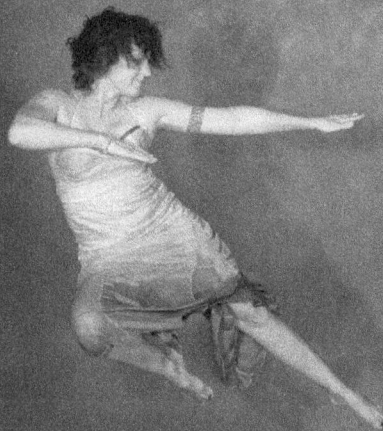
Choose Love

Over Fear